THE COMPLETE GUIDE
to Healing Foods

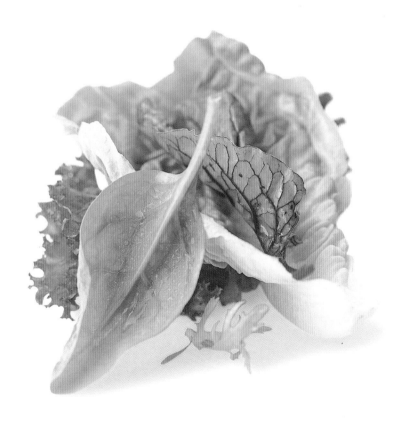

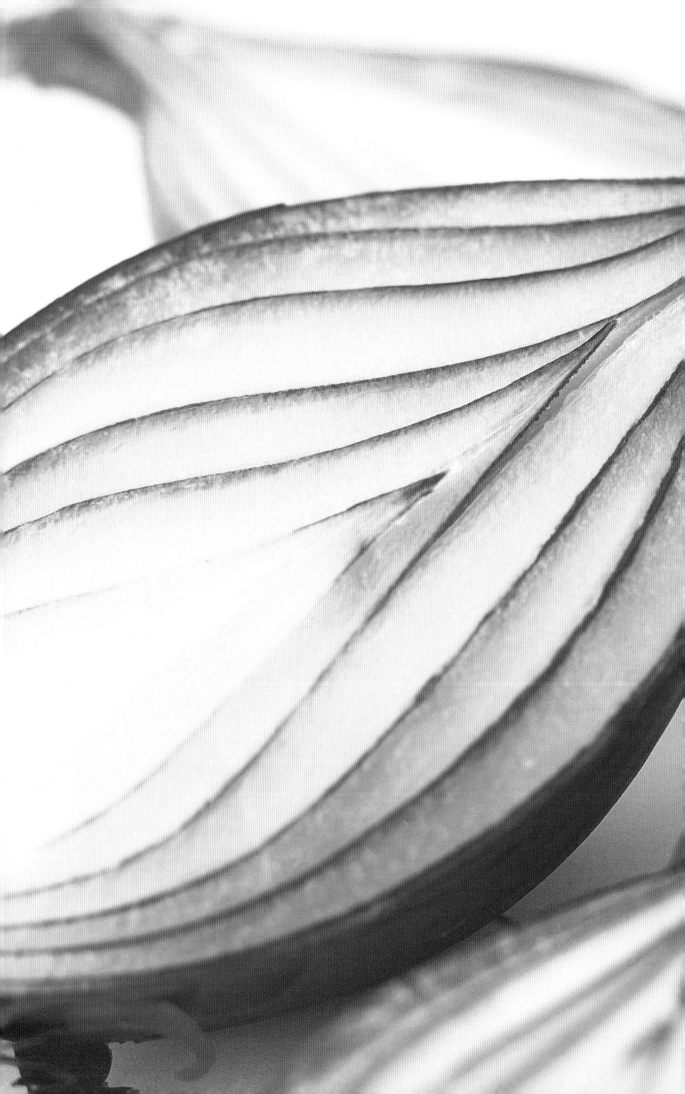

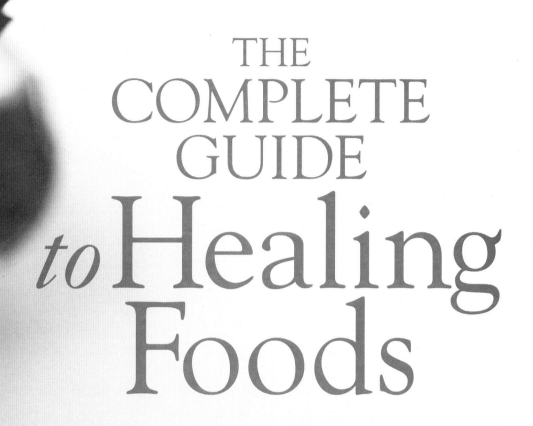

THE
COMPLETE
GUIDE
to Healing
Foods

AMANDA URSELL

A Dorling Kindersley Book

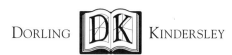

DORLING KINDERSLEY

LONDON, NEW YORK, SYDNEY, DELHI, PARIS,
MUNICH AND JOHANNESBURG

Produced for Dorling Kindersley by
Picthall & Gunzi Ltd,
21 Widmore Road, Bromley, Kent BR1 1RW

PROJECT DIRECTORS Christiane Gunzi
& Chez Picthall
EDITORS Louise Pritchard,
Lauren Robertson & Judith Sheppard
SENIOR DESIGNER Floyd Sayers
ART EDITOR Jacqui Burton
DTP Anthony Cutting

Dorling Kindersley:
SENIOR EDITOR Jude Garlick
SENIOR MANAGING EDITOR Krystyna Mayer
DEPUTY ART DIRECTOR Carole Ash
PRODUCTION MANAGER Maryann Webster
US PROJECT MANAGER Barbara Minton
US EDITOR Jane Perlmutter

Published in the United States by
Dorling Kindersley Publishing, Inc.
95 Madison Avenue,
New York, New York 10016

2 4 6 8 10 9 7 5 3

Library of Congress Cataloging-in-Publication Data
Ursell, Amanda.
    Healing power of food / Amanda Ursell.–1st
    American ed. p. cm.
    Includes bibliographical references and index.
    ISBN 0-7894-5163-8 (alk. paper)
    1. Nutrition–Popular works. 2. Diet therapy–
    Popular works. I. Title.
RA784 .U77 2000
613.2–dc21   99-086947

Reproduced in Singapore by Colourscan
Printed in Spain by Mateu Cromo, S.A. Pinto (Madrid)

see our complete catalogue at
www.dk.com

CONTENTS

INTRODUCTION 6

FOODS FOR BODY & MIND

FOOD PROFILES

INTRODUCTION

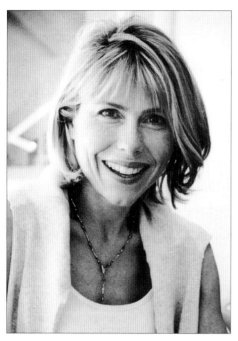

THE BENEFICIAL EFFECTS of certain foods on our health and well-being are increasingly recognized worldwide. The word nutrition is derived from the Latin word *nutrire*, meaning to nourish. While the foods and drinks that we consume give us immense pleasure, their main function is to provide the body with nourishment.

Throughout history in both the East and the West, healers have recognized the great importance of diet, and have shown a remarkable understanding of its health-promoting and potential healing powers. It is only relatively recently, however, with the development of sophisticated scientific tools, that scientists have begun to appreciate how and why this is the case. The explosion of interest in nutrition has led to some fascinating discoveries, many of which confirm the advice of ancient medical practitioners, and uncover new and exciting opportunities to understand just how we can improve health through dietary manipulation. It seems that, from conception through old age, the foods that we eat may affect everything, from our intelligence to our height, and from our fertility to our ability to fight diseases and our susceptibility to ailments such as certain cancers, heart disease, or cataracts in later life.

Scientists are now discovering that proteins, fats, carbohydrates, vitamins, minerals, and fiber are not the only important substances to be found in foods. The most recent research suggests that essential plant chemicals, or phytonutrients, present in fruits, vegetables, and grains may be important in helping to maintain health and to prevent, and even possibly help to cure, certain human diseases. Some research has indicated that vitamins and minerals may have roles in preventive health at levels beyond current recommended daily intakes.

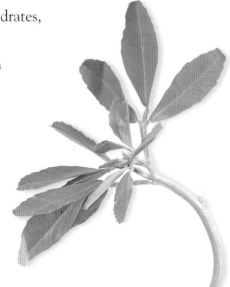

Achieving the right balance between enjoying foods and drinks and supplying our bodies with not just adequate, but optimum nourishment is the key to good nutrition. To that end, nutritionists are providing evidence to support the fact that in some cases, and at certain times of life, we may benefit from supplementing our diets with specific nutrients that help support various body systems and treat illness. It is important to remember, however, that no nutrient works alone. The nutrients found in the foods and drinks that we consume interact as a dynamic whole in order to nurture the body, so a well-balanced diet is the basis of good nutrition.

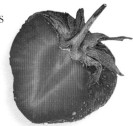

This book helps you to become familiar with the nutritional building blocks of a healthy diet, and advises you on how to establish basic healthy food intakes to suit your age and your body's special needs at each life stage. In addition, it provides information about the specific healing properties of more than 80 foods, explaining, for example, why broccoli is thought to be one of the top cancer-preventing vegetables. The book also contains specific nutritional and dietary advice, and, in the ailments section, outlines how foods can be used to relieve symptoms, to help treat the causes, and to prevent the progression of many diseases.

Whether you need information on avoiding infections such as the common cold, or you want to know how to deal with ailments such as heartburn, cystitis, or anemia, this book helps you to help yourself to a fit and healthy life. The world is constantly evolving, and the world of nutrition is no exception. Scientists all over the globe are constantly adding to knowledge that could help us and future generations to heal both our bodies and our minds.

Amanda Ursell

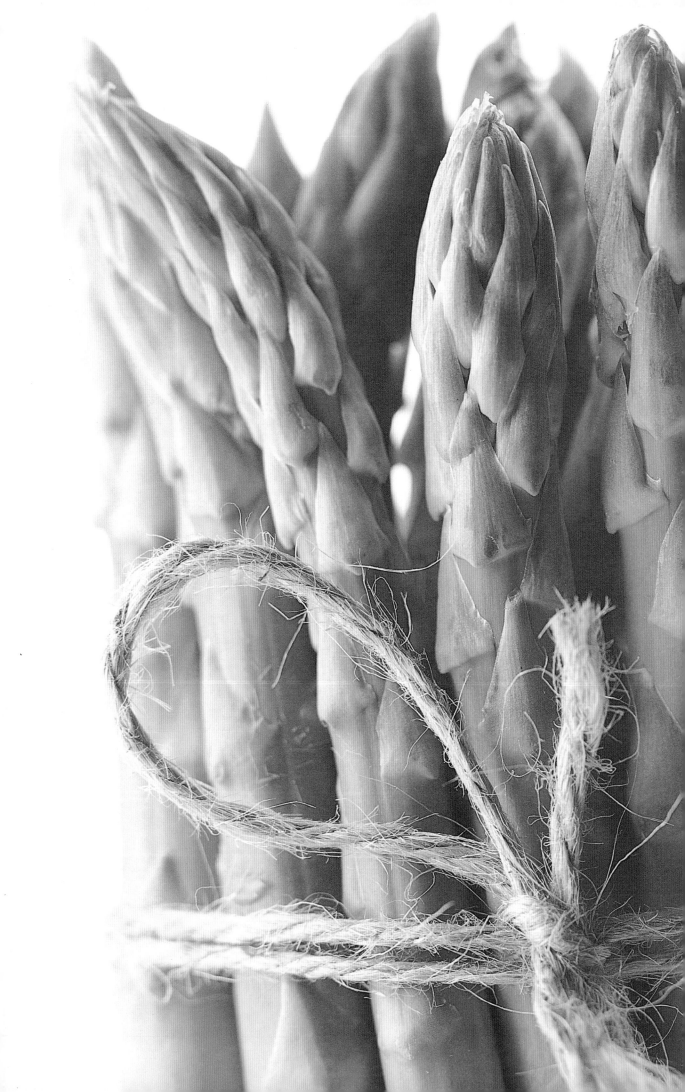

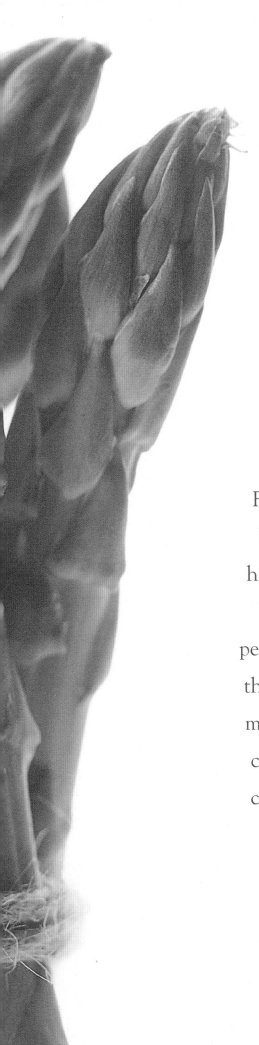

Foods for body & mind

For centuries, traditional healers have known that foods can have powerful healing effects on both body and mind. To understand how foods are able to perform such a role, it is useful to look at the building blocks from which they are made. This section introduces the main constituents of foods, such as proteins, carbohydrates, vitamins, and minerals, and explains their importance in a healthy, balanced diet.

FOOD AS MEDICINE

LONG BEFORE THE DEVELOPMENT of modern pharmacology in the 1800s, people looked to foods and plants as a way of maintaining health and curing ills. The body has long been viewed as being delicately balanced, and foods have traditionally been used to restore or maintain that balance. Today, research is confirming the central role that food and drink plays in a person's physical and mental well-being.

AYURVEDIC MEDICINE

This holistic system of healing has been practiced for thousands of years in India and Sri Lanka. According to Ayurvedic beliefs, the mind, body, and spirit are interconnected, and good health is dependent on maintaining a balance among the three. There is also a connection made between what people eat and drink and their state of health.

Ayurvedic medicine is based on the belief that well-being is affected by three vital energies, or doshas: "Pitta," which is fire and water; "Vata," which is air and ether; and "Kapha," which is earth and water. Foods have the ability to increase or pacify each dosha (*see opposite*). It is thought that the influences attached to a food are consumed along with its physical properties. The qualities and form of a food are thought to affect well-being in several ways, some obvious and others subtle.

CHINESE MEDICINE

Chinese doctors have been teaching their patients the art of balancing food intakes for centuries. In the Chinese system of medicine, the world is divided into five elements: water, metal, earth, fire, and wood. These relate to parts of the body, emotions, tastes, and seasons. Foods are classified according to five flavors: sweet, pungent, sour, bitter, and salty. They are divided according to temperature: hot, such as ginger and peppers; warm, such as sunflower seeds; neutral, such as mushrooms and figs; cool, such as tofu and eggplant; and cold, such as watermelon. A well-formulated diet is one that balances the body's yin and yang (*see left*), and life energy, or qi ("chee").

ANCIENT GREECE

Following the Chinese tradition, foods were classified in ancient Greece for healing purposes according to their temperature and taste. In 420 BC, Hippocrates divided foods into four categories: hot, such as onions and mustard; cold, such as lettuce; damp, such as grapes; and dry, such as asparagus. The properties of

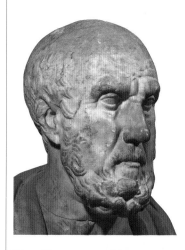

THE FATHER OF MEDICINE

Hippocrates is considered to be the father of modern medicine. He practiced his skills on the Greek island of Kos in the fifth century BC. His theories about maintaining health depended on the right balance of foods, and getting plenty of exercise and fresh air. Hippocrates was the first person to propose treating "like with like," prescribing remedies that would produce similar symptoms to the illness. This method of treatment, the cornerstone of homeopathy, is based on the idea that the effects of the treatment and the illness will cancel each other out, resulting in a return to good health.

YIN & YANG PROPERTIES

The principle of yin and yang is based on the idea that all objects or phenomena in the world can be understood as one of a pair of opposites. Chinese medicine strives to achieve balance, partly through the use of herbs and foods. It is usual to treat someone whose yin or yang is out of balance with foods of the opposite designation, which is believed to restore harmony and balance.

YANG FOODS	YIN FOODS
Sweet	Bitter
Pungent	Sour, salty
Warming	Cooling
Ascending energy	Descending energy

YANG CONDITIONS	YIN CONDITIONS
Heat	Cold
Dry skin	Moist skin
Depleted body fluid	Excess body fluid

foods were believed to balance the state of the four body humors, which were phlegm, blood, black bile, and yellow bile, and the four body temperaments, which were phlegmatic, sanguine, melancholic, and choleric. These were related to the seasons of the year. People were diagnosed according to their temperament and the season. For example, hot, dry foods, such as almonds and coriander, were advised for the treatment of mucus in a phlegmatic person during winter.

In the second century AD, Galen, a Greek physician, expanded Hippocrates' classifications. Galenic principles of medicine later spread to the Arab world, where, after the fall of Rome in the fifth century, they were amalgamated with Egyptian theories and folk beliefs. This rich mix became the basis of medicine in the West by the 12th century.

MEDICINE IN THE WEST

In the early Middle Ages, knowledge of ancient Greek medical practices was kept alive in the monasteries. This knowledge was combined with traditional folk medicine and herbal remedies, which had been passed on by word of mouth from one generation to the next. By 1530, Hippocratic teachings had again become popular, influencing the Swiss physician and alchemist Philippus Paracelsus, who pioneered the idea of specific treatments for particular diseases. In the 1600s, the British herbalist Nicholas Culpeper translated Latin medical texts to make traditional cures accessible to more people. As time passed, however, factors such as the Church's mistrust of herbalism and the developmemt of science brought about increasing conflict between doctors and herbalists, leading to the gradual decline of herbal medicine. In the 1800s, modern medicine, with its use of drugs, began to emerge. A doctor's training included little, if any, detail of how food affected health, a practice that continues in many medical schools.

A DECLINE IN TRADITION

With increasing industrialization and urbanization, people became more dependent on processed foods, which may lack some of the nutrients necessary for good health and a balanced diet. This, combined with the modern pharmaceutical approach to curing illness, saw the continued decline of traditional cures using foods and plants, and a detachment from the concept that what people eat is directly related to their health. However, interest in the relationship between health and nutrition has enjoyed a resurgence during the second half of the 20th century.

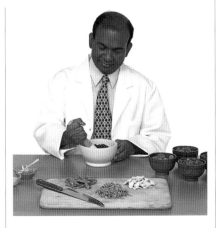

AYURVEDIC PRINCIPLES

According to Ayurvedic medicine, too much energy in one "dosha," or vital energy (*see page opposite*), can cause an imbalance in the body. Eating certain foods can redress the balance and return the body to its normal healthy state.

- **YOGURT** and cheese increase "Pitta."
- **COTTAGE CHEESE** and ice cream decrease "Pitta."
- **PEARS, DRIED FRUITS**, and watermelon increase "Vata."
- **BANANAS, CHERRIES**, and berries decrease "Vata."
- **POTATOES** and tomatoes increase "Kapha."
- **ASPARAGUS**, green beans, and lentils decrease "Kapha."

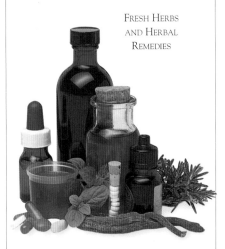

FRESH HERBS AND HERBAL REMEDIES

HERBALISM IN THE WEST

Herbalism is a holistic healing system based on the idea of balance that many traditional systems use. Although plant-based herbal remedies take longer to affect the body than pharmaceutical medicines, they tend to have fewer side effects and interfere less with the body's natural processes. Conventional medicine is becoming more open to herbalism, and some practitioners consider the two to be complementary.

NUTRITIONAL SCIENCE

IN 1747, BRITISH NAVY doctor James Lind examined 12 sailors aboard HMS *Salisbury*. He described the sailors as having scurvy, which was common among sailors at the time, with symptoms such as "putrid gums, the spots, and lassitude, with weakness of their knees." Lind divided the sailors into twos, prescribing each pair a different medicine: Cider; a mouthwash; vinegar; sea water; nutmeg and a medicinal powder; and oranges and lemons. Within six days, the two men who had eaten the oranges and lemons were fit for duty; the others were no better.

THE SCIENCE OF NUTRITION

Lind's experiment sparked much interest among medical practitioners at the time. It was clear that something in the citrus fruits had cured the debilitating, and potentially fatal, condition of scurvy. By the 1830s, more links had been discovered between food intakes and disease. For example, it was learned that bowing, rickety legs in poorly nourished children could be treated with cod liver oil and butter. In 1897, Dutch scientists found that the disease known as beriberi had been caused in one instance by a diet that relied too heavily on white rice, and could be cured by switching to whole-grain rice, which, unlike refined rice, retains its nutritious outer husks. As the science of nutrition has become firmly established, many more links have been found between the nutritious properties of foods and their role in disease prevention.

THE DISCOVERY OF VITAMINS

In 1912, the British biochemist Frederick Gowland Hopkins isolated substances in food that he described as "accessory food factors." He realized that, in addition to proteins, fats, and carbohydrates, they were essential for human health. The Polish scientist Casimir Funk named these substances "vital amines," later shortened to "vitamins." Vitamin A, found in egg yolk and cod liver oil, was discovered in 1913, and other discoveries followed. As each vitamin was identified, it was labeled with a letter and given a chemical name reflecting its physical nature.

MODERN NUTRITIONAL HEALING

Over the course of the 20th century, scientists isolated the vitamins and minerals in foods and identified their functions in the body. Most recently, research has investigated the effects that plant phytonutrients appear to have on the body. These plant substances are believed to help guard against illness.

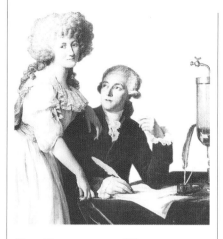

THE FOUNDER OF NUTRITION

The French chemist Antoine Lavoisier, who worked in conjunction with his wife Marie, is credited with being the founder of the science of nutrition. At the end of the 18th century, he and Pierre Laplace, a physicist, carried out experiments and concluded that "life is a process of combustion," showing that people need energy in order to live. The body burns "fuel" in the form of food, generating energy. Later, scientists calculated the energy content of various types of food in the diet and determined how many calories humans need daily in order to maintain a healthy weight.

ENERGY SOURCES

Carbohydrates, proteins, and fats are the main sources of energy in the diet, and this is measured in calories. Some energy sources, such as fats and alcohol, are high in calories and intakes of these should therefore be restricted.

NUTRIENT	CALORIES PER GRAM
Carbohydrates	4
Protein	4
Fats	9
Alcohol	7

RECOMMENDED INTAKES

Recommended daily intakes are guidelines for the nutrients that should be included in the diet every day. Standards may differ slightly between countries, but the concept is broadly universal. In the US, the term Reference Daily Intake (RDI) has replaced Recommended Daily Allowance (RDA). The number of calories recommended, or the energy requirement, is a guideline based on averages; some individuals may have very different requirements.

For example, there is a substance in soybeans that seems to help guard against breast cancer, and there are indications that phytonutrients in general may help to fight heart disease.

It is now possible to look globally at diet and disease patterns in order to study how the consumption of certain types and combinations of foods contributes to the health of different populations. This information contributes to research into the prevention and treatment of disease.

Modern laboratory-based research techniques and experiments have revealed how nutrients may affect health; how increased intakes of certain vitamins and minerals may benefit some people; at which stages of life people should take extra care to consume certain nutrients; and how certain components in foods may help to fight specific problems, such as high blood pressure, infertility, and a large number of other ailments.

THE ROLE OF DIETICIANS

Dieticians, or nutritionists (*see page 246*), are trained to translate the science of nutrition into everyday information about food consumption. In many countries, dieticians are the only legally recognized experts in nutrition and dietetics. Dieticians are able to devise diets that help to maintain good health, aid in the treatment of disease, and may help to prevent disease. A well-balanced diet represents the cornerstone of dietetic practice.

In some cases, dieticians may recommend nutritional supplements for certain individuals. For example, they may advise women who are planning to have a baby to take a daily supplement of 400mcg of folic acid in order to help reduce the risk of giving birth to a child with spina bifida. Elderly people may be prescribed vitamin D supplements to aid calcium absorption for maximizing bone strength.

OPTIMUM NUTRITION

Some nutritionists believe that recommended intake levels of vitamins and minerals ignore individual requirements, which are based on each person's genetic tendencies, lifestyle, social and emotional pressures, and age. These nutritionists believe that by improving the intakes of certain nutrients through personalized supplementation, individuals will experience improvements in their mental clarity and concentration, IQ levels, physical performance, the quality of their sleep, and resistance to infection. Supplementation may help to protect against disease and extend healthy lifespans. Some current research seems in part to support this view of nutritional health.

ESSENTIAL NUTRIENTS

The body needs the following nutrients to maintain health and provide energy.

- **BIOTIN** is needed for the metabolism of proteins and fats.
- **CALCIUM** is needed for strong bones and teeth, and for hormone secretion.
- **CARBOHYDRATES** provide energy, fiber, and many B vitamins.
- **CHLORIDE** is needed for water balance.
- **CHROMIUM** helps to control blood sugar levels.
- **COPPER** is needed for growth.
- **FATS** are a source of energy, fat-soluble vitamins, and essential fatty acids.
- **FLUORIDE** assists in bone and teeth formation.
- **FOLATE** is needed for red blood cell production and spinal-cord development.
- **IODINE** helps to regulate metabolism.
- **IRON** is needed for red blood cell production and oxygen transportation.
- **MAGNESIUM** strengthens bones and teeth, and promotes healthy muscles.
- **MANGANESE** assists the utilization of calcium and potassium.
- **MOLYBDENUM** aids enzyme functions.
- **PHOSPHORUS** is needed for bone health and energy release in body cells.
- **POTASSIUM** is needed for water balance and nerve and muscle health.
- **PROTEIN** maintains the body tissues.
- **SELENIUM** is an essential component of an enzyme that protects body cells.
- **SODIUM** maintains water balance.
- **VITAMIN A** helps growth and normal development, skin, and night vision.
- **VITAMIN B$_1$ (THIAMINE)** aids carbohydrate metabolism.
- **VITAMIN B$_2$ (RIBOFLAVIN)** is needed for fat and protein metabolism.
- **VITAMIN B$_3$ (NIACIN)** promotes healthy skin and metabolism.
- **VITAMIN B$_5$ (PANTOTHENIC ACID)** is essential for energy metabolism.
- **VITAMIN B$_6$** is required for protein metabolism and healthy nerves.
- **VITAMIN B$_{12}$** is essential for nerve function and healthy red blood cells.
- **VITAMIN C** helps to absorb iron and keeps connective tissues healthy.
- **VITAMIN D** helps to regulate calcium absorption and to maintain healthy bones and teeth.
- **VITAMIN E** protects cell membranes.
- **VITAMIN K** is needed for blood to clot and for metabolism.
- **ZINC** is involved in the immune system, taste, and bone health.

EATING FOR HEALTH

URRENT MAINSTREAM thinking in the West is that most foods can be enjoyed as part of a healthy diet. It is just a matter of getting the balance right. This means eating more of some foods, such as fruits, vegetables, and grains, and less of others, such as foods that contain high levels of fat or sugar.

EATING TO PREVENT DISEASE

Health experts believe that by including a wide range of fruits, vegetables, and grains in the diet, the vitamin, mineral, phytonutrient, and fiber content of the diet will improve. It is thought that these nutrients and plant substances may help to protect against the risk of heart disease, certain cancers, and degenerative diseases of aging, such as cataracts. Reducing the total amount of calories in the diet that come from fats could help to reduce the risk of heart disease and obesity, while consuming some essential fats, such as those found in oily fish, may help to protect against heart disease and inflammatory diseases, such as rheumatoid arthritis and psoriasis.

A balanced diet can also help to reduce cholesterol levels. Most of the cholesterol in the blood is made by the liver and is carried in the blood by two proteins: low-density lipoprotein (LDL) and high-density lipoprotein (HDL). High levels of LDL cholesterol may accumulate in blood vessels, blocking them and possibly causing a heart attack. Reducing the amount of saturated fats eaten can reduce the circulating levels of LDL cholesterol. Eating foods containing unsaturated fats rather than the saturated fats found in fatty meats, whole-milk dairy products, and many processed foods can be helpful. In those with normal cholesterol metabolism, the cholesterol found in foods such as shrimp has little effect on cholesterol levels, so these foods are not necessarily bad for the health (*see page 23*).

High blood pressure and the risk of stroke may be reduced by lowering salt intake. Cutting down on snack foods such as potato chips, canned vegetables, salted meats, and prepackaged meals will help, as will using less salt in cooking and at the table.

HOW MUCH FOOD DO PEOPLE NEED?

The amount of food an individual needs is based on the amount of energy (calories) that person's body requires. The Estimated Average Requirement (EAR), or recommended daily calorie intake, provides the average person with a guide to the amount of food necessary daily for maintaining a healthy weight. Some people may have special energy needs for a variety of reasons:

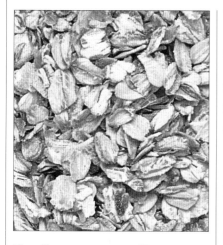

THE IMPORTANCE OF FIBER

Also called roughage, fiber comes from plant foods such as fruits, vegetables, and grains. Although it does not provide any nutrients, it has many benefits. Soluble fiber, which is found in legumes, oats, and some fruits, has been found to reduce cholesterol levels. Insoluble fiber, which is found in grains and vegetables, adds bulk to stools, speeding their movement through the colon. This is thought to protect against constipation and cancer of the colon. Diets in the West tend not to contain as much fiber as they should: It is recommended that at least an ounce of fiber is consumed a day.

Fruits and vegetables: Eat a wide variety of foods from this group

Bread, other grains, and potatoes: Choose high-fiber varieties

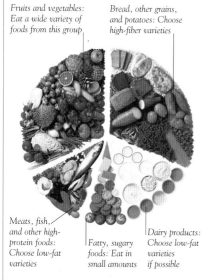

Meats, fish, and other high-protein foods: Choose low-fat varieties

Fatty, sugary foods: Eat in small amounts

Dairy products: Choose low-fat varieties if possible

A BALANCED DIET

The diagram above can be used to help to make healthy eating easier. This pictorial guide has been created to show the proportions in which foods should be consumed. Eating these proportions of foods helps to provide the right balance of proteins, carbohydrates, vitamins, minerals, and essential fats.

Women tend to need fewer calories than men, and older adults burn less energy than adolescents and young adults. Weight can also be a factor: If an individual is heavier than the average healthy weight for a person of his or her height, then less energy is needed to achieve and maintain that healthy weight. Level of activity is also a factor, since the more active a person is, the greater his or her energy needs are. However much energy an individual requires, the proportions of food from different groups should remain the same, as shown in the balanced diet for healthy eating diagram (*see opposite*).

EATING A BALANCED DIET

The balanced diet diagram (*see opposite*) applies to most people. It does not apply to children under the age of two years, who need whole milk and dairy products. Between the ages of two and five, children gradually begin to eat the same foods as the rest of the family, at which time the diagram will apply. Those under medical supervision or with special dietary requirements should check with a doctor to see if the diagram applies to them.

Five servings a day (totaling at least 14oz/400g) of fresh or frozen fruits and vegetables are recommended. Fruit juice or dried fruits can also contribute to these servings. Some vegetables are best eaten raw, while others must be cooked. The water used to cook them can be used as a nutritious stock in place of ready-made stock cubes, which contain sodium. To retain maximum nutritional value, vegetables can be served in their skins, and chopped just before they are cooked.

Starchy foods, such as breads and other grains and potatoes, should make up a large part of the diet, with between five and nine servings per day. Unrefined foods, such as brown rice, provide more fiber, vitamins, and minerals than refined varieties.

Meats, fish, and protein alternatives, including eggs, soybeans, and nuts, are important parts of the diet. Choose lean and reduced-fat varieties of these foods whenever possible. Three to five servings per day are recommended. It is advisable to include fish in the diet two or three times a week, with one portion consisting of oily fish. Dairy foods, such as cheese, are good sources of protein and calcium, but they tend to be high in fat, so low-fat varieties are preferable.

Foods containing fat and sugar should be eaten in small quantities. Whole-milk dairy products and cooking oils fall into this category. The body needs a certain amount of fat in order to survive, but this is best gained from unprocessed foods, such as nuts and seeds containing essential fats.

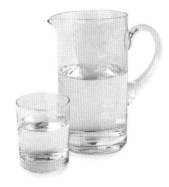

THE IMPORTANCE OF WATER

An essential nutrient, water makes up 50–60 percent of body weight. It is continually eliminated through the breath, sweat, and urine, and must be replaced every day through the consumption of foods and drinks. Exact needs depend on climate and levels of individual activity. At least 6 cups (1.5 liters) of water should be drunk daily, with another 4 cups (1 liter) for every hour of strenuous physical activity.

SODIUM CHLORIDE (SALT)

Current average intakes of salt, about 8–10g per day, are more than the body needs and may increase the risk of high blood pressure and stroke. Food manufacturers add salt when food is processed, and some sodium is naturally present in foods. Instead of adding salt when cooking foods, they can be flavored with herbs, spices, vinegar, and mustard. Intakes of no more than 6g of salt per day are recommended.

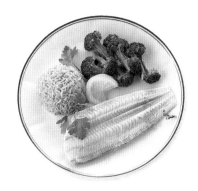

IMPROVING ABSORPTION

Eating combinations of foods can improve the absorption of nutrients: for example iron in fish is absorbed better with the help of beta carotene in broccoli.

• IRON in vegetables and grains is best absorbed when combined with meats or fish, or foods containing vitamin C.

• CALCIUM absorption is helped by vitamin D, found in oily fish, eggs, some fortified breakfast cereals, and butter.

CARBOHYDRATES

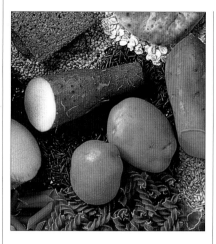

THE SUBSTANCES KNOWN AS carbohydrates provide the body with its main source of energy. They include sugars and starches and range from honey to oats. Other substances classed as carbohydrates include cellulose and glycogen.

Carbohydrates, in whatever form they are eaten, are broken down into simple sugars that are absorbed into the bloodstream and provide energy to drive all of the body's cellular functions, including those of the brain, nervous system, and muscles.

With the exception of lactose, the sugar found in milk, all dietary carbohydrates that are nutritionally significant to humans come from the plant world. Any carbohydrates that plants do not immediately need are converted into food reserves, which can be in the stalks, roots and tubers, seeds, or leaves.

HOW MUCH TO EAT

The total amount of food needed daily varies from person to person, according to an individual's age, gender, size, and lifestyle. "Slow-release" carbohydrates (*see opposite*), such as oats and pasta, should make up a significant part of the diet.

- **TWO TO THREE** portions of fresh fruits, such as apples, pears, peaches, bananas, and citrus fruits, should be eaten daily.

- **TWO TO THREE** portions of green leafy vegetables and root vegetables should be eaten daily. Foods in this group include watercress, spinach, carrots, sweet potatoes, cabbage, and green beans.

- **FIVE OR MORE** portions of whole-grain products, such as wholewheat pasta, rice, and breads, and oats, barley, millet, maize, or wheat, should be eaten each day.

- **FOODS WITH** added sugar, refined white flour products, and overcooked or burned foods should be limited.

Carbohydrates, such as fruits, whole grains, and vegetables, should make up the main part of the daily diet.

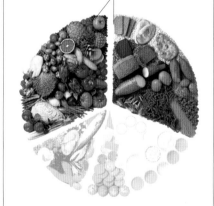

DIGESTION OF CARBOHYDRATES

Glucose can be absorbed directly into the bloodstream. Other carbohydrates must first be broken down into simple sugars before they can be used as an energy source. With regard to energy, it makes no difference whether the source of carbohydrate is a slice of bread or a piece of candy. The differences lie in the other nutrients found in a food. Oats supply nutrients such as B vitamins, minerals, and some protein. In addition, a bowl of oats is digested more slowly than candy, which is strictly a source of carbohydrate.

The digestion of carbohydrates starts in the mouth, where enzymes in the saliva start to break down the starches. Simple carbohydrates can pass straight into the bloodstream from the stomach, but most other carbohydrates, such as starches, must first pass through the small intestine, where they are broken down into simple sugars before they are absorbed into the bloodstream. Levels of blood sugar (glucose) are strictly controlled by the hormones insulin and glucagon. When blood sugar levels rise after a meal containing carbohydrate, insulin is released from the pancreas. This restores blood sugar levels to safe amounts by promoting the absorption of sugars into the blood. The sugars are then converted into cellular energy.

The speed at which a carbohydrate is digested and absorbed into the bloodstream, and energy generated, is determined by its glycemic index, or GI (*see page 18*). It was once thought that all starchy foods were digested slowly and that all sweet foods were digested quickly. However, some starchy foods, such as rice, have surprisingly high GIs and are rapidly digested, whereas sugar and honey, for example, are not as quickly absorbed as was

NATURAL FILLERS

Carbohydrates are natural appetite suppressants. It is difficult to eat too many carbohydrates, because satiation centers in the brain seem to be triggered more quickly when people eat carbohydrate foods than when they eat fatty foods.

TYPES OF CARBOHYDRATE

Carbohydrates consist of molecules of carbon, hydrogen, and oxygen. Different final compounds are formed depending on how many molecules there are and how they are joined. These can be as diverse as the sugar found in fruits and honey, the starch in potatoes and bananas, and the fiber in wheat and oats.

SIMPLE CARBOHYDRATES

These are sugars that tend to taste sweet, form crystals, and dissolve in water. They occur naturally in fruits, some vegetables, and honey, and can be processed from sugar beet and cane to create table sugar. There are two main types: monosaccharides and disaccharides.

COMPLEX CARBOHYDRATES

Complex carbohydrates are known as polysaccharides. Their molecules are composed of many units of simple sugars, which are joined together in chains of hundreds, or even thousands. Complex carbohydrates include starches and many types of fiber.

MONOSACCHARIDES

- **Glucose,** often called blood sugar, is the most important carbohydrate in the blood. When people refer to blood sugar levels, they mean glucose.
- **Fructose** is the simple sugar found in fruits, some vegetables, and honey.
- **Galactose** is found in lactose, or milk sugar, which is a disaccharide.

DISACCHARIDES

- **Sucrose,** or table sugar, is made up of one glucose and one fructose molecule. Once eaten, the body breaks apart the two sugars.
- **Lactose** is found in milk. It is made up of one glucose and one galactose molecule.
- **Maltose,** or malt sugar, is made up from two glucose molecules and is found in malted foods.

STARCHES

- **Rice, wheat, corn**, oats, bananas, potatoes, beans, and peas are included in this group. Many of these foods must be cooked before the starch can be easily digested.
- Not all starch is broken down in digestion. Some passes into the large intestine, where bacteria consume it, increasing the size and bulk of the stools.

FIBERS

- **Cellulose** makes up much of the cell walls of plants. It cannot be digested by the human body, but it helps to bulk up the stools and keep the intestines healthy.
- **Pectin** is a water-soluble form of fiber that is found in apples, pears, and oats. Pectin helps to regulate the absorption of simple carbohydrates into the blood.

---

previously thought. Eating foods that have a low to medium GI may help to control hunger, appetite, and blood sugar levels. High GI foods can be appropriate, for example, for a person with diabetes who has sudden low blood sugar levels, or an athlete during and after training.

PROBLEMS WITH METABOLISM

People with diabetes are not able to produce sufficient insulin, and they may have to take insulin pills or inject insulin and eat regular amounts of carbohydrates every day to keep blood sugar levels stable. Other people lack an enzyme called lactase, which is needed to break down lactose into its constituent molecules of glucose and galactose.

Many people in Asia, Africa, and the Middle East have little or no lactase, so when they eat milk products, such as cheese, yogurt, or cream, the lactose is not digested and absorbed, but moves unchanged into the large intestine. Here, the lactose is feasted on by bacteria, causing excessive production of gas and severe stomach cramps. People with lactose intolerance need to replace calcium-rich dairy products with other foods that supply this mineral, such as canned fish (*see page 118*), since calcium is needed for teeth and bone health.

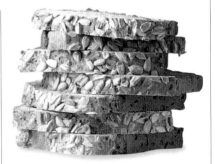

CARBOHYDRATES FOR ENERGY

An average active woman needs to eat about 10oz (300g) of carbohydrates daily, while an average active man needs about 1lb (400–450g) of carbohydrates daily. After strenuous exercise, the glycogen reserves (*see page 18*) in the body must be replaced as quickly as possible. These reserves should be replenished to provide the body with energy. Approximately 1lb (400g) of reserved glycogen is burned up during the following activities:

- 90–180 minutes of endurance exercise, such as jogging
- 45–90 minutes of circuit training
- 30–45 minutes of intense activity, such as high-impact aerobics

GLYCEMIC INDEX

The glycemic index (GI) indicates how quickly the sugars in foods are absorbed into the bloodstream. Glucose is the most rapidly absorbed, and appears in the bloodstream almost immediately after consumption. Its GI is 100. The higher the GI of a food, the quicker blood sugar levels rise after eating it.

FOODS	LOW	MEDIUM	HIGH
Soybeans	18	—	—
Cherries	22	—	—
Fructose	23	—	—
Plums	24	—	—
Grapefruit	25	—	—
Kidney beans	27	—	—
Peaches	28	—	—
Skim milk	32	—	—
Yogurt	33	—	—
Apple juice	41	—	—
Pasta	41	—	—
Cooked cereal	42	—	—
Lactose	46	—	—
Baked beans	48	—	—
Peas	48	—	—
Rye bread	50	—	—
Popcorn	—	55	—
Mangoes	—	55	—
Raisins	—	56	—
Orange juice	—	57	—
Honey	—	58	—
Sucrose	—	65	—
Bagel	—	—	72
Pumpkin	—	—	75
Brown rice	—	—	76
Cornflakes	—	—	77
Jelly beans	—	—	80
Baked potatoes	—	—	85
Glucose	—	—	100

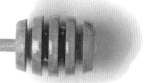

HONEY

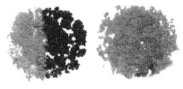

MUSCOVADO   DEMERARA
SUGARS   SUGAR

IS HONEY BETTER THAN SUGAR?

In terms of nutrition, honey and brown sugars such as demerara and muscovado differ very little from white sugar. Honey may contain traces of minerals. The glycemic index (GI) of honey is slightly less than that of sugar, but both are still considered to be medium GI foods.

CARBOHYDRATE RESERVES

The body has almost unlimited potential to store excess fat from the daily diet, but it is not possible to build up large deposits of carbohydrates. There is only about one hour's worth of glucose in the bloodstream at any one time. However, the body is able to keep some carbohydrates in reserve. Such reserves are made up of glucose and are stored in the liver and muscle. These stores are known as glycogen, or animal starch. About 4oz (100g) of glycogen is stored in the liver and 10oz (300g) in the muscle. This reserve can supply about half of an adult's daily glucose needs. Excessive amounts of carbohydrate cannot be stored as glycogen, so the liver converts any surplus to fat.

CARBOHYDRATES & WEIGHT GAIN

In the second half of the 20th century, many people in the West have been eating less; yet, ironically, they seem to have gained weight. The reason for this is partly due to the fact that they lead more sedentary lives, which means that they burn off fewer calories. It may also be because the diets of people in the West contain a different balance of nutrients than they did previously. Diets have fewer carbohydrates and more fat. This is a very important factor, because carbohydrates have fewer than half the calories, weight for weight, than fats. Eating one gram of carbohydrates provides just under four calories, whereas the same weight of fat provides nine calories. This explains how, even if they consume a reduced volume of food, people still gain weight. Eating more carbohydrates and fewer fatty foods, such as fried foods, could help to redress the balance.

CARBOHYDRATES & TOOTH DECAY

Eating sugary foods at mealtimes should not, in theory, increase the risk of tooth decay, especially if the teeth are brushed immediately after meals. The increased saliva that is produced upon eating helps to wash away sugar from around the teeth. Eating and drinking both sugary and starchy foods between meals is a different matter. Some of the sugar and starch sticks to the teeth, which leads to the formation of plaque. The plaque nourishes bacteria that are naturally present in the mouth, and acid is formed as a result. The acid attacks the enamel on the teeth and decay sets in. If it is not possible to clean the teeth after a snack, then chewing gum, especially varieties containing the substance known as xylitol, can help to increase saliva flow and prevent the proliferation of bacteria (see page 207), lessening the risk of tooth decay.

ALCOHOL

Ethyl alcohol, or ethanol, has been produced by most of the world's civilizations. It is made by fermenting carbohydrate, and can be used to preserve foods, such as fruits, and to kill bacteria. Known for its ability to deaden the senses, both emotionally and physically, alcohol was given prior to surgery before the discovery of anesthetics. Alcoholic drinks, the strength of which varies, tend to increase the desire to eat and also decrease self-control. These effects, combined with the calorie content of the drink, can lead to weight gain.

HOW ALCOHOL IS DIGESTED

Alcohol is broken down in the body by an enzyme called alcohol dehydrogenase, which is present in the stomach lining and the liver. The breakdown of alcohol begins in the stomach. If alcohol is taken with food, the enzyme has more time to work on it in the stomach, and its effects on the body seem to be less. Alcohol that is not broken down in the stomach passes into the bloodstream and breaks down as it passes through the liver. In general, the liver is able to cleanse the body of about 6g of alcohol per hour, although this differs from one person to another. There are several reasons that men are able to tolerate more alcohol than women. Men have greater amounts of alcohol dehydrogenase in the stomach than women do, so they break down alcohol more quickly. Their blood alcohol levels therefore rise less rapidly than in women. In addition, men have more water in their body tissues than women do. There is therefore more fluid to dilute the alcohol, so it remains less concentrated in men's bodies than in women's bodies.

THE EFFECTS OF ALCOHOL

A "social drinker" might have two to three units of alcohol per day – a unit of alcohol being equivalent to one glass of wine – and be mildly to moderately affected by it. Someone who has an alcohol dependency often shows a remarkable tolerance of it, although this may diminish over time. People who regularly drink four to six units a day can develop a serious drinking problem, with adverse effects for themselves and for their families. An intake of two units impairs concentration and slightly affects balance. Five units profoundly affects reactions; there is a greater risk of accidents, and in most countries this amount is well over the legal limit for driving. Excessive intakes of alcohol can lead to stupor, oblivion, and even coma. Alcohol withdrawal causes nerve damage and symptoms such as tremors.

SAFE ALCOHOL UNITS PER WEEK

Men are advised to drink no more than 28 units of alcohol a week, and women no more than 21. However, some doctors advise a limit of two units per day. It is best to spread drinking evenly over the week and to avoid alcoholic "binges."

DRINK	MEN	WOMEN
Beer (pint)	14	10.5
Gin (shot)	28	21
Lager (pint)	14	10.5
Shandy (pint)	14	10.5
Sherry (glass)	28	21
Whiskey (shot)	28	21
Wine (glass)	28	21

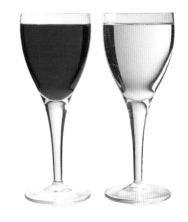

WINE
Wine was once used as an anesthetic. It is now believed that moderate consumption of red wine may help to reduce heart disease due to the wine's antioxidant properties. The flavonoids in red wine appear to lower levels of LDL cholesterol.

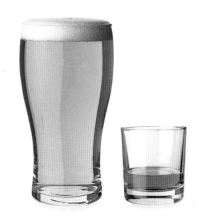

UNITS OF ALCOHOL
A pint of beer is equivalent to two units of alcohol, whereas a shot of a spirit such as gin or whiskey is equivalent to one unit. Regular intakes of two units of alcohol a day have been associated with a lower risk of coronary heart disease. However, evidence also suggests that even small intakes of alcohol increase the risk of breast cancer in women.

PROTEINS

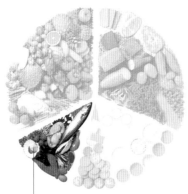

HOW MUCH TO EAT

Protein requirements vary: people with infections or those with physically demanding jobs need more protein than the average person. Requirements fall slightly after the age of 50.

- **MEN NEED** to eat about 2oz (55g) of protein a day, depending on body weight.
- **WOMEN SHOULD** eat about 1.5oz (45g) of protein a day.
- **PREGNANT WOMEN** need an extra daily protein intake of about 6g.
- **BREASTFEEDING WOMEN** need an extra 11g of protein a day for the first four months and 8g thereafter.
- **ATHLETES** may need to double their intakes when strength training.
- **INFANTS** experience fast rates of growth and have higher requirements of protein weight for weight than adults.

Protein, such as fish, lean meats, poultry, and legumes, should make up about 15 percent of the diet.

VEGETABLE PROTEIN SOURCES

The best vegetable protein is a grain known as quinoa, which originated in South America and was once the staple food of the Aztecs and Incas. Quinoa can be used in place of rice. Soy products are another excellent source of protein.

THE WORD PROTEIN is derived from the Greek word *protos*, meaning "first." Consisting of molecules called amino acids, proteins are the basic building blocks of the human body. A protein molecule looks much like a bead necklace made up of a combination of about 25 different amino acids. Amino acid molecules are made of atoms of carbon, hydrogen, and oxygen, plus a nitrogen-and-hydrogen, or amino, group. Protein comes from a variety of animal sources, including meats, fish, poultry, game, eggs, and dairy products; and plant sources, such as tofu, legumes, soy milk, nuts, seeds, and grains. Once protein has been eaten and digested, it is used throughout the body. It is a major component of every human cell and a cell's genetic material. Protein is found in muscles, bones, hair, and fingernails, and forms part of enzymes, hormones, and other substances that transport essential molecules in the bloodstream.

AMINO ACIDS

The body needs 22 different amino acids to maintain all of its protein-based structures and functions. Eight of these are known as essential amino acids, including tryptophan, lysine, and valine. These essential amino acids must be eaten in the diet in order for the body to function properly. The body can manufacture the remaining 14 amino acids, such as arginine, tyrosine, and hydroxyproline, from essential amino acids. The protein that comes from animal sources contains all the essential amino acids, and is considered to be of high biological value. Plant sources of protein lack some of the essential amino acids. A vegetarian or vegan diet that is free from animal protein requires a good mix of vegetable protein sources, such as nuts, legumes, grains, and seeds, in order to ensure that the essential amino acids are consumed regularly.

PROTEIN DIGESTION

Before the body can use the protein in foods, it must first break it down into amino acids. In this form, protein can be absorbed through the intestinal wall and into the bloodstream. In the stomach, a strong acid starts to change the form of the amino acids. When they reach the small intestine, special enzymes are released, which break down the strings of amino acids into small or single units, or "beads." Different enzymes are needed for protein digestion, depending on the source of the protein. A balanced diet, including sufficient amounts of vitamin B_6, is necessary for the production of these enzymes.

TYPES OF PROTEIN

Proteins are often described as being complete or incomplete. Complete proteins supply the essential eight amino acids. An incomplete protein does not.

Vegetarians need to ensure that they consume a wide variety of plant-based foods in order to include all of the essential amino acids in their diets.

COMPLETE PROTEINS

Meats, fish, eggs, cheese, and milk are sources of complete proteins, which contain all of the essential amino acids.

- Meats, including lamb, beef, and pork
- Fish
- Shellfish
- Poultry and game birds
- Eggs
- Milk
- Cheese
- Yogurt
- Other dairy products

ESSENTIAL AMINO ACIDS

The eight essential amino acids must be obtained from food. Infants also need a semi-essential amino acid called taurine.

- Isoleucine
- Leucine
- Lysine
- Methionine
- Phenylalanine
- Threonine
- Tryptophan
- Valine

NONESSENTIAL AMINO ACIDS

These amino acids can be manufactured by the body, so they do not have to be obtained from the diet.

- Alanine
- Arginine
- Asparagine
- Aspartic acid
- Cysteine
- Cystine
- Glutamine
- Glutamic acid
- Glutathione
- Glycine
- Hydroxyproline
- Proline
- Serine
- Tyrosine

APPETITE CONTROL

It is thought that protein foods play an important part in appetite control. Protein is believed to send messages quickly to the satiation centers in the brain that tell the body when it has eaten enough. Some weight-loss experts recommend eating the protein part of a meal first in order to trigger the satiation centers and prevent overeating. It is wise for everyone, especially those watching their weight, to select lean protein sources, to remove excess skin or fat, to use low-fat cooking methods, and to serve foods without adding fatty sauces and dressings.

PROTEIN DEFICIENCY

A lack of protein in the diet results in the body's using up its own protein reserves, mainly the muscles, in order to keep other important functions going. Muscle weakness, thinning hair, slow wound healing, and poor digestion are signs of low protein intakes. A weakened heart is also a sign of protein deficiency. In extreme and long-term cases, protein deficiency leads to fluid retention and distension of the stomach.

EXCESSIVE PROTEIN INTAKES

When more protein is eaten than is needed, the body removes the nitrogen part of the molecule and uses the remaining carbon, hydrogen, and oxygen elements as a source of calories. One gram of protein yields four calories. Excessive consumption of protein is a problem for people with liver disease (*see page 177*) or kidney disease (*see page 192*), and their intakes of this nutrient must be closely controlled.

PROTEINS FOR REPAIR

If a person is injured, his or her body will need extra protein in order to enable it to make new tissues (*see page 167*) and to compensate for a higher rate of metabolism. Bone fractures increase protein needs, since the bone has what is called a "protein matrix," on which calcium and other minerals are laid.

SOURCES OF PROTEIN

It is advisable to eat at least two foods that are sources of protein every day. A varied range of foods such as milk, meats, poultry, and fish will supply most people's needs. Vegetarians need a wide variety of cereals, legumes, nuts, and seeds.

FOODS	PORTION	PROTEIN
Lean grilled rump steak	5.5oz (155g)	44g
Lean grilled pork chop	5oz (135g)	26g
Lean roast lamb	3oz (85g)	25g
Lean roast chicken	3oz (85g)	19g
Lean roast turkey	3oz (85g)	25g
Lean roast ham	2oz (50g)	9g
Lean roast duck	3.5oz (100g)	25g
Grilled cod steak	5oz (130g)	27g
Steamed salmon steak	5oz (135g)	23g
Grilled tuna steak	1.5oz (45g)	10g
Boiled egg	2oz (60g)	8g
Semi-skim milk	2½ cups (1 pint)	19g
Low-fat yogurt	¾ cup (150g)	7g
Cheddar cheese	⅔ cup (40g)	10g
Cottage cheese	½ cup (110g)	16g
Wholewheat bread	2 slices	6g
Bran flakes	⅓ cup (25g)	3g
Boiled brown rice	1½ cups (165g)	4g
Baked beans	1⅓ cup (200g)	10g
Soybeans	¾ cup (100g)	14g
Tofu	3.5oz (100g)	8g
Peanuts	¼ cup (30g)	7g
Sesame seeds	1tbsp (15g)	4g

FATS

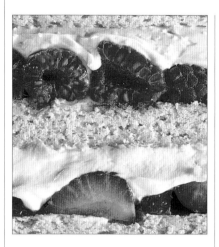

HOW MUCH TO EAT

A healthy diet should derive no more than 35 percent of its calories from fats, which for an average man is about 3oz (90g) of fat per day and for a woman approximately 2.5oz (70g) per day.

- **LEAN MEATS** trimmed of fat, skinned poultry, and low-fat instead of whole-milk dairy products are recommended.

- **FATTY MEATS** and whole-milk dairy products should be eaten in moderation.

- **MEAT PRODUCTS**, such as meat pies and burgers, have a high fat content. The diet should contain only limited amounts of such foods.

- **CAKES, COOKIES,** and fatty fried foods should be eaten in small amounts only.

- **FATS AND OILS** should be used only sparingly in cooking and in dressings.

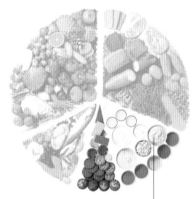

Fats, which include vegetable oils and animal fats, should make up about 35 percent of the daily diet.

DIETARY INTAKE

Almost 25 percent of total intakes of fats in the West is derived from meats and meat products. Cookies, cakes, and desserts supply almost 20 percent, fat spreads 16 percent, and milk and milk products 15 percent. French fries and roasted potatoes plus salty snacks make up the remaining sources of fats.

THE BODY'S MOST concentrated sources of energy are fats. Fats may be visible in foods, for example in butter, margarine, and sunflower oil, or around a piece of meat, or they are invisible, as in cheese, fried foods, cakes, and cookies. Fats are concentrated sources of energy, or calories, and supply the body with fat-soluble vitamins and essential fatty acids. They are often thought of as different from oils, but in terms of chemical composition they belong to the same group.

THE STRUCTURE OF FATS

Fats and oils are made up of molecules of fatty acids and glycerol. A fatty acid molecule is a chain of units containing carbon atoms. Each carbon atom has the ability to attract two hydrogen atoms. The number of hydrogen atoms that become attached determines whether the fatty acid is saturated, monounsaturated, or polyunsaturated. The more hydrogen atoms there are attached to the carbon chain, the more saturated the fats and the more solid they are at room temperature; the fewer hydrogen atoms attached, the more likely it is that the fats will be liquid and classified as an oil. Polyunsaturated fats have the smallest number of hydrogen atoms.

THE BALANCE OF FATTY ACIDS

All fats are made up of a combination of the three types of fatty acid. A fat is said to be saturated, monounsaturated, or polyunsaturated, depending on which type of fatty acid is present in the largest proportion. Butter has mostly saturated fats and is solid at room temperature. The colder butter becomes, the harder it gets. Olive oil contains mainly monounsaturated fatty acids and is liquid at room temperature. It gets thicker when chilled. Sunflower oil contains mostly polyunsaturated fatty acids and it is also liquid at room temperature. Sunflower oil remains liquid even when chilled.

FATTY ACIDS & CHOLESTEROL

A diet that is rich in saturated fats tends to increase the body's production of low-density lipoprotein (LDL) cholesterol and therefore raises cholesterol levels. High cholesterol is a risk factor for heart disease (*see pages 152 and 154*). Polyunsaturated fatty acids do not affect cholesterol levels. Monounsaturated fatty acids seem to reduce LDL cholesterol production. It is thought that diets containing predominantly monounsaturated fatty acids may help to protect against heart disease.

TYPES OF FAT

Fats are classified as saturated, monounsaturated, or polyunsaturated, according to the types of fatty acid of which they are composed. Meats and butter contain mostly saturated fats, whereas olive oil contain mostly monounsaturated fats. Sunflower and sesame seeds are high in polyunsaturated fats.

SATURATED FATS

Saturated fats, such as those found surrounding cuts of meat, are solid at room temperature. Diets rich in saturated fats appear to raise the amount of cholesterol. Saturated fats intakes should be kept to ten percent or less of the total.

- Meats with visible fat, such as lamb chops
- Cream
- Butter
- Cheese
- Coconut and coconut oil
- Cakes and cookies
- Lard

MONOUNSATURATED FATS

Unsaturated fats, found in oily fish, nuts, seeds, and oils extracted from these nuts and seeds, tend to be liquid at room temperature. Monounsaturated fats and oils appear to help lower levels of cholesterol.

- Olives
- Olive oil
- Canola oil
- Peanut oil
- Margarines made from olive oil and canola oil

POLYUNSATURATED FATS

Unsaturated fats, found mainly in oily fish, nuts, seeds, and oils extracted from nuts and seeds, tend to be liquid at room temperature. Polyunsaturated fats appear to have a neutral effect on cholesterol levels.

- Fish oils
- Sunflower seeds
- Sunflower oil
- Sesame seeds
- Sesame oil
- Nuts

CHOLESTEROL

The body can manufacture cholesterol, but small amounts are also absorbed directly from meats and full-fat dairy products. Foods such as eggs and shrimp are also known to be rich cholesterol sources. It has traditionally been thought that eating these foods raises cholesterol, so increasing the risk of heart disease. However, new research indicates that for most people who have normal fat and cholesterol metabolism this is not the case, and that cholesterol is actually raised by saturated fatty acids, and not by cholesterol in foods. This finding suggests that the inclusion of a modest amount of cholesterol in the diet is advisable, because it can have a beneficial effect on the body and may help to reduce the risk of strokes.

FATS & CALORIES

For every gram of fat or oil that is eaten, the body is supplied with nine calories. This is double the number of calories that is provided by the same weight of protein or carbohydrate foods. For this reason, diets that are rich in fats are also rich in calories and can lead to weight gain. It is thought that the more fats that are eaten, the greater the production in the brain of a hormone called galanin, which seems to increase the desire for fats. As more fats are eaten, the body produces more galanin and so craves even more fats. When too many calories are consumed in the form of fats and oils, the body converts them into body fat rather than burning them up for energy, and stores the fat in fat cells, which leads to weight gain.

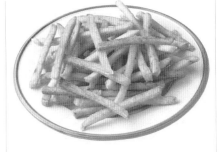

WHY WE LIKE FATS

Fats help to make foods palatable. They carry flavors and give foods a pleasant feel in the mouth, which is why potato chips and french fries are so popular. Some fats consumed in reasonable quantities are an essential part of a healthy diet. This is especially the case when the fats are derived from plant and marine sources, such as nuts, seeds, and fish. They supply the body with essential fatty acids.

When fats are mixed with sugars, they become particularly palatable and, as a result, it is easy to overindulge in foods such as cakes, cookies, and pastries. Fats are thought not to trigger the satiation centers in the brain, thereby making it easy to overeat without really being aware of the excess. This passive overeating of fats is thought to play a role in the increasing problem that obesity poses in the West. It is worth noting that, through gradually reducing the amount of fats consumed in the diet, the taste buds eventually readjust and fatty foods seem less appealing. This can help to break the cycle of overeating (*see page 178*).

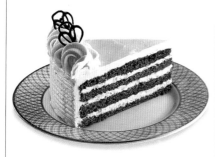

TRANS FATS

Many processed baked goods, such as cakes and cookies, which use cheap, hard margarines in their manufacture, have a high content of trans fats. When oils are processed to make margarine, they undergo a process that adds hydrogen to some of the carbon chains of the fatty acids, making them more saturated. This makes the product solid at room temperature. During this process substances known as trans fats are formed. These behave in the body in the same way as saturated fats and can therefore raise cholesterol and possibly increase the risk of heart disease. Margarines rich in polyunsaturated fats consist of only five to seven percent trans fats, while hard margarines contain about 40 percent trans fats.

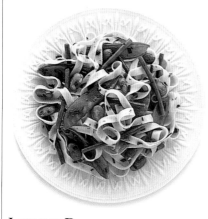

LOW-FAT DIETS

Some health experts believe that people should aim to eat far fewer fats in their diets, consuming only 15–20 percent of their total calories from fats in order to keep weight down and reduce the risk of heart disease. Consuming no more than 20 percent of calories in the form of fats is the equivalent of approximately 2oz (50g) of fats a day for men and 1 3/4 oz (42g) a day for women. Very-low-fat diets are promoted by some specialists to reverse or prevent heart disease. Combined with giving up smoking, reducing stress, and getting moderate exercise, such diets may reduce the need for surgery, angioplasty, or cholesterol-lowering drugs.

ESSENTIAL FATTY ACIDS

Some fatty acids in the diet are absolutely essential to health. These essential fatty acids, or EFAs, are found in plant and fish oils. Linoleic acid is found predominantly in nuts and seeds and oils made from these foods, while alpha-linolenic acid is mostly found in the oils from fish such as salmon and mackerel. These fatty acids are also known as omega-6 and omega-3 essential fats. They cannot be made by the body and so, like vitamins and minerals, must be eaten in the diet. Essential fatty acids are vital components of cell walls throughout the body, especially in the brain and eyes. Inadequate intakes may result in leaky cell walls and the cell itself becoming dehydrated. Essential fatty acids are also needed for the production of hormonelike substances called prostaglandins, which regulate continuous activities around the body, for example the control of blood pressure. Prostaglandins produced from EFAs are also capable of decreasing inflammatory processes and may therefore help to relieve the symptoms of rheumatoid arthritis and psoriasis. It is thought that a high intake of trans fats (*see lefthand column*) and saturated fats can actually stop the body making proper use of essential fatty acids, so it is important to keep intakes of foods that contain the largest amounts of trans fats to a minimum.

FISH OILS

Fish oils contain two derivatives of alpha-linolenic acid known as eicosapentaenoic acid, or EPA, and docosahexaenoic acid, or DHA. Good intakes of both EPA and DHA are believed to make the blood less sticky and less prone to clotting. They also seem to lower certain blood fats, although not cholesterol, as is often claimed. People who regularly eat oily fish, such as salmon, herring, and mackerel, have lower risks of heart disease than people in countries where fewer amounts of oily fish are consumed. Daily consumption of oily fish has been shown to relieve psoriasisand other inflammatory conditions, as well as helping to improve the functioning of the immune system.

FAT-SOLUBLE VITAMINS

Some vitamins are fat-soluble and are found only in fats and oils. Vitamin A, for example, is present in milk, butter, cheese, egg yolk, some oily fish, the oils derived from the livers of fish such as cod, halibut, and shark, and in the livers of animals. Vitamin D is present naturally in foods similar to those containing vitamin A. These include butter, eggs, some oily fish, and cod liver oil. Most vitamin D, however, is made under the skin through the action of sunlight converting a substance known as pre-vitamin D into the active form. Vitamin E is found in large amounts in the oils of nuts and seeds and in the oily germ of whole-grain cereals. Vitamin K is found in soybeans and oils, and in the colostrum of human breast milk. Much of the vitamin K needed by the body is made in the bowel through the action of bacteria. Vitamins A, D, E, and K are stored in the body and it is possible that excessive intakes could become toxic. Some people who do not absorb fats well, due to illness or medication such as laxatives, may need to take dietary supplements of these vitamins.

LIPOPROTEINS

Fats and oils are also known as lipids, and a substance composed of a fat combined with a protein is a lipoprotein. Lipoproteins act as cholesterol carriers in the blood. The body makes four types of lipoprotein: very-low-density lipoprotein, known as VLDL; low-density lipoprotein, known as LDL; high-density lipoprotein, known as HDL; and chylomicrons. Chylomicrons are microscopic droplets of fat in the blood. Cholesterol is often referred to as LDL or HDL cholesterol.

About 65 percent of total cholesterol is carried by LDL. It is deposited in the cells of body tissues, including those in the arteries around the heart and brain. High levels of LDL lipoprotein tend to be associated with an increased risk of heart disease. HDL, on the other hand, carries less cholesterol and more protein. It transports cholesterol from the body tissues to the liver for breakdown and excretion from the body. Higher levels of HDL are therefore considered to be protective against heart disease. Eating a diet that is low in fats, especially saturated fats, but which regularly contains amounts of fish oils and supplies good quantities of soluble fiber from oats, legumes, apples, and pears helps to lower circulating levels of LDL.

BENEFITS OF FATS

In addition to providing a dense source of energy, fat-soluble vitamins, and essential fatty acids, fats have other vital roles. Some fats are necessary in the diet to provide insulation. A layer directly under the skin performs this vital function. Similarly, fats act as protective padding around vital organs, such as the kidneys, helping to protect them from injury and providing physical support. Fats are also crucial in the structure of every cell wall, as well as helping to insulate nerve fibers and allow electrical impulses to travel along the nerves.

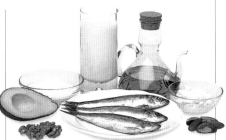

PREGNANCY & BREASTFEEDING
Foods such as seeds, nuts, and oily fish are rich in essential fatty acids and are important for pregnant and breast-feeding women. These foods ensure the development of the baby's brain during pregnancy and in the first months of life.

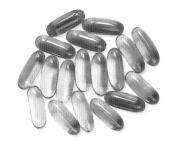

EVENING PRIMROSE OIL
Oil from the seeds of the evening primrose plant is known to be one of the few sources of an omega-6 fatty acid derivative known as gamma-linolenic acid (GLA). Clinical trials have shown that increased intakes of GLA can alleviate mild forms of eczema and cyclical breast pain. GLA is converted into prostaglandins, which are thought to alleviate premenstrual syndrome.

SKIM MILK   WHOLE MILK

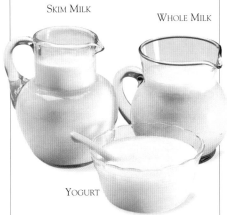

YOGURT

CHILDREN & FATS
Children below the age of two should be given whole milk, and should not be encouraged to eat a low-fat diet. They require fats to fuel growth and physical activity. Once over five years, children should follow the same kind of healthy eating plan as adults, obtaining about 35 percent of their calories from fats.

VITAMINS

THESE ORGANIC SUBSTANCES are present in small amounts in foods, and are a necessary part of the human diet. A lack of any of the 13 main vitamins may mean that the body cannot function at optimum levels, and may lead to a corresponding deficiency disease. Although it was recognized by physicians in ancient times, including Hippocrates in the 4th century BC, that certain foods prevented certain diseases, scientists only isolated some of the substances responsible – vitamins – and identified their chemical structures in the early 20th century.

FAT- & WATER-SOLUBLE VITAMINS

The fat-soluble vitamins are A, D, E, and K. These vitamins need fats for their absorption into the body. Intakes of these vitamins that exceed the body's immediate needs are stored in the body. Prolonged, high intakes of fat-soluble vitamins may cause problems such as nausea or hair loss. The water-soluble vitamins are C and those belonging to the B group. Excess water-soluble vitamins are expelled from the body in the urine.

BIOTIN

A lack of biotin is rare, but if it occurs it leads to fatigue, muscle pains, dry and scaly skin, anemia, and hair loss. It is needed for protein and fat metabolism. Biotin is made by bacteria in the intestines. Good dietary sources include liver, kidneys, egg yolks, dairy foods, cereals, nuts, fish, fruits, and vegetables.

FOLATE & FOLIC ACID

Folate, or vitamin Bc, as it is also known, is found in beets, green leafy vegetables, black-eyed peas and other legumes, brussels sprouts, and whole-grain foods. This vitamin is involved in the production of red blood cells and the synthesis of the genetic material DNA. It also has a role in the immune system. A lack of folate in the diet, decreased absorption, several pregnancies, the use of certain drugs, and large amounts of alcohol can all lead to folate deficiency, which quite quickly affects the production of red blood cells, causing a form of anemia. Folate also helps to reduce the risk of babies being born with spina bifida, and to lower levels of homocysteine, a substance that, when in excess, is thought to increase the chances of developing heart disease. Folate is not always well-absorbed from foods, and women planning a pregnancy are therefore advised to take a daily 400mcg supplement of the synthetic form of folate, known as folic acid.

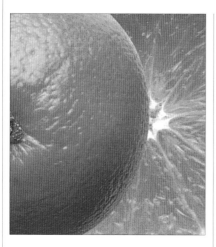

THE NAMING OF VITAMINS

The word vitamin derives from the Latin *vita*, meaning life, and *amines*, meaning nitrogen compounds. When first discovered, each vitamin was given a letter, for example C. Once its chemical structure had been determined, it was given a specific name. There are now 13 known vitamins.

• THE NAMING SYSTEM can sometimes be confusing. Vitamin B, for example, is not one vitamin but a group of several vitamins. The first few B-group vitamins were given numbers, but as more were discovered, some were just given chemical names, such as niacin.

• SOME VITAMINS go under other names for different reasons. For example, vitamin A may be referred to as retinol or beta carotene. Beta carotene is not the same substance as vitamin A, but can be converted into vitamin A by the body.

• THE LABELS on packaged vitamin supplements sometimes give the vitamins' chemical names rather than their common names. A selection of these chemical names is given on page 38.

RECOMMENDED VITAMIN INTAKES

The recommended daily intakes of vitamins are established by government agencies and international bodies, and figures for individual vitamins may vary slightly from country to country.

VITAMIN	MEN	WOMEN	CHILDREN
Vitamin A (mcg)	700	600	500
Vitamin C (mg)	40	40	30
Vitamin D (mcg)	–	–	–
Vitamin E (mg)	Over 4	Over 3	–
Vitamin B_1 (mg)	1	0.8	1.0
Vitamin B_2 (mg)	1.3	1.1	1.0
Niacin (mg)	17	13	12
Vitamin B_6 (mg)	1.4	1.2	1.0
Vitamin B_{12} (mcg)	1.5	1.5	1.0
Folate (mcg)	200	200	150
Pantothenic acid (mg)	3–7	3–7	3–7

HOW STORAGE & COOKING AFFECT VITAMINS

The levels of most vitamins decrease during the storage and cooking of foods. Exposure to air, heat, or water generally has an adverse effect on vitamins. The observation of some simple rules when storing and cooking fruits and vegetables can significantly reduce the loss of nutritional value in these foods.

HEAT

Heat is applied through boiling, steaming, baking, pressure cooking, stir-frying, pan frying, broiling, baking, roasting, barbecuing, or microwaving. The application of dry heat may cause fewer vitamin losses than using hot water.

• Vitamins B_1, B_6, B_{12}, C, E, folate, and pantothenic acid are all decreased through exposure to heat. Cooking should be reduced to the shortest times possible.

AIR

Some vitamins in foods are prone to oxidation when exposed to the air. Storing foods in conditions that are colder than room temperature tends to reduce the rate of oxidation.

• Vitamins B_6, C, E, and folate are all destroyed by exposure to air. Foods that contain vitamin E should be stored in airtight containers and consumed within recommended periods. Nuts and seeds will turn rancid when stored for too long, which is a sure sign that vitamin E has been destroyed. Store foods that are rich in vitamin C in a cool place.

WATER

Water-soluble vitamins are prone to dissolving in the water used for cooking. The larger the quantity of water used in the cooking process, the greater the loss. Using the cooking liquid to make a sauce or gravy can help to retain the vitamins that have been leached out of the food.

• Vitamins B_1, B_2, B_6, B_{12}, biotin, and C all dissolve in water. Cooking methods using the least amount of water preserve these vitamins best; for example microwaving, steaming, and stir-frying.

VITAMIN A

Vitamin A, or retinol, is found naturally only in animal sources of food, including liver, whole milk, butter, and eggs.

It is needed to keep the linings of the eyes, nose, mouth, and throat smooth and supple, and to help fight infections.

Vitamin A can be made in the body from beta carotenoids, the orange pigment found in yellow, red, orange, and green vegetables. Vitamin A is stored in the liver and most adults have large enough reserves of this vitamin to last for months, if not years. If intakes are very low, damage to the eyes, which can be permanent, is a clear sign of deficiency.

VITAMIN B_1 (THIAMINE)

A lack of vitamin B_1, or thiamine, leads to anxiety, loss of appetite, a tendency to tire quickly, and disturbed sleep. These symptoms are due to the absence of thiamine in the production of energy from food in the body, especially from carbohydrates. Wholewheat products, legumes, wheat germ, bran, eggs, and whole-grain rice are good suppliers of thiamine, but milled rice and refined grains are poor sources.

VITAMIN B_2 (RIBOFLAVIN)

This vitamin is needed for energy production, especially from proteins and fats. A lack of riboflavin leads to cracks and sores around the mouth. Riboflavin is found in whole-grain wheat products, fortified breakfast cereals, fresh legumes, fish, liver, meats, eggs, milk, and cheese, as well as in yeast extracts.

SYMPTOMS OF DEFICIENCIES

The body can store only limited amounts of water-soluble vitamins, so a regular intake is needed. Deficiency of these nutrients is more likely than deficiency of fat-soluble vitamins, which can be stored for considerable lengths of time. The following list summarizes common symptoms of vitamin deficiencies:

• BIOTIN Fatigue, poor appetite, nausea, scaly skin, muscle pains

• FOLATE Weakness due to anemia, sore mouth and tongue

• VITAMIN A Night blindness, dry and scaly skin, poor growth in children

• VITAMIN B_1 (THIAMINE) Muscle weakness

• VITAMIN B_2 Cracks around the mouth, sore tongue

• VITAMIN B_3 (NIACIN) Scaly skin, inflammation of the mouth, general weakness, weight loss

• VITAMIN B_5 (PANTOTHENIC ACID) Fatigue, nausea, headache, muscle cramps, stomachache

• VITAMIN B_6 Skin disorders, cracks at the corners of the mouth, depression

• VITAMIN B_{12} Anemia, sore mouth and tongue, diarrhea, general weakness

• VITAMIN C Poor wound healing, vulnerability to bruising, bleeding gums

• VITAMIN D Rickets, muscle spasms, osteomalacia (weak, softened bones)

• VITAMIN E Anemia and nerve problems leading to diminished eyesight and difficulty in walking

• VITAMIN K Poor blood clotting

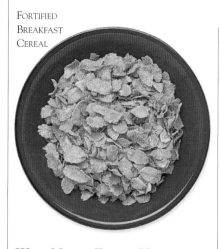

FORTIFIED
BREAKFAST
CEREAL

WHO NEEDS EXTRA VITAMINS?

For most people, eating a varied diet will provide adequate amounts of vitamins. Some countries, such as the US, now fortify most cereal products with folic acid. This measure aims to reduce levels of the chemical homocysteine in people's blood and so reduce the risk of heart disease. As well as identifying diseases associated with a particular vitamin deficiency, nutritionists have targeted certain groups of people who may also need extra vitamins.

• WOMEN PLANNING a pregnancy should increase their folic acid intake with a 400mcg daily supplement to reduce the possibility of spinal-cord defects in developing babies.

• PREGNANT women need to increase intakes of vitamins A, B_2, and C and, in the last three months of pregnancy and during breastfeeding, vitamins A (*see also* page 39), B_1, B_2, B_3, B_{12}, C, and D.

• PEOPLE AGED OVER 65 and pregnant and breastfeeding women are advised to take a 10mcg daily supplement of vitamin D, and to increase their intakes of foods containing this vitamin.

• INFANTS NEED about 8mcg of vitamin D a day in their diets until they are three years of age.

• PEOPLE WHO EAT large quantities of polyunsaturated oils need commensurate amounts of vitamin E. It is thought that 0.4mg of this vitamin is required for each gram of polyunsaturated fat in the diet.

• PEOPLE WHO ARE EXPOSED to very little sunshine should consider taking a 10mcg daily supplement of vitamin D and increasing their intake of foods containing this vitamin.

• VEGETARIANS, VEGANS, and others who avoid animal products should find alternative sources of vitamin B_{12}.

• SMOKERS ARE BELIEVED to use up more vitamin C than nonsmokers, so their daily intake of this vitamin should be increased by at least 80mg a day.

VITAMIN B_3 (NIACIN)

Niacin is the name used to describe two naturally occurring nutrients – nicotinic acid and nicotinamide. Niacin is essential for the production of energy from food. It prevents the deficiency disease known as pellagra, which causes problems with the skin such as dermatitis, and prevents problems with the nervous system such as depression. Niacin is found in significant amounts in liver, kidneys, red meats, fish, yeast extracts, and peanuts. Legumes, dried fruits, and other nuts are also moderately good suppliers of this vitamin.

VITAMIN B_5 (PANTOTHENIC ACID)

A deficiency of this B vitamin is rare but can lead to skin problems, numbness and tingling, and a burning sensation in the feet. It is needed for protein and fat metabolism and healthy skin and hair, and is widely found in animal foods, whole grains, and legumes. Pantothenic acid is found in all body tissues and is essential for the smooth running of the metabolic system, growth and development, and the burning of fat stores for energy.

VITAMIN B_6

Three forms of vitamin B_6 are found in foods. Pyridoxine is most common in vegetable foods, while pyridoxal and pyridoxamine are found in animal food sources. These three forms are interchangeable in tissues and play a vital role in the metabolism of proteins and the manufacture of red blood cells and antibodies. They are also needed for the health of the nervous system. Vitamin B_6 is found in almost all foods. Good amounts are present in meats, liver, fish, whole-grain cereals, peanuts, potatoes, green cabbage, peas, and bananas.

VITAMIN D

There are two forms of vitamin D: vitamin D_2, known as ergocalciferol, and vitamin D_3, known as cholecalciferol. These are converted into substances involved in maintaining calcium balance in the body. Strict vegetarians have a greater risk of deficiency than nonvegetarians, since vitamin D can be found only in a narrow range of foods including certain oily fish, such as mackerel, sardines, and pilchards, as well as egg yolks, butter, and some fortified breakfast cereals. Vitamin D is also made under the skin through the action of ultraviolet radiation from the sun. Prolonged low intakes of this vitamin, combined with very little exposure to sunshine, lead to bone problems. These take the form of rickets in children and weak bones in adults.

VITAMIN B12

Also called cyanocobalamin, this vitamin is necessary for the production of red blood cells and the genetic material DNA, and is involved in maintaining the health of the nervous system. Vitamin B_{12} is made by bacteria, fungi, or algae and reaches the human diet via animals that have fed on these nutrients. The main sources are liver, kidneys, meats, poultry, fish, and dairy products. Plant sources of this vitamin are rare, so vegetarians tend to rely on fortified foods and supplements. A deficiency of vitamin B_{12} can lead to anemia, depression, and severe neurological problems.

VITAMIN C

Also called ascorbic acid, vitamin C is needed to keep collagen, which acts rather like cement between cells, in good condition. A lack of this vitamin results in the collagen literally breaking down. This means that old wounds may reopen, teeth become loose, gums start to bleed, and the walls of tiny blood vessels may break down and start to leak. Vitamin C is also needed by the immune system, and it plays a role in the production of hormones and the absorption of iron in the intestine. Since vitamin C cannot be stored, regular intakes are necessary through the diet. High intakes (the so-called "megadoses" of up to about a gram) are claimed to help prevent colds, and may play a role in helping to fight certain cancers.

VITAMIN E

Vitamin E is comprised of compounds known as tocopherols, which are needed to protect the lipids, or fats, in cell walls from damage. They are able to do this because of their antioxidant properties. Vitamin E also appears to have anti-inflammatory effects and to be capable of stimulating the immune system and DNA synthesis. High intakes of vitamin E are believed to help prevent heart disease. Good sources are avocados, nuts, seeds, wheat germ, vegetable oils, whole-grain breads, and cereals.

VITAMIN K

Vitamin K was named by Danish scientists who discovered that it was associated with coagulation, the ability of blood to clot. Vitamin K is involved with the production of proteins in the liver that are part of the coagulation process. There are different forms of vitamin K. For example, vitamin K_1 occurs naturally in cabbage, cauliflower, and spinach, while vitamin K_2 is made by bacteria in the large intestine. Vitamin K deficiency is rare.

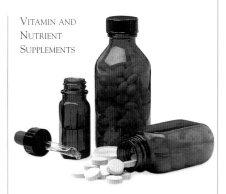

VITAMIN AND NUTRIENT SUPPLEMENTS

VITAMIN INTERACTIONS

The action of vitamins may be enhanced by the intake of other nutrients. This is because some nutrients come in a form that is not easily absorbed by the body. If these vitamins are taken in conjunction with certain other vitamins that aid their absorption, their beneficial effects can be fully realized. Conversely, some foods and drinks can be detrimental to the absorption of vitamins by the body.

• **VITAMIN A** Adequate intakes of vitamins C and E help to maintain the levels of vitamin A in the body. Excess intakes of alcohol may cause deficiencies of this vitamin. Too much of the minerals copper, iron, and manganese can also deplete vitamin A stores.

• **B COMPLEX VITAMINS** If consumed in large quantities, caffeine can flush water-soluble vitamins out of the body faster than usual. Taking the contraceptive pill can lower blood levels of B vitamins.

• **VITAMIN B_{12}** Adequate intakes of folate and the amino acid methionine help to protect vitamin B_{12}.

• **BETA CAROTENE** This is best absorbed by the body when fat is eaten in the same meal. For example, a small amount of olive oil in a dressing could enhance the absorption of carotene from a salad including grated carrot.

• **VITAMIN D** Large intakes of the minerals iron, copper, and manganese are capable of oxidizing vitamin D and increase the risk of deficiency.

• **VITAMIN E** Sufficient intakes of the mineral selenium and vitamin C help preserve levels of vitamin E. Large intakes of copper, iron, and manganese are able to oxidize vitamin E and deplete body stores of this vitamin.

• **FOLATE** Including adequate amounts of folate in the diet helps to protect iron stores in the body.

MINERALS

THERE ARE 16 MINERALS that are considered essential to human life. Some of their most important functions include developing and maintaining the skeleton, ensuring water balance, and forming blood. Minerals are needed in small but regular amounts, and although a lack of them can cause disease, large intakes of certain minerals can also be dangerous.

Minerals are substances composed of one type of atom and have their origins in nonliving things, such as rocks and metal ores. These substances are integrated into the soil in which plants are rooted. About one percent of the diet consists of minerals, which are obtained by eating plant foods directly, and via the animals that feed on these plants.

In the past, deficiency diseases caused by a lack of minerals could be plotted geographically. For example, people living inland, away from good sources of iodine in seafood, developed goiter due to iodine deficiency. Today, localized deficiencies include forms of malnutrition that can affect very young children in the tropics, where selenium levels in the soil are low. Modern agricultural methods and the addition of minerals to water and staple foods have helped to eliminate many such geographical pockets of mineral deficiency.

MAJOR MINERALS & TRACE ELEMENTS

Nutritionists divide minerals into two groups: Major minerals and trace elements. The classification distinguishes the amounts needed in order to maintain body reserves. The major minerals (calcium, chlorine, magnesium, phosphorus, potassium, and sodium) are needed by the body in larger amounts than the trace elements (chromium, copper, fluorine, iodine, iron, manganese, molybdenum, selenium, and zinc). Sulfur is also a major mineral, but is not referred to often since it is an integral part of certain proteins. If a diet has adequate protein it also has adequate sulfur. In a typical diet, 60–80 percent of inorganic material is made up of the major minerals, with the trace elements making up the rest.

CALCIUM

Babies start life with approximately 30g of calcium in their bones. During growth into adulthood, about 1,170g of calcium need to accumulate. In an adult body, 99 percent of the calcium is laid down within the protein structure of bones and teeth, giving them both strength and rigidity. Once peak bone density is achieved by the age of 20, good intakes of calcium are needed

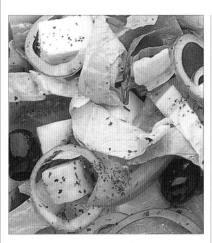

SOURCES OF MAJOR MINERALS

Many foods are good dietary sources of the major minerals, and a balanced diet should provide the necessary nutrients for most people. Some examples include:

- **CALCIUM** Milk, cheese, yogurt, nuts, legumes, whole grains, tofu, tahini, calcium-enriched soy milk
- **CHLORIDE** Sodium chloride, more commonly known as table salt
- **MAGNESIUM** Milk, cheese, legumes, nuts, fish, wholewheat bread, potatoes
- **PHOSPHORUS** Milk, cheese, legumes, nuts, egg yolks
- **POTASSIUM** Vegetables, fresh and dried fruits, legumes, nuts, instant coffee
- **SODIUM** Processed and manufactured foods, baked foods, breakfast cereals
- **SULFUR** Meats, cheese, milk, nuts

SOURCES OF TRACE ELEMENTS

The trace elements are essential to life but are only required in very small amounts. Whole-grain cereals, green leafy vegetables, and seafood are good sources of most of the trace elements.

- **CHROMIUM** Whole-grain cereals, vegetables, meats, fish, legumes, nuts
- **COPPER** Meats, fish, shellfish, nuts, whole-grain cereals, wheat germ
- **FLUORIDE** Fish, seafood, sea vegetables, tea, drinking water
- **IODINE** Seafood, iodized sea salt, milk
- **IRON** Meats, liver, game, dark oily fish, poultry, green leafy vegetables, nuts, seeds, dried fruits
- **MANGANESE** Whole-grain cereals, green leafy vegetables, legumes
- **MOLYBDENUM** Whole-grain cereals, legumes, organ meats, green leafy vegetables
- **SELENIUM** Whole-grain cereals, seafood, legumes, Brazil nuts
- **ZINC** Oysters and other shellfish, meats, whole-grain cereals

THE ABSORPTION OF MINERALS

The absorption and metabolism of minerals rely to some extent on the presence of other dietary components. The presence of certain nutrients can enhance the absorption and metabolism of some minerals, while excessive intakes of other nutrients and substances can decrease the absorption and metabolism of other minerals. This highlights the potential problem of "megadosing" on nutrients.

SUBSTANCES INCREASING ABSORPTION

- **Calcium** Vitamin D, lactose (in milk), and copper can be combined with calcium for optimal absorption. Essential fatty acids, found in oily fish, also enhance calcium absorption.
- **Iron** For iron to be most effectively absorbed, it can be combined with foods containing vitamin C, folic acid, beta carotene, and copper.

- **Phosphorus** Foods that contain calcium, copper, vitamin D, and the lactose found in milk aid the absorption of phosphorus.
- **Zinc** Protein aids the absorption of zinc.

SUBSTANCES DECREASING ABSORPTION

- **Calcium** Whole-grain cereals, rhubarb, spinach, and carbonated cola drinks can disturb calcium balance.
- **Copper** Iron and zinc can decrease copper absorption.
- **Iodine** Thiocyanates, organic goitrogens, and potassium may reduce the absorption of iodine.
- **Iron** Whole-grain cereals, rhubarb, spinach, and tea reduce absorption of iron.

- **Magnesium** Rhubarb and spinach impair the absorption of magnesium.
- **Manganese** Absorption of manganese is blocked by calcium and phytates.
- **Phosphorus** Iron and aluminum should not be combined with phosphorus.
- **Zinc** Whole-grain cereals, alcohol, excess sugar, iron, and calcium impair zinc absorption.

on a daily basis to ensure that the skeleton remains strong. The remaining one percent of calcium in an adult body is found in tissues and body fluids, where it is essential for regulating the flow of water in and out of cells, for sending messages between cells, and for the maintenance of muscle cells. Good sources of calcium include milk and dairy products, oily fish with bones, nuts, seeds, tofu, and green leafy vegetables.

CHLORIDE

Chlorine combines with other chemicals to form chlorides, such as sodium chloride, or common salt. Chloride is found in the fluids both inside and outside the cells of the body. Chlorine is also a constituent of hydrochloric acid, which aids digestion in the stomach. Dietary sources include salt, breads, cereals, and a vast array of manufactured foods.

CHROMIUM

Chromium is needed for enhancing the action of insulin, a hormone that is involved in the control of the concentration of glucose in the blood. The main sources of this trace element in the diet are whole-grain cereals and vegetables.

COPPER

Copper is needed for the formation of many enzymes, especially those involved in the development of blood and bone. It helps to strengthen the body's defense system, and it is also involved in nerve transmission. Good sources of copper include meats, especially organ meats, whole-grain cereals, and wheat germ.

MINERAL SYMBOLS

The chemical symbols for the minerals are usually self-explanatory, since they are simply abbreviations of the chemical names – for example, P for phosphorus, Ca for calcium, or Mg for magnesium. Some current symbols, however, are derived from a previous version of the mineral's name and some are taken from the Latin name.

- **COPPER** Cu (from *cuprum*)
- **IRON** Fe (from *ferrum*)
- **POTASSIUM** K (from *kalium*)
- **SODIUM** Na (from *natrium*)

RECOMMENDED MINERAL INTAKES

These figures are for average intakes only. Young children, adolescents, people in late middle age, and women at certain times of life may have more specific mineral requirements. Too much fluoride should be avoided.

MINERAL	MEN	WOMEN	7–10 YEARS
Calcium (mg)	700	700	550
Chlorine (mg)	2,500	2,500	1,800
Chromium (mcg)	25	25	–
Copper (mg)	1.2	1.2	0.7
Fluoride (mg)	–	–	–
Iodine (mcg)	140	140	110
Iron (mg)	8.7	14.8	9
Magnesium (mg)	300	270	200
Manganese (mg)	–	–	–
Molybdenum (mcg)	50–400	50–400	0.5–1.5
Phosphorus (mg)	550	550	450
Potassium (mg)	3,500	3,500	2,000
Selenium (mcg)	75	60	30
Sodium (mg)	1,600	1,600	1,200
Zinc (mg)	9.5	7	7

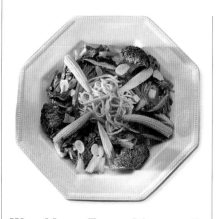

WHO NEEDS EXTRA MINERALS?

It is possible that through eating a varied diet an adequate supply of minerals can be obtained. Some people may, however, benefit from supplements.

• WOMEN are advised to increase their intake of calcium by 550mg a day when breastfeeding, and to have 440mg extra phosphorus. They also need 6mg more zinc per day for the first four months of breastfeeding, and a slightly increased intake of copper and iodine.

• WOMEN OF CHILDBEARING AGE who experience heavy menstrual bleeding need to pay particular attention to their iron intakes. This is even more important if their diet contains little or no red meats, poultry, or fish.

• VEGETARIANS should take extra care to include fortified sources of iron in their diets – for example breakfast cereals, as well as plant sources, such as green leafy vegetables, nuts, and seeds – since common sources of iron in the diet are typically meats, poultry, and fish.

• VEGANS need to pay particular attention to calcium intakes, especially during the first 20 years of life. Fortified soy milk products are good sources, as are green leafy vegetables, sesame and sunflower seeds, tahini, and tofu.

• ELDERLY PEOPLE can be prone to confusion if potassium is lacking in their diets. Extra fruits and vegetables can help to boost the potassium intakes.

• MEN who exclude red meats and seafood from their diets may require additional zinc supplements. Zinc is found in nuts and seeds but, like the iron from plant sources, it is less efficiently absorbed into the blood than the zinc from animal foods.

• PEOPLE living in countries where selenium-diminished wheats are used in breadmaking flour may have lower selenium intakes than are recommended. These people may benefit from eating selenium-rich foods, such as seafood, meats, organ meats, eggs, and dairy products, and from selenium supplements.

FLUORINE

Fluorine is found as fluoride in drinking water. It is stored in bones and teeth, helping to give them strength. Fluorine is also added to toothpaste as fluoride because of its ability to help reduce the risk of decay. Excess fluoride can result in staining of the teeth.

IODINE

This is a constituent of thyroid hormones, which regulate many cell activities and are also involved in protein synthesis, tissue growth, and reproduction. While a lack of iodine leads to goiter and affects mental abilities, too much can be toxic. The best natural sources of this mineral include seafood and milk.

IRON

This trace element is vital for the production of hemoglobin in blood, which transports oxygen from the lungs to every cell in the body. A lack of iron in the diet leads to a depletion of iron reserves in the body and may eventually cause the condition known as anemia (*see page 160*). Iron is also associated with the functioning of several enzymes. Women and girls in particular are prone to low intakes and low reserves of iron. Large intakes can also cause health problems. The form known as haem iron, which is found in meats, fish, and poultry, is more easily absorbed than the form known as nonhaem iron, which is derived from plants. Plant sources of iron include nuts, seeds, and green leafy vegetables.

MAGNESIUM

This mineral is essential for the development and maintenance of strong bones and teeth, for the transmission of nerve impulses, and for the action of muscles. It is also needed for the production of many of the enzymes that trigger reactions throughout the body and for the replication of the human genetic material DNA. Milk, breads, grains, and potatoes supply magnesium. It is part of the green plant pigment chlorophyll and is therefore found in green vegetables. A lack of magnesium leads to muscle weakness, nerve disorders, and palpitations.

MANGANESE

Involved in enzyme reactions, manganese influences the body's use of calcium and potassium and helps to maintain the structure of cells. Common sources of manganese include whole-grain cereals, nuts, tea, fruits, and vegetables.

MOLYBDENUM

Associated with certain enzymes that break down proteins, molybdenum is widely found in vegetables and legumes. This trace element is important for a healthy reproductive system and intakes should be maintained during pregnancy.

PHOSPHORUS

Some 80 percent of phosphorus is found in the bones, where it helps to give rigidity, and in teeth. In other tissues it is needed for the metabolism of carbohydrates and for energy reserves. Phosphorus is essential for the structure and functioning of cell walls, and for healthy cell growth and reproduction. It is found in dairy products, grains, and meats. Excessive intakes of phosphorus may upset the calcium balance in the bones.

POTASSIUM

This mineral is mostly found inside cells and, like sodium, is important in the maintenance of the balance of fluids in the body. It is found in all fruits and vegetables and fruit juices. A lack of potassium can lead to mental confusion and muscular problems. Good intakes may help to reduce blood pressure.

SELENIUM

Selenium plays a role in converting fats and proteins into energy, and may help to reduce the risk of heart disease and cancer. Low intakes may affect male fertility and may result in nutritional disorders. Very low intakes may lead to heart failure. Selenium is found in cereals grown on selenium-rich soil, in Brazil nuts, seafood, and meats. Large intakes of selenium can result in a breakdown of the structure of the nails.

SODIUM

Sodium is needed to help regulate the amounts of fluid in the body. The correct balance of fluids is essential to life. Sodium is found dissolved in fluids inside the cells, between cells in blood plasma, in lymph glands, in secretions such as sweat, and in the urine. Sodium is most frequently found in the diet as sodium chloride, or salt. Excessive intakes may raise blood pressure.

ZINC

This trace element is needed for healthy bones, the activation of enzymes, the release of vitamin A, growth, the immune system, male fertility, and insulin release. Rich sources of zinc include oysters, other shellfish, red meats, and whole-grain cereals.

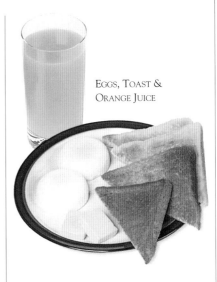

EGGS, TOAST &
ORANGE JUICE

ENHANCING ABSORPTION

The absorption and digestion of some minerals can be enhanced by combining them with other components in the diet.

- **EGGS AND TOAST** for breakfast supply iron. Absorption is enhanced by drinking orange juice, which contains vitamin C.

- **RED MEATS** are rich in easily absorbed iron. Absorption may be further improved by serving with carrots or sweet potatoes, which are rich in beta carotene.

- **CANNED FISH** are rich in vitamin D. The softened bones should be eaten with the flesh because these supply calcium.

- **TOAST MADE FROM** whole-grain bread supplies zinc. Adding baked beans will provide additional protein.

- **ESSENTIAL FATTY ACIDS** from oily fish are believed to enhance the absorption of calcium from the digestive tract.

PHOSPHORUS & CALCIUM

Phosphorus helps the body to absorb calcium into the bones. Too much may retard calcium retention and lead to demineralization. A good ratio of one part phosphorus to four parts calcium is easily achieved in a healthy and balanced diet containing dairy products, nuts, seeds, vegetables, fruits, starchy foods, and protein. Excessive amounts of phosphorus are consumed in a diet that contains large amounts of processed foods, such as meat products (for example, canned meats), processed cheese, instant soups and desserts, and cola drinks in particular.

PLANT NUTRIENTS

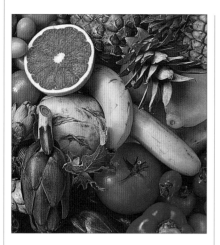

I N ADDITION TO FATS, proteins, carbohydrates, vitamins, and minerals, scientists have discovered that plants also contain substances known as phytochemicals, or phytonutrients. There are literally thousands of these plant chemicals present in grains, fruits, and vegetables. They have specific roles to play, such as protecting the plant from strong ultraviolet rays, infections, and pollution. When people eat fruits, vegetables, and grains, they may acquire the benefits of phytonutrients.

DISCOVERING PHYTONUTRIENTS

Many thousands of plant chemicals, or phytonutrients, have now been identified. It is in the laboratory that their identification takes place. Researchers painstakingly identify the compounds in foods, then start working out how they react and interact. In the case of soybeans, the phytonutrients thought to play a role in protecting against breast cancer have been identified as isoflavones, substances that are very similar in structure to the human hormone estrogen. Once identified, plant chemicals are tested in the laboratory to see what they are capable of doing under artificial conditions. Scientists have yet to prove that phytonutrients protect against particular diseases, but the evidence suggests that increasing consumption of fruits, vegetables, and other plant foods is a positive step for health. That it could be lifesaving adds an exciting new dimension.

CAN PLANTS PREVENT DISEASE?

Scientists have been able to relate high intakes of specific foods in particular countries with low rates of certain diseases. In countries such as Japan, for example, where soy-based foods such as tofu are eaten regularly, there are lower rates of breast cancer than elsewhere. Research has indicated that if Japanese women move to other countries where their intake of soy products falls, the occurrence of breast cancer among them increases. Studying this kind of association can help researchers to identify what the protective factors may be.

PHYTONUTRIENTS & HEART DISEASE

Certain phytonutrients are believed to help prevent heart disease. It is likely that some, such as a red pigment called lycopene that is present in tomatoes, protect blood vessels from cholesterol buildups in arteries by means of their antioxidant functions. Other plant chemicals may help to keep blood pressure under control or blood free from clots.

HOW MUCH TO EAT

Many specialists recommend that in order to ensure a good intake of phytonutrients, a wide variety of fruits, vegetables, and cereal products is eaten on a regular basis. In practice, this means trying to consume at least five servings of fruits and vegetables each day. These can be fresh or frozen and, in some cases, such as carrots and legumes, canned. Fruit and vegetable juices count as servings.

• EACH SERVING is assumed to weigh about 3oz (80g), making a total daily intake of about 14oz (400g) of fruits and vegetables. Selecting different colors of fruits and vegetables is a simple method of ensuring a variety of phytonutrients.

• GRAINS should be included in most meals if possible. Whole-grain varieties are the most likely to contain protective phytonutrients and include wholewheat bread, wholewheat pasta, brown rice, buckwheat, and bulghur wheat. Whole-grain breakfast cereals also contribute to the dietary intake.

• BEANS AND OTHER LEGUMES are rich in plant chemicals and can be eaten as an alternative source of protein to meats, fish, and poultry. Using legumes as the main source of protein once a day will significantly boost phytonutrient intakes.

• NUTS AND SEEDS supply a range of phytonutrients such as lignans, as well as many vitamins, minerals, proteins, and essential fats. Some sunflower, pumpkin, and sesame seeds, as well as a variety of nuts, should be eaten on a regular basis.

• HERBS AND SPICES are good sources of various phytonutrients and are easy to add to the ingredients in any meal.

COMMON PHYTONUTRIENTS

Scientists have only recently begun to understand the contribution that phytonutrients make to human health. Increasing numbers of these substances are being identified and their properties investigated. The groups listed on this page are just a selection of the many phytonutrients that researchers have analyzed.

CAROTENOIDS

These seem to protect against heart disease and cancer by reducing damage to HDL cholesterol and encouraging healthy cell growth while discouraging cancerous cells.

FLAVONOIDS

Flavonoids may help to fight heart disease by preventing a buildup of cholesterol in arteries. They may block cancer-causing substances and suppress cancerous changes.

ISOFLAVONES

These plant estrogens seem to mimic human estrogen. They have antioxidant effects and are thought to help reduce the risk of heart disease and cancer.

ISOTHIOCYANATES

These phytonutrients seem to help to neutralize free radicals and increase the activity of cancer-fighting enzymes. They may reduce the risk of lung cancer.

LIGNANS

These chemicals have weak estrogenic effects and appear to limit cancerous changes. They also act as antioxidants and may help to protect against heart disease.

PHENOLIC COMPOUNDS

These are thought to be able to counteract the effects of pollutants such as cigarette smoke. They are antioxidants and may help to control cancerous changes to cells.

SAPONINS

Saponins seem to help to inhibit tumor formation and aid fat digestion. They may help to reduce levels of fats in the blood and possibly reduce the risk of heart disease.

TERPENES

These seem to interfere with cancer-causing substances, and in particular they may also help prevent tooth decay and reduce the risk of stomach cancer.

PHYTONUTRIENTS & CANCER

It is possible that some phytonutrients can provide protection against various types of cancer. The suspected mechanisms that are involved in this protection are numerous. Certain phytonutrients, such as bioflavonoids, may block cancer-causing substances from reaching the tissues and cells that they normally target. They might, on the other hand, help to prevent blood vessels from reaching a newly-formed cancer and, in effect, starve it to death. Some phytonutrients may work by triggering enzymes that remove cancer-causing substances from the body, while others may help to prevent cells that have been exposed to such substances from becoming malignant and replicating out of control. Certain phytonutrients, such as chlorophyll, may be capable of protecting the body against cancer simply by strengthening the immune system so that it can successfully resist invading cancers; others, such as isoflavones, may block off sites where naturally occurring body hormones might otherwise attach and trigger cancerous growth.

WHERE TO FIND PHYTONUTRIENTS

Many thousands of phytonutrients have now been identified. So far only a limited number of these have been thoroughly researched. They are present in all fruits, vegetables, grains, and legumes, as well as in drinks such as tea, coffee, wine, and juices. The amount of phytonutrients present may vary according to soil quality in the area where a plant is grown.

BEST FOOD SOURCES

The following list provides examples of the immense variety of phytonutrients and their common dietary sources.

- BETA-CRYPTOXANTHIN Mangoes, papayas, peaches
- CAROTENOIDS Carrots, sweet potatoes, mangoes, apricots
- COUMARINS Oranges, grapefruits, flax seeds, green vegetables, green tea
- ELLAGIC ACID Strawberries, raspberries, blackberries
- FLAVONOIDS Apples, onions, grapes
- INDOLES Green leafy vegetables
- ISOFLAVONES Soybeans, tofu, soy milk, whole grains, chickpeas, millet, sorghum
- ISOTHIOCYANATES Broccoli and other cruciferous vegetables
- KAEMPFEROL Radishes, kale, leeks, endive, broccoli, tea
- LENTINAN Mushrooms
- LIGNANS Whole grains, seeds, berries
- ORGANOSULFURS Garlic, onions
- PHENOLIC COMPOUNDS Citrus fruits, tomatoes, peppers, tea, wine
- PHYTOENE Mangoes, pumpkins
- SAPONINS Soybeans
- TERPENES Citrus fruits
- ZEAXANTHIN Red and yellow peppers

FOOD SUPPLEMENTS

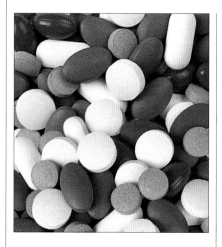

WHEN TO TAKE SUPPLEMENTS

The best way of remembering to take supplements is to make them part of a daily routine, so that taking them becomes a regular habit. In most cases, extra nutrients are needed during the day, so the morning is a good time to take them. Calcium is an exception. It may be more beneficial to take this in the evening, since this is when calcium is being replaced in the bones. It is also thought to help with sleep. Supplements should usually be taken with food, since they are absorbed better in this way. Some supplements are most effective when combined with others.

• **IRON** supplements work best when taken with vitamin C, since this vitamin helps to increase iron absorption.

• **VITAMIN B** supplements work best when they are in a vitamin B complex.

• **VITAMIN C** is absorbed better when combined with bioflavonoids, which increase its effectiveness. It is best to use supplements that include both nutrients.

• **VITAMIN E** is most effective when it is taken with vitamin C.

THERE IS GROWING EVIDENCE to suggest that, even if a person eats a balanced diet, he or she does not necessarily receive all the nutrients needed to maintain a healthy body. There are times when extra intakes of food supplements can be beneficial, such as during adolescence, pregnancy, and old age. Those who are chronically ill, on restrictive diets, or on long-term weight-reduction programs, may also benefit from supplements. Research is beginning to reveal that taking large amounts of certain vitamins, minerals, and even some phytonutrients may help people to fight diseases and other health problems.

OPTIMUM NUTRITION

Some scientists and nutritionists believe that the current recommended daily intakes (RDIs) for vitamins and minerals are too low. These RDIs (*see page 12*) are set at levels that are known to prevent deficiency disease. For example, the recommended intake of vitamin C at 40mg a day ensures that the disease scurvy will not develop. There is a school of thought, however, that believes that, rather than consuming nutrients at levels that are known to prevent deficiency, people should be taking them at levels that promote optimal health. This would mean that an intake of between 400mg and 1,000mg of vitamin C a day should be taken in order to achieve and maintain the best possible health. Intakes of vitamin C at these high levels are believed to boost the immune system and fight off infections such as colds, help to bolster cancer-fighting systems in the body, and help to combat the signs of aging.

ESSENTIAL SUPPLEMENTS

Some supplements are recommended by both traditional and optimum nutritionists. For example, folic acid supplements of 400mcg a day should be taken by women who are planning to conceive, in order to help reduce the risk of spinal defects such as spina bifida in the baby. Supplements of vitamin B_{12} are advisable for all strict vegetarians since this vitamin is hard to find in nonmeat foods unless they are fortified. Vitamin D supplements are recommended for people who have little exposure to sunlight during the summer months, and therefore have little opportunity to make this vitamin in their skin. People over 65 years old, as well as pregnant and breastfeeding women, are advised to take 10mcg of vitamin D per day. Infants should also receive vitamin D at levels of 8mcg a day until they are at least three years old.

OPTIMUM INTAKES

Intakes at the levels shown below are thought by some nutritionists to not only fight disease and infection but to promote optimal health (*see right*).

VITAMINS & MINERALS	MEN 25–50	MEN 51+	WOMEN 25–50	WOMEN 51+
Vitamin A (mcg)	1,000	2,000	800	2,000
Vitamin B_1 (mg)	7.5	9.2	7.1	9
Vitamin B_2 (mg)	2.5	2	2.5	2
Vitamin B_3 (mg)	30	25	30	25
Vitamin B_6 (mg)	10	25	10	20
Vitamin B_{12} (mcg)	2	3	2	2
Vitamin C (mg)	400	800	400	1,000
Calcium (mg)	1,500	1,500	1,500	1,500
Vitamin E (mg)	400	800	400	800
Folic acid (mg)	800	1,000	800	1,000
Selenium (mg)	200	200	200	200
Zinc (mg)	20	20	20	20

NON-NUTRITIONAL SUPPLEMENTS

There is a vast array of food supplements available from health-food stores, pharmacies, and supermarkets. It is advisable to find the highest-grade versions of these products that use standardized extracts and have been tested in the laboratory. Certain brands of the products listed here have well-researched benefits.

ANTHOCYANIDINS

Taken from bilberries and the skins of red grapes and cranberries, these strongly antioxidant extracts appear to help to improve the suppleness of collagen, keeping the arteries and veins flexible and the skin firm. They may be useful for a healthy complexion.

CO-ENZYME Q

Normally manufactured in the body, co-enzyme Q, or Co-Q, improves the ability of cells to use oxygen. Research has shown that taking Co-Q in supplement form may help to improve oxygen flow to the heart in people who have problems such as angina pectoris.

PHYTOESTROGENS

Capsules containing isoflavones from soy flour and other sources, such as red clover, are now available, and are thought to help protect premenopausal women against breast cancer. They have also been shown to help reduce menopausal symptoms such as hot flashes.

SAW PALMETTO

Studies show that extracts from saw palmetto berries can reduce symptoms of the benign growth of the prostate gland. Saw palmetto seems to inhibit the enzyme that converts testosterone into a form that causes prostate enlargement. It is therefore a useful supplement for men.

ECHINACEA

Rich in phytonutrients, supplements of echinacea are believed to support the immune system. Capsules or drops can be taken at the onset of a cold or flu.

GARLIC

Garlic contains allicin in its active form, which helps to lower cholesterol levels. Supplements may help to reduce the risk of thrombosis and hardening of the arteries.

GINKGO BILOBA

Standardized extracts of gingko biloba have been shown to improve the circulation, which makes it a useful supplement for people who have heart disease.

HYPERICUM

Extracts of hypericum can improve mood and relieve mild depression. Hypericum has been used to treat seasonal affective disorder (*see page 234*).

BENEFICIAL SUPPLEMENTS

There are several reasons for supplementing the diet. At times of growth or an excessive use of energy, the body may use up its natural reserves of a particular nutrient, in which case it may be necessary to replenish those reserves with a supplement. Supplements can also be used to boost the levels of a nutrient in the body in order to guard against future deficiency. Adolescent girls and women who follow a strict vegetarian diet may benefit from taking iron supplements of 15mg a day. Women who have had a baby, or are planning several pregnancies in quick succession, are likely to run down their bodies' reserves of iron, and may benefit considerably from taking extra iron in the form of supplements.

Calcium intakes in many teenagers are known to fall significantly below currently recommended levels. The strengthening of bones can be achieved only until the age of 20. After this time, the final adult bone strength is set. The teenage years are therefore very important for the formation of strong bones for the rest of life. If intakes of calcium-rich foods, such as dairy products, are low, daily calcium supplements of 800–1,500mg can be very helpful.

Male infertility appears to be an increasing problem in the West. The mineral selenium is now known to play an important role in the production of sperm. In some countries,

WHEN NOT TO SUPPLEMENT

Some nutritional supplements interact with prescribed drugs. Others are affected if they are taken with substances such as coffee, so it is important to check with a doctor before taking any supplements to make sure that they are appropriate.

• CALCIUM interacts with tetracycline antibiotics, and supplements should not be taken at the same time as a course of these antibiotics.

• FISH OILS may disturb the action of the drug warfarin, which is prescribed for people with blood-clotting problems.

• FOLIC ACID is affected by phenytoin, an anticonvulsant drug, which increases the speed at which folate is broken down in the body. Extra folic acid is therefore required by those who are prescribed phenytoin.

• VITAMIN A SUPPLEMENTS should not be taken by pregnant women, since excessive intakes of this vitamin may cause birth defects.

• VITAMIN B SUPPLEMENTS are adversely affected by coffee and tea, so they should not be taken together.

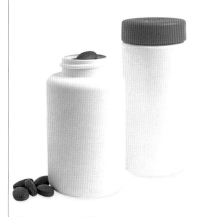

CHEMICAL NAMES

The labels on food supplements can be confusing, since they may use the chemical name instead of the more commonly recognized letter system of referring to vitamins and minerals.

• FOLIC ACID is the synthetic form of folate.

• VITAMIN A is retinol, retinyl palmitate, or beta carotene.

• VITAMIN B_1 is either thiamine, thiamine hydrochloride, or thiamine mononitrate.

• VITAMIN B_2 is riboflavin.

• VITAMIN B_3 is niacin or niacinamide.

• VITAMIN B_5 is pantothenic acid or calcium pantothenate.

• VITAMIN B_{12} is cyanocobalamin.

• VITAMIN C is ascorbic acid, calcium ascorbate, magnesium ascorbate, or sodium ascorbate.

• VITAMIN D is ergocalciferol or cholecalciferol.

• VITAMIN E may be known as d(I) alpha-tocopherol, tocopheryl

NUTRIENT BALANCE

It is advisable to take any mineral or vitamin as part of a multivitamin and mineral supplement. This will help to avoid any imbalances, since taking supplements of one particular nutrient can disturb the balance of others within the body.

• LARGE INTAKES of iron can affect the phosphorus balance and cause zinc imbalances. Large intakes of zinc can cause iron imbalances, and large intakes of both iron and zinc can adversely affect the copper balance.

• EXCESSIVE INTAKES of iron, copper, and manganese increase the oxidation of vitamins A, D, and E and thereby risk lowering levels of these nutrients.

• LARGE INTAKES of phosphorus may leech calcium from the bones.

• TOO MUCH CALCIUM and phosphorus can affect levels of manganese.

intakes of selenium are falling since there is now less selenium present in wheat-based foods, such as bread, than there used to be. In the US, however, this is not a problem since wheat is grown in soil rich in selenium. Supplements of 100–200mcg taken daily have been shown to improve male fertility and should be considered in areas where selenium intakes are low.

Evening primrose oil contains gamma-linolenic acid (GLA), which is usually made in the body from the essential omega-6 fatty acid linoleic acid, found in nuts and seeds. Some people are not able to make GLA within the body and seem to benefit from taking GLA directly in the form of evening primrose oil. When taken as a supplement, evening primrose oil has been shown to help reduce some symptoms of premenstrual syndrome, benign breast discomfort, hyperactivity in children and, when taken in combination with fish oil, to reduce the inflammation associated with rheumatoid arthritis.

Oils from oily fish supply the nutrients eicosapentaenoic acid (EPA) and docosahexaenoic acid (DHA) made in the body from the omega-3 essential fatty acid alpha-linolenic acid. Regular intakes of EPA and DHA provided by fish-oil supplements have been shown to help to reduce the vicosity, or "stickiness," of blood and therefore the risk of blood clots forming. They also appear to improve inflammatory-based conditions, such as rheumatoid arthritis and psoriasis, as well as Raynaud's syndrome. These supplements are particularly useful for people who do not like, or are unable to consume, oily fish, such as herrings, mackerel, salmon, and sardines, on a regular basis. Supplements of EPA and DHA are also thought to be useful for pregnant and breastfeeding women in order to ensure that their babies have adequate supplies of these substances, which are essential for the development of the brain and eyes.

Smokers require extra vitamin C, since the habit of smoking increases the metabolism of this vitamin. Intakes of 80mg a day of vitamin C are recommended by traditional nutritionists, while optimum nutritionists believe that even larger intakes of 1,000mg a day are more appropriate.

PHYTONUTRIENT SUPPLEMENTS

The growing interest in phytonutrients and their potential ability to prevent degenerative diseases, such as certain cancers, heart disease, and cataracts, has led to the development of synthetic versions of these substances being packaged and sold in supplement form. For example, it is now possible to buy quercetin and rutin, carotenoids and anthocyanidins, in the form of capsules and tablets. There is, as yet, no evidence to support the fact that, in these synthetic forms, phytonutrients have protective effects. When taken in sources of food, it is likely that their potentially protective effects are in part explained by their synergy with other phytonutrients, vitamins, and minerals.

WHAT'S IN A SUPPLEMENT?

Supplements in tablet form contain other substances in addition to their vitamin, mineral, or other nutritive content. For example, fillers such as dicalcium phosphate are added to bulk up the active ingredients, while binders such as cellulose, alginic acid, and sodium alginate are added to create the correct consistency. In some cases lubricants are also used, and these may include silica or magnesium stearate. Coatings are used to protect the tablets, making them smooth and easy to swallow. They come in various forms, such as zein or waxes. Most capsules are made from gelatin that is sourced from animal products. Some capsules are now available that are produced from a seaweed product called agar (*see page 71*), making them suitable for vegetarians.

TAKING SUPPLEMENTS

Unlike some medicines, dietary and health supplements should not be viewed as an instant solution. The body needs a steady, regular supply of nutrients, preferably from the diet, or from supplements, for metabolism and the growth and repair of body tissues, since not all nutrients are stored in the body. For someone who is unable to eat a varied diet, dietary supplements may be part of a regular and long-term routine. It is important to be aware that, although supplements may help to protect against some illness and aid recovery, they alone cannot always cure disease.

SUPPLEMENTS VERSUS A GOOD DIET

Everyone should aim to eat as varied and balanced a diet as possible to provide for their nutritional needs. Supplements are useful to "plug the gaps" if regular consumption of a balanced diet is not possible because of a lack of accessibility of the right kinds of food, or when nutritional requirements are increased at specific times in life or as a result of disease. Supplements supply micronutrients but cannot replace the macronutrients in the diet – those major components of foods that include carbohydrates, fats, and proteins.

RISK OF OVERDOSING

It is important to be aware that taking certain supplements in excessive quantities can have harmful effects.

• **BETA CAROTENE** Daily intakes of over 15mg of beta carotene can turn the palms of the hands and soles of the feet orange. This is because carotenoids are stored in body fat. The coloring is reversed once intakes are lowered.

• **VITAMIN A** Single doses of 300mg in adults and 100mg in children may be harmful. Regular intakes greater than 9,000mcg a day in men and 7,500mcg in women should be avoided. High intakes can lead to bone damage, loss of hair, double vision, and vomiting. In pregnant women, intakes of more than 3,330mcg a day may result in birth defects.

• **VITAMIN B$_1$** Long-term intakes of more than 3g a day can lead to headaches, insomnia, irritability, a rapid pulse, and general weakness.

• **VITAMIN B$_3$** Doses of nicotinic acid in excess of about 200mg per day cause dilation of blood vessels in the skin, and therefore flushing. Other blood vessels may also dilate, decreasing blood pressure.

• **VITAMIN B$_6$** It is possible that high doses of vitamin B may cause nerve problems, particularly in hands and feet.

• **VITAMIN C** When taken in quantities of over 1gm a day, vitamin C may lead to diarrhoea in some people. Those on high intakes of vitamin C should decrease intakes slowly. Quick withdrawal may cause scurvy because the body will have become used to high intakes.

• **VITAMIN D** Intakes above the recommended dosage should be avoided for infants, since this can lead to poor growth and development.

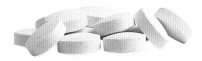

NUTRITIONAL SUPPLEMENTS IN TABLET FORM

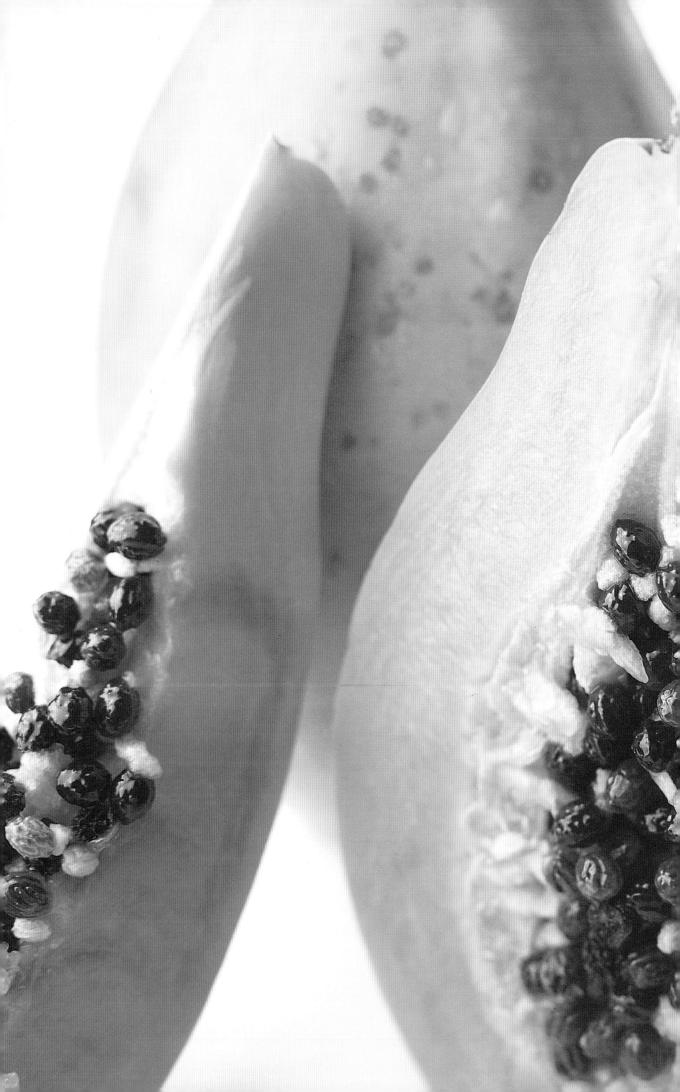

Food profiles

This section encourages a greater understanding of the beneficial effects that certain foods have on health. The traditional uses and nutritional composition of each food are listed, as are the latest scientific findings on the food's potential healing properties. The most valuable nutrients are listed according to their significance in relation to each food.

·······················STAR NUTRIENTS KEY·······························

Valuable nutrients found in each food profiled on the following pages are listed under **Star Nutrients & Phytonutrients**. Some have not yet been assigned official nutritional values and do not appear in the **Key Nutrients** charts for each food.

MINERALS

Ca	Cu	Fe	I	K	Mg	P	Se	Zn
Calcium	Copper	Iron	Iodine	Potassium	Magnesium	Phosphorus	Selenium	Zinc

VITAMINS

B₁	B₂	B₃	B₅	B₆	B₁₂
Vitamin B_1	Vitamin B_2	Vitamin B_3	Vitamin B_5	Vitamin B_6	Vitamin B_{12}

Bc	C	D	E	H
Folic Acid	Vitamin C	Vitamin D	Vitamin E	Biotin

VEGETABLES

THERE ARE HUNDREDS of varieties of vegetables throughout the world. They fall into many groups, and are increasingly recognized for their extraordinary health-giving benefits. Low in calories, yet high in bulking fiber, vegetables add a range of essential vitamins and minerals to the diet. They are the source of a host of protective phytonutrients that are increasingly believed to help prevent diseases including heart disease, certain cancers, cataracts, and spinal defects.

PROTECTIVE MEASURES

Over thousands of centuries of evolution, plants have developed ways of resisting and surviving the various stresses in their environment, including ultraviolet radiation from the sun, pollution, and invasion by bacteria, viruses, and insects. One method of self-protection was the development of protective plant chemicals, known as phytonutrients. If vegetables containing these substances are eaten, their protective qualities seem to be passed on to the consumers, helping people to fend off the threat of diseases and the stresses of modern living.

MAJOR BENEFITS

The specific energy content of vegetables varies. Some starchy varieties, such as potatoes, sweet potatoes, and parsnips, supply more than leafy vegetables, such as cabbages, spinach, and lettuce, but the overall contribution vegetables make to the caloric content of the diet is small. It would be necessary to eat $4^{1}/_{2}$–$6^{1}/_{2}$ lbs (2–3 kg) of vegetables to provide 1,000 calories. They supply virtually no protein and little fat. Many contain useful amounts of calcium and iron, good amounts of potassium, and small amounts of B vitamins. Vitamin C, folate (folic acid), and carotenes are the nutrients supplied in most significant quantities, along with fiber.

PHYTONUTRIENTS

With increasingly sophisticated analytical techniques, it has become possible to identify the chemicals, or phytonutrients, in vegetables that supply such valuable health benefits. Scientists have recently discovered, for example, the potential cancer-fighting effects of genistein and daidzein, the plant estrogen compounds found in soy products; the ability of allicin in garlic and onions to boost the immune system and to help fight infections; and the isothiocyanates in cruciferous vegetables, such as broccoli, that appear to suppress tumor growth.

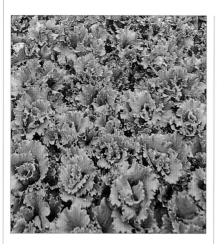

ORGANIC VEGETABLES

The organic production of vegetables is kinder to the environment than modern methods, but there is no evidence that it improves nutritional quality. Whether or not organic vegetables taste better than nonorganic is subjective. Organic production systems use microorganisms, soil flora and fauna, and other plants and animals in place of agrochemicals. Farmers using agrochemicals, however, are thought to be those most at risk from their side effects.

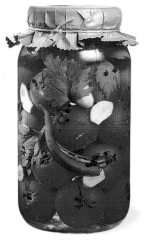

PICKLES & PRESERVES

Vegetables, sometimes with fruit, can be preserved in vinegar, either alone or in combinations, to make pickles, chutneys, and relishes. These can be sweet or sour, chunky or smooth, and can be eaten alone or as accompaniments to meats, cheese, and fish. Firm, young vegetables and fruits are preferred for pickling, and the smaller varieties are best when pickled whole. The vegetables are preserved by the acetic acid content of the vinegar, which protects them against spoilage from microorganisms. Baby onions, shredded cabbage, gherkins, cauliflower florets, and whole or sliced beets all make good pickles.

STORAGE, FREEZING & CANNING

Green leafy vegetables that are stored unrefrigerated in a warm climate can lose up to 20 percent of their vitamin C within the first two hours of picking, and up to 90 percent 24 hours after picking. The losses are less dramatic in temperate climates. The rate of loss of vitamin C levels out after an initial fall, and can be as little as eight percent over 14 days. The loss is mainly due to oxidation which, during storage, is mostly caused by enzymes released within the vegetables as a result of bruising, wilting, warm temperatures, and rotting. Storing vegetables in the regrigerator at home is advised in order to minimize the loss of nutrients. Vegetables that are fast frozen within two hours of harvesting, stored correctly, and cooked according to package instructions retain vitamin levels equal to, or better than, vegetables eaten soon after harvesting, and better than those bought in many supermarkets. The availability of beta carotene is improved by canning; most of the B vitamins, with the exception of vitamin B_1, and vitamin E remain remarkably intact. Vitamin C is, however, largely destroyed by this method of preservation, through the effects of both heat and oxygen left in the can after processing.

PREPARATION

Where possible, the trimming and peeling of vegetables should be minimal to retain as many nutrients and phytonutrients as possible. Tearing preserves more vitamins than cutting. Much of the fiber in potatoes is found in the skin, and the darker, outer leaves of cabbage and lettuce are the richest sources of carotenes. Preparation should be left as close to the time of consumption as possible to reduce exposure of cut surfaces to light and oxygen, which leads to the oxidation, and therefore deterioration, of unstable vitamins such as vitamin C.

COOKING

While many vegetables can be eaten raw, some must be cooked. Vitamins B_1, B_2, B_6, B_{12}, the B vitamin biotin, and vitamin C dissolve in water. Cooking methods using the least amount of water preserve these vitamins best. Steaming, microwaving, and pressure cooking have been shown to preserve on average about 73 percent of the vitamin C in broccoli, compared to 35 percent retained when it is boiled. Avoid frying vegetables, which adds fat and calories to these low-energy-density foods.

MAIN VEGETABLE GROUPS

There are many ways to classify the hundreds of edible vegetables now widely available. Some of the major and most popular groups are listed below.

- **BEANS** include runner, French, adzuki, lima, mung, and kidney.
- **BRASSICAS** include cabbage, brussels sprouts, cauliflower, broccoli, watercress, and mustard and cress.
- **LEAFY VEGETABLES** include spinach, Chinese cabbage, kale, and sorrel.
- **LEGUMES** include peas, soybeans, chickpeas, and lentils.
- **CHILIES AND PEPPERS** include several varieties of chilies and red, yellow, green, purple, and white peppers.
- **FRUIT-VEGETABLES** include eggplants, cucumbers, gherkins, and green, yellow, red, cherry, and plum tomatoes.
- **FUNGI** include porcini, field, shiitake, maiitake, and oyster mushrooms.
- **THE ONION FAMILY** includes onions, shallots, leeks, garlic, and chives.
- **ROOT VEGETABLES (TUBERS)** include rutabagas, turnips, salsify, carrots, parsnips, celeriac, beets, and radishes.
- **SALAD LEAVES** include lettuce, chicory, arugula, radicchio, and endive.
- **SEAWEEDS** include rock and marsh samphire.
- **SQUASHES** include pumpkins, summer squash, zucchini, and acorn squash.
- **STARCHY ROOTS** include potatoes, cassavas, sweet potatoes, and yams.
- **STEM AND STALK VEGETABLES** include celery, asparagus, and bamboo shoots.

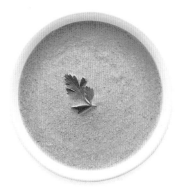

VEGETABLE SOUPS & JUICES

Eating canned or homemade soup is an enjoyable, nutritious, and easy way to consume vegetables. There is a growing interest in vegetable juices because of their high nutritional value. Raw vegetable juice contains, in a delicious and easily digestible form, the excellent vitamin and mineral content that can be lost when vegetables are cooked.

BRASSICAS

STAR NUTRIENTS & PHYTONUTRIENTS

C Ca Fe Carotenes, Indoles

The group of vegetables known as the brassicas contains a variety of plants that are consumed worldwide. These include broccoli, cabbage, cauliflower, kale, Brussels sprouts, turnips, and the more exotic kohlrabi, rutabaga, and bok choy. They are low in calories and supply many nutrients and "phytonutrients," including iron, carotenes, and the vitamins B, C, and E.

KEY BENEFITS

- CAN BOOST THE IMMUNE SYSTEM
- MAY HELP TO PREVENT CANCER
- MAY HELP TO PREVENT SPINA BIFIDA
- MAY HELP TO PREVENT HEART DISEASE

FOOD PROFILE

★ HOW MUCH TO EAT

- A 3oz serving of most brassicas supplies over 68 percent of an adult's total daily vitamin C requirement.

CHOOSING & STORING

- Buy flowering brassicas with firm, compact heads and closed flower buds.
- Choose small sprouts, which have a better flavor than large ones.
- Keep in a dark, cool place to conserve nutrients, flavor, and texture.

COOKING & EATING

- Most brassicas can be eaten raw.
- Cutting, chewing, and cooking brassicas release compounds called indoles, which may help to prevent estrogen-related cancers.

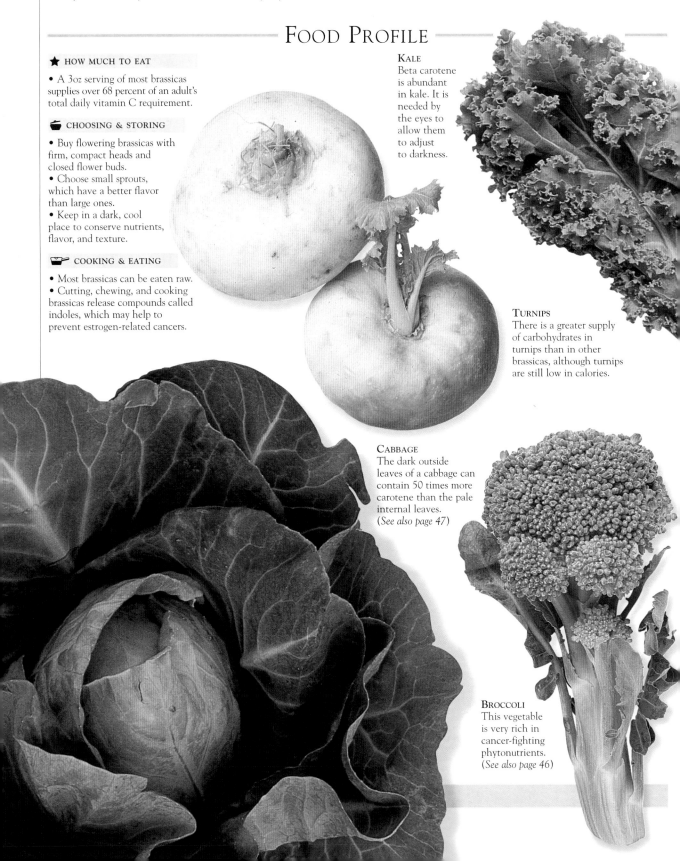

KALE
Beta carotene is abundant in kale. It is needed by the eyes to allow them to adjust to darkness.

TURNIPS
There is a greater supply of carbohydrates in turnips than in other brassicas, although turnips are still low in calories.

CABBAGE
The dark outside leaves of a cabbage can contain 50 times more carotene than the pale internal leaves.
(*See also page 47*)

BROCCOLI
This vegetable is very rich in cancer-fighting phytonutrients.
(*See also page 46*)

KEY NUTRIENTS *per 1–1¹/₄ cups*	CABBAGE	BROCCOLI	BRUSSELS SPROUTS	CAULIFLOWER	KALE	TURNIP	RED CABBAGE
Calories	26	33	42	34	33	23	26
Iron (mg)	1	2	1	1	2	0.2	1
Folate (mcg)	75	90	135	66	120	14	75
Vitamin C (mg)	49	87	115	43	110	17	49
Vitamin B₆ (mg)	0.2	0.1	0.4	0.3	0.3	0.1	0.04
Beta carotene (mcg)	385	575	215	50	3145	20	385
Vitamin E (mg)	1	1	1	0.2	2	–	–
Calcium (mg)	52	56	26	21	130	48	52
Potassium (mg)	270	370	450	380	450	280	270
Fiber (g)	2	3	4	2	3	2	3

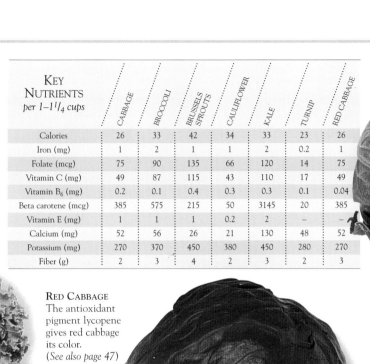

RED CABBAGE
The antioxidant pigment lycopene gives red cabbage its color.
(*See also page 47*)

CAULIFLOWER
Plant chemicals called glucosinolates give cauliflowers their mustardlike flavor. This is particularly strong when the vegetable is eaten raw.

BRUSSELS SPROUTS
Weight for weight, Brussels sprouts contain the most folate of all the brassicas.

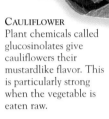

HEALING PROPERTIES

☑ TRADITIONAL USES
Cabbage leaves can be used by breast-feeding mothers to soothe painful nipples. The leaves can also be applied directly to wounds, arthritic joints, inflammations, and acne. In Chinese medicine, kale is believed to ease lung congestion, and its juice is used to treat gastric ulcers. Because of kohlrabi's neutral nature, it is given to balance blood sugar levels and to aid alcohol detoxification.

❊ SPECIFIC BENEFITS
Disease
Studies have shown that the antioxidant pigment beta carotene, which is the most abundant carotenoid in brassicas, may stimulate the immune system. It helps to increase the power of immune system cells, thereby improving the body's ability to defend itself against disease. The B vitamin, folate (and the man-made form of folate, known as folic acid), is also needed to produce antibodies and white blood cells. Brussels sprouts, kale, broccoli, cabbage, and cauliflower are all useful suppliers of folate.

Cancer
Research based on laboratory tests and population studies implies that broccoli, cabbage, and cauliflower may have cancer-fighting properties. Both vitamin C and the amino acid cysteine in these vegetables are thought to be involved. Brassicas also contain indoles, which may reduce the risk of breast cancer, and sulforaphane, which, via a chain reaction, is thought to be able to detoxify potential cancer-causing substances.

Spina Bifida
There is evidence that folate helps to prevent spina bifida, a defect of the spinal cord, from developing in unborn babies. The spinal cord develops within the first month of pregnancy, so women of childbearing age should ensure high dietary intakes of folate, as well as taking the recommended daily supplement of 400mcg of folic acid.

Heart Disease
Folate appears to be needed by the body in order to prevent levels of a substance called homocysteine from rising above normal. Raised levels of this substance can cause heart disease. Homocysteine is made from an amino acid as part of the body's normal metabolism. After carrying out some functions, it is converted back into an amino acid with the help of folate. About 60 percent of people fail to complete this reconversion and are left with a high level of homocysteine. Taking in more folate may help to prevent this.

CAUTION

People with goiter should not eat too many brassicas. Some glucosinolates in brassicas break down into isothiocyanates, which prevent the thyroid gland from absorbing iodine.

SEE ALSO CANCER, PAGE 214; HEART DISEASE, PAGE 152

BROCCOLI

STAR NUTRIENTS & PHYTONUTRIENTS

(C) (Bc) (Fe) (Ca) Beta carotene

O ne of the richest sources of iron in the vegetable world, broccoli has probably attracted more attention than any other vegetable regarding its potential cancer fighting properties. Broccoli belongs to the cruciferous family, which also includes cabbage, kale, and cauliflower. It not only supplies potential cancer preventing phytonutrients, but also provides a range of vitamins and minerals, including vitamins C and E, calcium, and iron.

KEY BENEFITS

- MAY HELP TO PREVENT VARIOUS KINDS OF CANCER
- CAN HELP TO PREVENT ANEMIA
- MAY REDUCE THE RISK OF COMMON INFECTIONS
- MAY BE BENEFICIAL TO SMOKERS

FOOD PROFILE

KEY NUTRIENTS
per 4oz (1³/₄ cups)

Calories	33
Iron (mg)	2
Fiber (g)	3
Beta carotene (mcg)	575
Folate (mcg)	90
Vitamin C (mg)	87
Calcium (mg)	56
Potassium (mg)	370
Vitamin E (mg)	1
Sodium (mg)	8

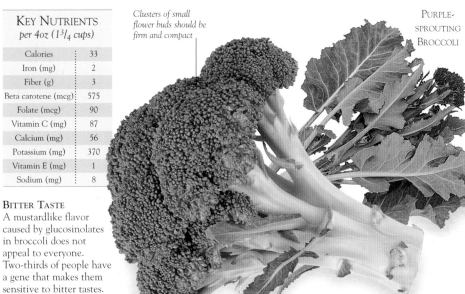

Clusters of small flower buds should be firm and compact

PURPLE-SPROUTING BROCCOLI

GREEN BROCCOLI

BITTER TASTE
A mustardlike flavor caused by glucosinolates in broccoli does not appeal to everyone. Two-thirds of people have a gene that makes them sensitive to bitter tastes. Serving broccoli in white sauce makes it more palatable.

★ **HOW MUCH TO EAT**

- An average 1-cup serving of broccoli supplies 2mg of the 10mg of iron recommended for adults daily. Eating two to three servings of broccoli a week amy boost iron levels and play a role in cancer prevention.

🍲 **CHOOSING & STORING**

- Buy fresh, compact, green or purple-sprouting broccoli.
  - Store broccoli unwashed, in the refrigerator for between one and two days. Alternatively, keep in a cool place and use as soon as possible.

🥘 **COOKING & EATING**

- Steam, boil, microwave, or stir-fry broccoli. Use in soups, add cooked to omelettes and pasta, or allow to cool, then use in salads.

HEALING PROPERTIES

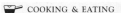

📋 **TRADITIONAL USES**
Chinese medicine usually recommends broccoli to treat eye inflammations and near-sightedness. Broccoli's "cooling nature" and slightly bitter flavor are said to give it its diuretic properties.

❖ **SPECIFIC BENEFITS**
Cancer
Ranked first in the National Cancer Institute's list of all-around cancer-fighting vegetables, broccoli has been the subject of much research. Broccoli is believed to play a role in protecting against cancers of the lung, stomach, mouth, ovaries, breast, cervix, colon, and prostate. It is rich in several potential cancer fighting substances such as indoles, glucosinolates, beta

carotene, and vitamin C. There is one particular substance, known as sulforaphane, that has been extensively examined in laboratories. Sulforaphane is a phytonutrient that stimulates the formation and function of "phase II" enzymes. These enzymes have been identified as being responsible for processing and removing cancer causing substances from cells under experimental conditions. It is speculated that these phase II enzymes may be able to perform this function in the human body.

Anemia
A good source of iron and beta carotene, broccoli may help to prevent anemia, especially in vegetarians.

Many women have iron reserves below the recommended level of 500mg. A significant proportion of women in the West have no iron reserves at all. This can result in full-blown anemia, which causes severe fatigue, an inability to concentrate, and an impaired immune system, making those affected much more susceptible to infection. Scientists believe that the body can absorb a third less iron from vegetables than it can from red meat, due to substances such as phytates that block iron absorption. They have recently revealed that the beta carotene in iron-rich vegetables such as broccoli may help to overcome this blockage and make the iron available.

Childhood Infections
Children with respiratory infections, measles, and gastroenteritis have been found to have a significant drop in blood levels of vitamin A. The beta carotene that broccoli provides is converted into vitamin A when the body's stores run low. Adding broccoli to children's diets may, in theory, help to reduce childhood infections.

Smoking
The phytonutrients called isothiocyanates present in broccoli may help to reduce the carcinogenic effects of cigarette smoke. Broccoli is also rich in vitamin C, which is required in increased amounts by smokers.

SEE ALSO ANEMIA, PAGE 160; CANCER, PAGE 214; CHILDREN & NUTRITION, PAGE 136; INFECTIONS, PAGE 212

CABBAGE

A cruciferous vegetable, the cabbage comes in several guises, including spring, flower, red, savoy, and head cabbage. All of these varieties contribute good amounts of vitamin C, folate, beta carotene, and fiber to the diet. Long recognized in traditional medicine for its healing powers, recent scientific study of the cabbage has now confirmed the wide diversity of its healing properties, which orthodox medicine has often found puzzling.

KEY BENEFITS

- MAY HELP TO PREVENT CANCER
- RELIEVES STOMACH ULCERS
- HELPS TO RELIEVE MASTITIS
- MAY HELP TO REDUCE THE RISK OF HEART DISEASE

FOOD PROFILE

KEY NUTRIENTS
per 1 cup (100g)

Calories	26
Fiber (g)	2
Potassium (mg)	270
Calcium (mg)	52
Vitamin C (mg)	49
Vitamin E (mg)	1
Iron (mg)	1
Vitamin B1 (mg)	0.2
Beta carotene (mcg)	385
Folate (mcg)	75

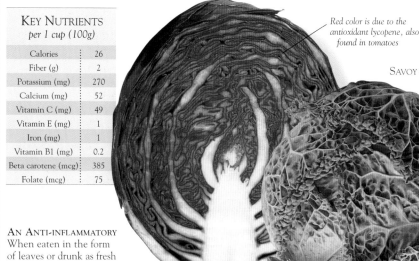

Red color is due to the antioxidant lycopene, also found in tomatoes

SAVOY CABBAGE

RED CABBAGE

AN ANTI-INFLAMMATORY
When eaten in the form of leaves or drunk as fresh cabbage juice, cabbages have anti-inflammatory effects inside the body. They also have this effect when the crushed leaves are applied externally to inflamed skin.

★ HOW MUCH TO EAT

- A ¾-cup serving of cabbage supplies the body with almost all the recommended daily intake of vitamin C. Regularly eating two to three servings a week of raw green cabbage may help to reduce the risk of cancer.

CHOOSING & STORING

- Look for a crisp, firm cabbage that feels heavy for its size.
- Store cabbage in a plastic bag or wrapped in a paper towel in the refrigerator. It should stay fresh for several days.

COOKING & EATING

- Cabbage is most nutritious when eaten raw. Before cooking, remove discolored leaves, then steam, microwave, or boil in the minimum amount of water to preserve the water-soluble and heat sensitive vitamin C.

HEALING PROPERTIES

🖉 TRADITIONAL USES
Cabbage has been used in folk medicine in the West for hundreds of years to help digestive and lung disorders and aches and pains. Applied externally, the leaves were used to treat wounds, ulcers, mastitis, inflamed joints, and acne. Cabbage was also taken to treat migraine and fluid retention. In Chinese medicine, cabbage is used to treat conditions with discharges of yellow mucus, and is recommended for constipation in the Far East.

✤ SPECIFIC BENEFITS
Breast and Prostate Cancers
Phytonutrients in cabbage known as indoles work on enzymes that can break down hormones involved in causing breast and prostate cancers. Under experimental conditions, indole-3-carbinol has been shown to inhibit the growth of breast cancer.

Bacterial Infections
Cabbage has long been known for its action against bacterial infections. Scientists believe that this may be attributed to phytonutrients known as glucosinolates.

Peptic Ulcers
For over 40 years, cabbage juice has been recognized as an effective treatment for stomach ulcers. It is thought that this effect can be attributed to the substance known as S-methylcysteine sulphoxide. For stomach or duodenal ulcers, one folk remedy suggests drinking half a cupful of fresh cabbage juice two to three times daily between meals for two weeks.

Mastitis
The anti-inflammatory properties of cabbage can help to relieve the pain of mastitis and engorged breasts during breastfeeding. The middle rib of the cabbage leaves should be removed and the leaves then gently crushed and applied directly to the skin.

Heart Disease
Red cabbage supplies the red antioxidant lycopene. Research has found that higher intakes of this antioxidant in the diet are associated with lower levels of heart disease in men.

OTHER FORM

Sauerkraut
Fermented cabbage that has been shredded and salted is known as sauerkraut. It is thought that sauerkraut stimulates digestion and it works well with foods that are filling. Sauerkraut is very salty and should be avoided by those with high blood pressure who have been advised to follow a low-salt diet.

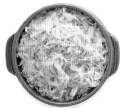

SAUERKRAUT

SEE ALSO CANCER, PAGE 214; PEPTIC ULCERS, PAGE 171; HEART DISEASE, PAGE 152; WOMEN & NUTRITION, PAGE 140

ARTICHOKES

STAR NUTRIENTS & PHYTONUTRIENTS
  Cynarin, Silymarin, Inulin
K   Fe

A thistle-like plant, the artichoke has been described as the aristocrat of the traditional kitchen garden, and it remains today a vegetable that people tend to eat on special occasions. Artichokes are rich in potassium and low in calories. They are also plentiful in the phytonutrient cynarin, which is believed to help reduce blood levels of cholesterol and triglyceride.

KEY BENEFITS
- MAY LOWER HIGH CHOLESTEROL AND FATS
- COULD PROTECT AGAINST HEPATITIS
- INCREASES THE AMOUNT OF BENEFICIAL BACTERIA IN THE LARGE INTESTINE
- MAY PROTECT AGAINST SKIN CANCER

FOOD PROFILE

KEY NUTRIENTS
per 1 small artichoke (100g)

Calories	18
Potassium (mg)	360
Iron (mg)	1
Folate (mcg)	21
Calcium (mg)	41
Pantothenic acid (mg)	0.3
Vitamin B$_1$ (mg)	0.1
Sodium (mg)	27
Beta carotene (mcg)	39
Fiber (g)	4

A KIND OF THISTLE
Artichokes belong to the thistle family. In the center of the artichoke is a thistle-like "choke." It must be removed before eating the artichoke flesh, or "heart." This is easy to do once the artichoke has been cooked.

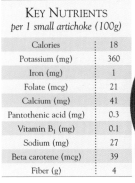

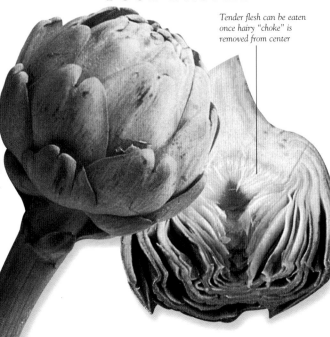

Tender flesh can be eaten once hairy "choke" is removed from center

★ HOW MUCH TO EAT
- An artichoke heart weighs about 2oz and supplies 180 of the 3,500mg of potassium needed on a daily basis. Eaten regularly, artichokes may help those with heart disease and high levels of cholesterol.

CHOOSING & STORING
- Choose heavy, plump artichokes with large, compact leaves that move when pressed.
- Store in the refrigerator for up to a week.

COOKING & EATING
- Trim, then soak upside down in salted water for an hour to dislodge dirt trapped between the leaves. Brush with lemon juice, then steam, microwave, or bake. Small artichokes may be eaten whole or sliced. With large artichokes, eat the heart and the soft parts of the leaves.

HEALING PROPERTIES

✔ TRADITIONAL USES
Many members of the thistle family have been used in the past to alleviate the symptoms of liver disease. Traditionally, artichokes were used in the West as a purifying tonic, helping the liver to eliminate toxins from the blood. Artichokes are recommended by herbalists for regenerating the constitution of the liver, which is particularly important in older people. The artichoke is also said to help restore and promote the flow of bile from the gallbladder, which helps the digestive system with the breakdown and metabolism of dietary fats. The kidneys are also believed to benefit from the artichoke's active constituents, which strengthen their metabolic functions.

✚ SPECIFIC BENEFITS
High Blood Cholesterol
Through the use of modern scientific methods, it has been discovered that the artichoke contains substances that appear to reduce blood cholesterol. The most widely studied active constituent is the phytonutrient cynarin which, when extracted from artichokes and given to people with high cholesterol levels, was found to be effective in lowering them. Studies are beginning to indicate that another artichoke extract known as monocaffeoylquinic acid may be even more effective.

High Blood Triglycerides
Experiments using the artichoke extracts cynarin and monocaffeoylquinic acid

have revealed that they may be able to reduce triglyceride levels in the blood.

Liver Disease
Cynarin and another substance in artichokes known as caffeic acid have been found to protect the liver from hepatitis infections when given as extracts to animals. These phytonutrients also appear to help the liver regenerate itself after it has been damaged or when parts have been removed.

Constipation
Artichokes may help to relieve constipation, since the complex carbohydrate that they contain known as inulin is nondigestible to humans, and has a laxative effect. In elderly patients who were

given inulin, it was found that their constipation decreased significantly, with only mild feelings of discomfort.

Bowel Cancer
The inulin in artichokes has been found to increase the beneficial bifidobacteria in stools and decrease enterobacteria and enterococci. This could promote a healthier environment in the bowel and could possibly reduce the risk of bowel cancer.

Skin Cancer
In experimental situations, the antioxidant in artichokes called silymarin has been shown to protect against skin cancer. It is as yet unknown if eating artichokes regularly would prove to be protective against skin cancer.

SEE ALSO CANCER, PAGE 214; CONSTIPATION, PAGE 175; HIGH BLOOD CHOLESTEROL, PAGE 154; LIVER DISEASE, PAGE 177

ASPARAGUS

Cultivated as a gourmet vegetable, it is the young, unemerged shoots of the asparagus plant that are eaten. With its bitter and mildly pungent flavor, asparagus is well known for its diuretic properties and is rich in potassium, the trace element needed for maintaining good water balance in the body. A serving of asparagus is also an excellent source of the B vitamin folate.

KEY BENEFITS

- STIMULATES THE KIDNEYS AND HELPS TO RELIEVE WATER RETENTION
- MAY HELP TO PREVENT HEART DISEASE AND HIGH BLOOD PRESSURE
- MAY HELP TO PREVENT CATARACTS

FOOD PROFILE

KEY NUTRIENTS
per 4–5 spears (100g)

Calories	25
Potassium (mg)	260
Folate (mcg)	175
Vitamin B$_1$ (mg)	0.2
Vitamin E (mg)	1
Iron (mg)	1
Zinc (mg)	1
Phosphorus (mg)	72
Fiber (g)	2
Vitamin C (mg)	12

A NATURAL DETOXIFIER
The many active plant chemicals in asparagus give it a bitter, mildly pungent flavour and make it an excellent detoxifier. Often eaten to combat the effects of over-indulgence, one particular constituent, asparagine, may help to build healthy new cells.

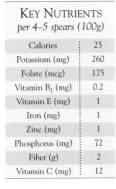

★ HOW MUCH TO EAT

- Five average-sized spears of asparagus weigh approximately 5oz and supply more than the daily requirement of folate that is reommended for both men and women.

CHOOSING & STORING

- Buy fresh, locally grown asparagus. Choose straight green or white spears.
- Do not store. Eat on the day of purchase.

COOKING & EATING

- Snap the stalks where they begin to thicken. Trim the asparagus, then steam whole, preferably upright, in 2.5in of water. Cover, then cook until tender. Serve with vinaigrette.

HEALING PROPERTIES

☑ TRADITIONAL USES

Medical applications of asparagus can be traced back thousands of years to ancient China, where it was first used as a "cooling" remedy to treat chronic bronchitis, lung congestion, and tuberculosis. Asparagus was also used to improve femininity in "aggressive" women, to ease menstrual difficulties, and to help purge the excesses of sweet, refined, intoxicating foods. In ancient Greece, asparagus was prescribed to stimulate and strengthen kidney function. Hippocrates prescribed asparagus for his overweight patients and those with blemished skin. In Ayurvedic medicine, asparagus is given to treat indigestion. As a home remedy, it has long been used to help to relieve various kidney and bladder problems, rheumatism, and gout. Asparagus has also been used in folk medicine to help to restore failing eyesight, ease toothache, and even to relieve the pain of bee stings.

✳ SPECIFIC BENEFITS

Bloating
It is the combination of the active ingredients in asparagus, which include asparagine, asparagose, chelindonic acid, coniferin, and potassium, that cause a diuretic effect. For the treatment of water retention caused by heart failure, and to treat hypertension (high blood pressure), doctors commonly prescribe diuretic drugs. Less serious cases of water retention, such as premenstrual bloating, may benefit from several servings of asparagus in the ten days before menstruation.

High Blood Pressure
The cause of high blood pressure is often unknown but there is usually a very strong hereditary tendency. High blood pressure can, in part, be caused by decreased blood flow through the kidneys. With less blood being processed by the kidneys, less water is removed and the blood volume and pressure remains higher than normal. Modern medicine uses specific drugs to treat high blood pressure, but in the past asparagus was used to help relieve symptoms and to prevent complications such as heart disease and migraines. If high blood pressure runs in the family, a diet that is low in salt and regularly includes asparagus could prove to be useful in its prevention.

Cataracts
The antioxidant glutathione is low in people who develop cataracts. An ancient herbal remedy called hachimijiogan increases levels of glutathione in the eye, which helps to prevent cataracts. Asparagus contains glutathione, and may have a similar effect.

CAUTION

Canned asparagus contains a large amount of added salt.

SEE ALSO BLOATING, PAGE 179; CATARACTS, PAGE 202; HIGH BLOOD PRESSURE, PAGE 155

CELERY

Grown for its crispy stalk, celery is native to Europe. It was first recorded in 850 BC in Homer's *Odyssey* and has been cultivated for its medicinal properties for thousands of years. Consisting of 95 percent water, this fibrous vegetable contains little protein, fat, or sugar, but it does supply a wide range of minerals and vitamins, and is known for its diuretic properties.

KEY BENEFITS

- USEFUL IN WEIGHT-LOSS EATING PLANS
- MAY HELP TO RELIEVE HIGH BLOOD PRESSURE
- KNOWN FOR ITS CALMING EFFECT
- USED TO TREAT RHEUMATOID ARTHRITIS

FOOD PROFILE

KEY NUTRIENTS
per 1 large stalk (100g)

Calories	7
Fiber (g)	1
Cellulose (g)	0.5
Potassium (mg)	320
Vitamin C (mg)	8
Calcium (mg)	41
Beta carotene (mcg)	50
Vitamin B$_1$ (mg)	0.1
Selenium (mg)	3
Vitamin E (mg)	0.2

POWERFUL INGREDIENTS
The seeds, root, fruit, and essential oils of celery are concentrated sources of biologically active substances. The stalks share these medicinal properties but have less powerful effects.

CELERY STALKS

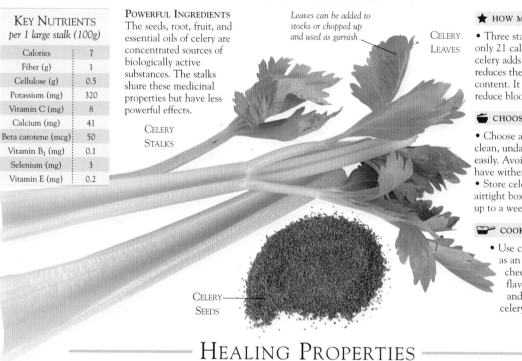

Leaves can be added to stocks or chopped up and used as garnish

CELERY LEAVES

CELERY SEEDS

★ HOW MUCH TO EAT

- Three stalks of celery supply only 21 calories. Eaten regularly, celery adds bulk to the diet and reduces the overall caloric content. It may also help to reduce blood pressure.

CHOOSING & STORING

- Choose a compact head with clean, undamaged stalks that snap easily. Avoid thick stalks that have withered leaves.
- Store celery unwashed, in an airtight box in the refrigerator for up to a week.

COOKING & EATING

- Use celery raw in salads or as an accompaniment to cheese. Celery also adds flavor and bulk to soups and casseroles. To cook celery, braise or microwave.

HEALING PROPERTIES

🗎 TRADITIONAL USES
In ancient Greece, celery was used by Hippocrates to stimulate digestion and to eliminate excess fluids from the body. In Chinese medicine, celery is said to have a "cooling" nature with a sweet and bitter flavor. It is therefore used to benefit the stomach, spleen, and pancreas, and to calm an aggravated liver. It is also used for eye inflammations and burning urine. In addition, celery's blood purifying properties help those with acne and canker sores. Western herbalism has traditionally recommended celery as a cleansing tonic after the winter months. The juice of celery is used in herbal medicine to treat urinary tract infections.

▣ SPECIFIC BENEFITS
Weight Problems
The very low caloric value of celery means that it is possible to eat large volumes of this vegetable yet consume extremely small numbers of calories and virtually no fat. For this reason it is good to include celery in its raw or cooked state in meals and snacks. In addition to its low calorie content, celery may be able to help overeaters to end a meal. This is probably because of its slightly bitter flavor, which is caused by the glycoside called apiin.

High Blood Pressure
The phytonutrient known as 3-n-butyl phthalid is found in celery. Phthalides are capable of regulating the hormones that control blood pressure in

the body. Tests carried out on small numbers of people with high blood pressure revealed that treatment with an extract of celery containing the active phthalid constituent reduced the severity of this hormonal problem in the majority of those studied.

Stress and Anxiety
Scientists have investigated the phytonutrients called phthalides in celery and found that in addition to their diuretic action, phthalides also have anticonvulsant and tranquilizing effects on the central nervous system. These findings may help to explain why celery has long been recommended by herbalists in the West for its calming effect on people.

Rheumatoid Arthritis
Celery is said to be effective in the treatment of rheumatoid arthritis. No studies have been conducted to prove or disprove this, but there is much anecdotal evidence to suggest that both the juice and whole stems may be useful. It is possible that celery's neutralizing effects in the body, combined with the silicon that it is said to contain, helps to renew joints and connective tissue.

CAUTION

It is advisable to avoid long exposure to the sun or tanning beds after eating large amounts of celery, as this may cause a reaction in the skin due to substances in celery called psoralens.

SEE ALSO HIGH BLOOD PRESSURE, PAGE 155; RHEUMATOID ARTHRITIS, PAGE 197; STRESS AND ANXIETY, PAGE 231

AVOCADOS

Strictly speaking, the avocado is a fruit, but since it is used mainly for savory dishes, it is referred to as a vegetable. With a history that can be traced back to 7000 BC, it was enjoyed by the Aztecs and Incas for its soft texture and possibly its health giving properties. Unusually for a vegetable or fruit, avocados are rich in oils and vitamin E. They also contain several B vitamins.

KEY BENEFITS
- MAY PLAY A ROLE IN THE PREVENTION OF HEART DISEASE
- USEFUL FOR BOOSTING THE IMMUNE SYSTEM IN THE ELDERLY
- COULD HELP TO IMPROVE MALE FERTILITY

FOOD PROFILE

KEY NUTRIENTS
per 1 large avocado (100g)

Calories	190
Monounsaturated fat (g)	12
Polyunsaturated fat (g)	2
Total fat (g)	20
Vitamin E (mg)	3
Potassium (mg)	450
Copper (mg)	0.2
Vitamin B₆ (mg)	0.4
Pantothenic acid (mg)	1
Fiber (g)	3

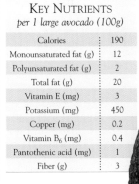

ALMOST PERFECT
The avocado is highly nutritious, and in nutritional terms, is said to be an almost complete food. Avocados are high in calories and fats, and they should be eaten in moderation by weight watchers. Most of the fat is monounsaturated, so it does not increase blood cholesterol levels.

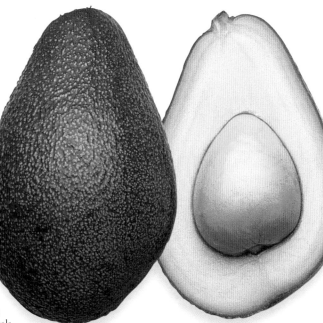

★ **HOW MUCH TO EAT**
- Half an avocado supplies about 4mg of vitamin E. Adults are advised to take a minimum of 30 international units (iu).

CHOOSING & STORING
- Select well-shaped avocados without bruises or blemishes. For immediate use, buy avocados that yield when pressed around the neck.
- To ripen firm avocados, store with a banana in a paper bag for a few days.

COOKING & EATING
- Cut in half lengthwise, then twist to separate the halves, and remove the pit.
- Serve in the skin or scoop out to make dips or cold soups. Alternatively, peel, slice, or cube, then add to salads.

HEALING PROPERTIES

⧉ TRADITIONAL USES
According to traditional Chinese medicine, the "cooling" nature of avocados helps to harmonize the liver while lubricating the lungs and intestines. Known to be a source of copper, it is also used to aid the formation of red blood cells. Easily digested and absorbed, avocados are recommended for nursing mothers and as a remedy for ulcers. Their reserve of monounsaturated fat and vitamin E has given them a name for beautifying the skin and helping wounds and burns to heal. Research in the West suggests that avocados can help to depress the secretion of the hormone insulin via a sugar called manoheptulose. They may therefore be useful for satisfying hunger.

⊞ SPECIFIC BENEFITS
Heart Disease
Researchers have concluded that high levels of vitamin E taken in the form of supplements or from foods such as avocados are associated with a reduced risk of cardiovascular disease. This is likely to be because low-density lipoprotein (LDL) cholesterol (*see page 25*) is protected by vitamin E from damage by free radicals in the blood. If damaged, it appears that LDL cholesterol is likely to create build ups in the blood vessels. Stopping LDL damage thereby helps to reduce cardiovascular problems. While many foods contain vitamin E, much of it is eliminated or destroyed during processing. Avocados have the advantage of

requiring no processing. While many scientists may recommend that vitamin supplements offer the best protection against heart disease, a diet that is rich in the natural, easily absorbable form of vitamin E may also be highly beneficial.

Infections in the Elderly
Studies have shown that vitamin E supplements given to elderly people are of benefit to their immune systems. This may be due in part to vitamin E's ability to reduce the number of harmful substances in the body that normally increase on aging. Avocados provide vitamin E in a palatable form. Including them in the diet of elderly people may help to protect them from infections.

Infertility in Men
It appears that vitamin E plays an important role in improving sperm counts and mobility. Together with vitamin C, it seems to play a role in stopping the sperm from clumping together and increases their mobility, so that they can swim to the egg more easily. Increasing intakes of foods rich in vitamin E and taking a supplement of about 600mg a day may improve levels of fertility in men.

Parkinson's Disease
Recent studies investigating the food choices of people with a form of Parkinson's disease has revealed that diets that are rich in vitamin E may offer some protection against this illness. This idea still needs testing.

SEE ALSO HEART DISEASE, PAGE 152; INFECTIONS, PAGE 212; INFERTILITY IN MEN, PAGE 227; PARKINSON'S DISEASE, PAGE 236

SQUASHES & PUMPKINS

STAR NUTRIENTS & PHYTONUTRIENTS

C K Beta carotene, Fiber

Vegetables of the genus of plants known as *Cucurbita* have long, trailing stems, and include squashes, pumpkins, and summer squash. Immature fruits of squashes with soft skins are described as summer squashes. Winter squashes are mature with a hard skin. Vegetables in this group contain beta and alpha carotene, which give them their color, and the antioxidant vitamins C and E.

KEY BENEFITS

- MAY PREVENT CANCER OF THE PROSTATE
- COULD HAVE A ROLE IN REDUCING DAMAGE TO THE RETINA AND LENS OF THE EYE
- HELP TO STRENGTHEN THE IMMUNE SYSTEM
- MAY REDUCE THE RISK OF HEART DISEASE

FOOD PROFILE

★ HOW MUCH TO EAT

- A 1¹/₄-cup serving of butternut squash may help to fight cancers. It may also help to protect the eyes from cataracts and boost night vision.

🍲 CHOOSING & STORING

- Choose clean, unblemished vegetables that feel heavy.
- Store whole vegetables in a cool, well ventilated place.
- Store cut pieces with their seeds intact and peel still on, in plastic kitchen wrap, in the refrigerator.

🍲 COOKING & EATING

- Remove the seeds and peel from large vegetables. Cut into chunks and boil, steam, or bake.
- Cook zucchini and small summer squash whole.

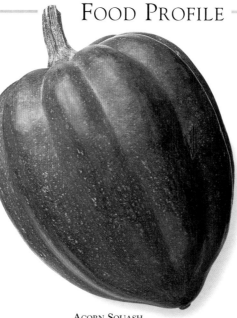

ACORN SQUASH
The antioxidant carotenoid known as beta cryptoxanthin is present in acorn squashes.

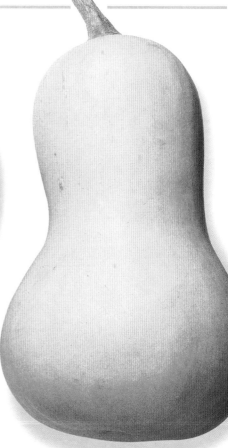

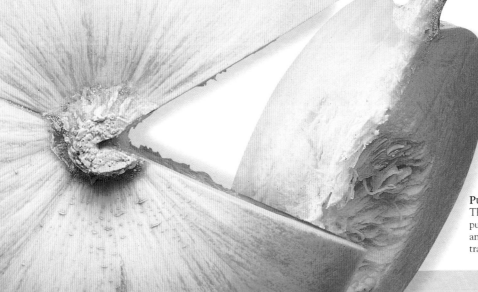

PUMPKIN SEGMENT

BUTTERNUT SQUASH
Substances called coumarins are present in butternut and all other squashes. These substances can detoxify enzymes that may lead to cancer development.

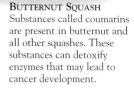

PUMPKIN SEEDS

PUMPKIN
The pigment lycopene is found in pumpkins. The seeds are rich in iron and zinc, and contain selenium, a trace element vital to male fertility.

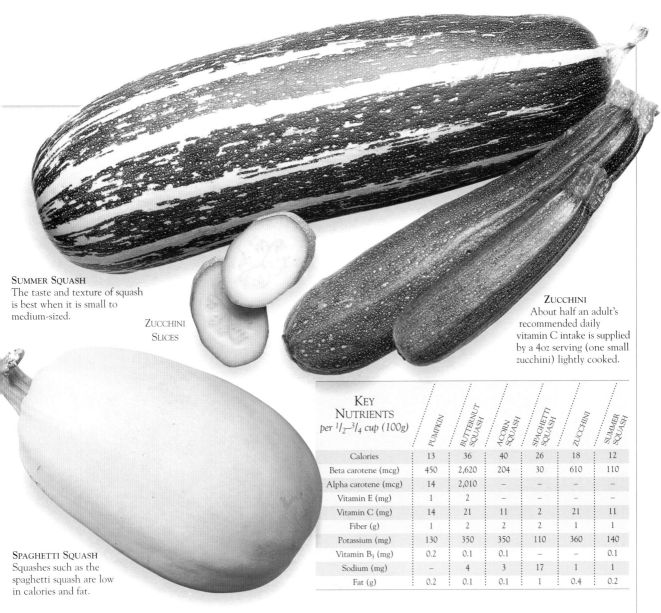

SUMMER SQUASH
The taste and texture of squash is best when it is small to medium-sized.

ZUCCHINI SLICES

ZUCCHINI
About half an adult's recommended daily vitamin C intake is supplied by a 4oz serving (one small zucchini) lightly cooked.

SPAGHETTI SQUASH
Squashes such as the spaghetti squash are low in calories and fat.

KEY NUTRIENTS per $^1/_2$–$^3/_4$ cup (100g)	PUMPKIN	BUTTERNUT SQUASH	ACORN SQUASH	SPAGHETTI SQUASH	ZUCCHINI	SUMMER SQUASH
Calories	13	36	40	26	18	12
Beta carotene (mcg)	450	2,620	204	30	610	110
Alpha carotene (mcg)	14	2,010	–	–	–	–
Vitamin E (mg)	1	2	–	–	–	–
Vitamin C (mg)	14	21	11	2	21	11
Fiber (g)	1	2	2	2	1	1
Potassium (mg)	130	350	350	110	360	140
Vitamin B₃ (mg)	0.2	0.1	0.1	–	–	0.1
Sodium (mg)	–	4	3	17	1	1
Fat (g)	0.2	0.1	0.1	1	0.4	0.2

HEALING PROPERTIES

TRADITIONAL USES
In traditional Chinese medicine, pumpkin is said to have "cooling" properties and to relieve dysentery, eczema, and water retention. It is also thought to help regulate blood sugar levels and to help stimulate the pancreas into action. For this reason, people who have diabetes and hypoglycemic problems are advised to eat pumpkin regularly. Pumpkin and pumpkin seeds are capable of destroying intestinal worms and dislodging and discharging mucus from the lungs, bronchi, and throat. Various squashes are also attributed, in Chinese medicine, with the ability to dislodge worms from the gut. Watery, summer zucchini are said to have a "cooling" and refreshing effect on the body and to act as a diuretic, thus helping to relieve water retention. They are most effective when eaten with their skins on. Also in Chinese medicine, squash juice is documented as being used in the treatment of burns when applied directly to the skin, while pumpkin juice is used as a laxative, and also as an effective supplement to the body's natural processes of detoxification.

SPECIFIC BENEFITS
Prostate Cancer
The regular consumption of yellow and green vegetables, including pumpkins, may reduce the risk of prostate cancer in men over 60 years of age. Beta and alpha carotene, which are found in pumpkins, butternut squashes, and zucchini, are believed to help to protect the prostate from cancer by "mopping up" substances that trigger the disease. These may either already be present in the body naturally, or may have been introduced to it through environmental pollution.

Cataracts
Elderly people with only a low level of the antioxidant beta carotene in their blood are more at risk of developing eye problems, such as cataracts and macular degeneration, than those with a high level of beta carotene. Adding pumpkin chunks to soups and stews is a digestible and palatable way for people to increase their intakes of beta carotene.

Colds and Influenza
Exposure to colds and influenza viruses has been shown to reduce levels of antioxidants, including vitamins C, E, and beta and alpha carotene. Pumpkins, zucchini, and squashes all supply these antioxidants and may help to protect against common colds and strains of influenza.

Heart Disease
The pigment lycopene, vitamin E, vitamin C, and beta carotene, all of which are found in squashes and pumpkins, are thought to reduce the risk of heart disease. These substances may help to prevent damage to the artery walls, caused by low-density lipoprotein (LDL) cholesterol (see page 25).

SEE ALSO CANCER, PAGE 214; CATARACTS, PAGE 202; COLDS & INFLUENZA, PAGE 184; HEART DISEASE, PAGE 152

ROOT VEGETABLES

STAR NUTRIENTS & PHYTONUTRIENTS

STAR NUTRIENTS & PHYTONUTRIENTS

   Fiber, Carotenes

This group contains a wide variety of vegetables, such as the salad roots beets and radishes, the composite root crops turnips, rutabagas, and salsify, and the *Umbellifer* roots carrots, parsnips, and celeriac. In addition to these, there are also the common starchy root crops such as potatoes, yams, cassavas, and arrowroot. The roots have varying nutritional values.

KEY BENEFITS

- MAY PREVENT BLOOD CLOTS AND BLOCKAGES, REDUCING THE RISK OF HEART DISEASE
- COULD HELP TO PREVENT VARIOUS CANCERS
- PROTECT AGAINST THE DAMAGE CAUSED BY NICOTINE INHALED THROUGH SMOKING

FOOD PROFILE

★ HOW MUCH TO EAT

- A ²/₃-cup serving of parsnips supplies almost 25 percent of an adult's daily fiber requirement.
- A ³/₄-cup portion of boiled beet supplies over 50 percent of an adult's recommended daily intake of the B vitamin folate.
- ²/₃ cup of carrots supply 6mg of beta carotene. There is no recommended daily intake for beta carotene, but some experts believe that adults should take in 10mg a day.

🥄 CHOOSING & STORING

- Look for firm, unblemished roots that are not sprouting.
- Make sure that the leaves of any root vegetables are fresh and green and not wilting.
- Most root vegetables keep well once they have been trimmed and placed in the refrigerator.

🍲 COOKING & EATING

- Root vegetables can be boiled, steamed, microwaved, or baked.
- Some root vegetables, such as carrots and radishes, can be eaten raw.

PARSNIPS
This familiar root vegetable supplies niacin, a B vitamin needed for energy metabolism. It also contains some folate and vitamin C.

POTATOES
Although supplying only 11mg of vitamin C per 4oz, potatoes are usually eaten in large quantities, so they make an important contribution to vitamin C intakes.

BEETS
This vegetable is known to purify the blood. The sweet taste of beet comes from its natural sugars. (*See also page 57*)

RUTABAGAS
With just 11 calories per cooked ³/₄-cup serving and virtually no fat, a rutabaga is a very filling low-calorie food.

RADISHES
The substances that give radishes their distinctive peppery taste are said to help relieve mucus conditions.

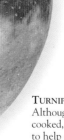

TURNIPS
Although usually eaten cooked, turnip is believed to help clear up lung congestion if eaten raw.

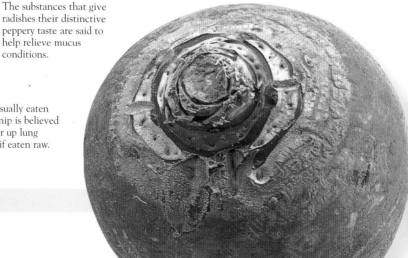

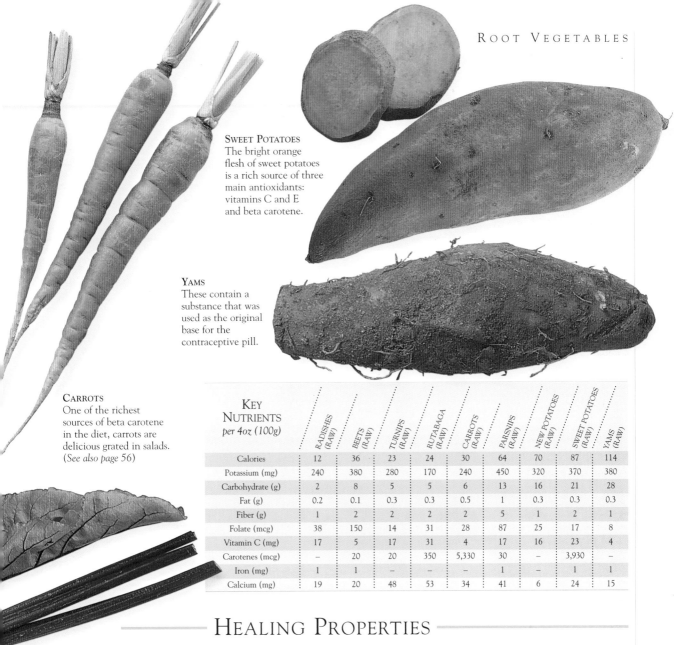

SWEET POTATOES
The bright orange flesh of sweet potatoes is a rich source of three main antioxidants: vitamins C and E and beta carotene.

YAMS
These contain a substance that was used as the original base for the contraceptive pill.

CARROTS
One of the richest sources of beta carotene in the diet, carrots are delicious grated in salads. (*See also page 56*)

KEY NUTRIENTS per 4oz (100g)	RADISHES (RAW)	BEETS (RAW)	TURNIPS (RAW)	RUTABAGA (RAW)	CARROTS (RAW)	PARSNIPS (RAW)	NEW POTATOES (RAW)	SWEET POTATOES (RAW)	YAMS (RAW)
Calories	12	36	23	24	30	64	70	87	114
Potassium (mg)	240	380	280	170	240	450	320	370	380
Carbohydrate (g)	2	8	5	5	6	13	16	21	28
Fat (g)	0.2	0.1	0.3	0.3	0.5	1	0.3	0.3	0.3
Fiber (g)	1	2	2	2	2	5	1	2	1
Folate (mcg)	38	150	14	31	28	87	25	17	8
Vitamin C (mg)	17	5	17	31	4	17	16	23	4
Carotenes (mcg)	–	20	20	350	5,330	30	–	3,930	–
Iron (mg)	1	1	–	–	–	1	–	1	1
Calcium (mg)	19	20	48	53	34	41	6	24	15

HEALING PROPERTIES

🌿 TRADITIONAL USES

An all-around detoxifier, radishes are said in the East to help prevent viral infections such as colds and influenza. They are good for clearing the sinuses and treating sore throats. A tablespoon of grated radishes eaten daily for several weeks has long been recommended by traditional healers in the West as a treatment for kidney and bladder stones. Beets have traditionally been used in Chinese medicine, in combination with carrots, to regulate hormones during menopause. They are also used to treat liver ailments and constipation, and to reduce uric acid production. Turnips are said to promote sweating. Parsnips have been used in the East for their diuretic properties and to help clear the liver and gallbladder of obstructions. They are also said to have mild analgesic properties. Potatoes have been prescribed for arthritis and rheumatism because they neutralize body acids. Sweet potatoes have been used in the East to treat night blindness due to their high content of beta carotene. The Mexican wild yam is a natural contraceptive. It contains diosgenin, precursor to the hormone progesterone, which was used as the basis for the contraceptive pill before it was made synthetically. Yams also relax muscles, and extracts are used in eczema creams. Some species of yam are used in China to treat urinary disorders; others are used to soothe the stomach.

✚ SPECIFIC BENEFITS

Heart Disease
It has been revealed that a regular intake of root vegetables is associated with the prevention of blood clots and blockages in blood vessels, which can be the cause of heart disease. Large intakes of root vegetables may therefore decrease cardiovascular related deaths.

Cancer
Evidence suggests that the regular consumption of raw vegetables, especially carrots, may help to decrease the risk of stomach and lung cancers, and possibly oral and rectal cancers. Beta carotene seems to have the strongest effect, followed by vitamin C, then vitamin E. It is thought that these nutrients soak up and perhaps deactivate potential carcinogens, thus preventing cancer inducing damage to DNA. For this reason, sweet potatoes are believed to protect against the dangers of nicotine and to guard against uterine and lung cancer. Other carotenoids and active phytonutrients, such as alpha carotene in beets and lutein in potatoes, may also have this protective effect against some types of cancer.

CAUTION

Do not eat potatoes that have sprouted or are green. They contain an alkaloid substance called solanine. The symptoms of solanine poisoning include gastro-intestinal disturbances and neurological disorders.

SEE ALSO CANCER, PAGE 214; HEART DISEASE, PAGE 152

CARROTS

STAR NUTRIENTS & PHYTONUTRIENTS

E K Beta carotene, Alpha carotene, Fiber

This crisp root vegetable, with its distinctive orange flesh, is naturally sweet and bursting with the protective antioxidant pigment beta carotene. Carrots also contain alpha carotene, which has antioxidant properties as well. Cooking carrots improves the accessibility of their beta carotene to the body, especially when they are served with a small amount of fat, such as butter.

KEY BENEFITS

- MAY HELP TO PREVENT CANCERS OF THE MOUTH, STOMACH, LUNG, AND RECTUM
- APPEAR TO FIGHT LISTERIA INFECTIONS
- INCREASE IRON ABSORPTION

FOOD PROFILE

KEY NUTRIENTS
per ¹/2 cup (100g)

Calories	30
Carotene (mcg)	5,330
Calcium (mg)	34
Folate (mcg)	28
Potassium (mg)	240
Carbohydrate (g)	6
Fiber (g)	2
Fat (g)	0.5
Vitamin E (mg)	1
Vitamin C (mg)	4

FULL OF CAROTENES
Carotenes are the antioxidant pigments in carrots and other vegetables that give them their bright color. If the body's reserves of vitamin A are low, beta carotene is converted into vitamin A in the intestinal wall and liver.

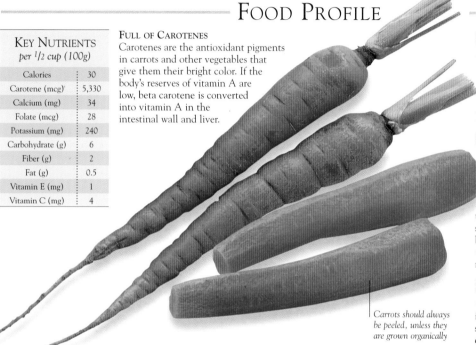

Carrots should always be peeled, unless they are grown organically

★ HOW MUCH TO EAT

- A ²/3-cup serving of carrots supplies 6mg of beta carotene. There is no recommended daily intake for beta carotene, but some experts believe that about 10mg should be taken daily.

CHOOSING & STORING

- Look for firm, smooth, well-shaped, bright orange carrots. Avoid those with cracks or soft or wet areas. Older carrots contain less carotenoids than young ones. If young carrots still have their tops, these should be bright green in color.
- Store carrots unwashed in the refrigerator for about a week.

COOKING & EATING

- Eat raw whole, sliced, or grated in salads. Alternatively, boil, steam, or microwave. Add to casseroles, stews, and soups.

HEALING PROPERTIES

🌿 TRADITIONAL USES
In Chinese medicine, carrots are used to stimulate the elimination of wastes and to dissolve gallstones. Carrots are also said to eliminate putrefactive bacteria in the intestines, and to contain an essential oil that is effective against ringworm. Eating two or three raw carrots a day for several days can fight off unwelcome infestations. Carrot juice is known by herbalists in the West for its diuretic action and as a treatment for heartburn.

⬛ SPECIFIC BENEFITS
Stomach and Lung Cancers
Carrots are one of the richest known sources of beta carotene. This antioxidant has the ability to soak up and make harmless the dangerous

by-products of metabolism and pollution known as free radicals. Left unattended, these are thought to be able to damage cells and start cancerous changes. A summary of the most well-conducted trials looking at beta carotene intakes has led experts to conclude that good intakes probably protect against cancers of the lung and stomach. Carrots may also protect against cancers of the mouth and rectum.

Food Poisoning
Some ready-made salads contain dangerously high levels of the food poisoning bacteria known as *Listeria monocytogenes*. Tests on ready-prepared carrots inoculated with *Listeria* revealed that carrots can

reduce *Listeria* levels. The antibacterial substance in carrots that has this effect has not yet been identified.

Iron Deficiency
Beta carotene has been shown to increase the absorption of iron from breakfast cereals threefold. It is possible that beta carotene joins forces with iron and keeps it in a soluble form so that phytates in cereals that block iron absorption are overridden. Increasing consumption of carrots to improve beta carotene intake may therefore also improve iron absorption.

Night Blindness
The traditional belief that carrots help you to see in the dark is well founded. Night blindness is usually due to a

lack of the substance visual purple, which requires beta carotene for its formation. The beta carotene in carrots helps to ensure that visual purple can be produced.

Sexual Problems
The ancient Greeks drank carrot juice as an aphrodisiac. Research suggests that carrots may contain a compound that stimulates sexual appetite. Research is continuing into this area.

CAUTION

Excessive consumption of carrots can lead to beta carotene deposits just under the skin, giving it a yellowish tinge. While harmless, the pigmentation can be aesthetically unappealing.

SEE ALSO ANEMIA, PAGE 160; CANCER, PAGE 214; FOOD SAFETY, PAGE 242

BEETS

This salad root is a relative of the wild sea-beet commonly found around European and Asian shorelines. Until the Romans began cultivating the vegetable for the root itself, only the beet leaves were eaten. By the 1400s, beets had become popular in English cuisine. Low in calories, raw beets are an excellent source of folate and a useful source of iron.

KEY BENEFITS

- MAY HELP WOMEN TO REDUCE THE RISK OF BABIES BEING BORN WITH SPINA BIFIDA
- MAY REDUCE THE RISK OF HEART DISEASE
- MAY HELP TO KEEP CHOLESTEROL LEVELS STABLE
- USEFUL REFUELING FOOD FOR TIRED MUSCLES

FOOD PROFILE

KEY NUTRIENTS
per 1/3 cup (100g)

Calories	36
Potassium (mg)	380
Fat (g)	0.1
Carbohydrate (g)	8
Fiber (g)	2
Folate (mcg)	150
Iron (mg)	1
Carotene (mcg)	20
Calcium (mg)	20
Vitamin C (mg)	5

Deep red color is due to the pigment betanin, widely used as a food coloring

FRESH RAW BEET

COOKED BEET

SWEET BEET
Beets are low in calories considering their sweetness and are said to taste as sweet as sugar. Probably as a consequence of their sweet taste, they are often acceptable to children.

★ **HOW MUCH TO EAT**
- Three small boiled beets that weigh a total of 4oz supply about 53 percent of the recommended daily amount of folate.

🍲 **CHOOSING & STORING**
- Choose firm, clean, smooth fresh beets with a rich red color and no soft, wet patches. Small beets are the most tender.
- Store beets for four to five days in the refrigerator.

🍳 **COOKING & EATING**
- Rinse, but avoid scrubbing, as this damages the skin. To cook, simmer for an hour, adding 1 tablespoon of salt for every 2lbs of beets. Otherwise bake or roast.
- Use cold in salads or add to soups. Beet leaves can be prepared and cooked in the same way as spinach.

HEALING PROPERTIES

📓 TRADITIONAL USES
The ancient Greeks and Romans used red beets to relieve a fever. In medieval Europe, the juice of beets was recommended when little else could be tolerated. The beet's purifying qualities have long been recognized by naturopaths. It stimulates the liver, kidneys, gallbladder, spleen, and bowel. In addition, naturopaths believe that beets stimulate the lymphatic system and strengthen the immune system, helping to fight colds. In Chinese medicine, beets are said to strengthen the heart, sedate the spirit, purify the blood, and treat sluggishness of the liver. It is given to women to regulate hormonal problems in menopause.

✴ SPECIFIC BENEFITS
Spina Bifida
Pregnant women and those planning to have a baby are strongly encouraged to increase their intake of folate through a daily supplement of folic acid, and through foods that are rich in folate, such as beets. Extra folate in the diet appears to reduce the risk of spina bifida in the unborn child. Cooking a beet decreases its folate, but a 2/3-cup serving still provides 110mcg, making it one of the richest food sources of this vitamin. In pickled beets almost all of the folate is destroyed.

Heart Disease
The high folate content of beets may make this vegetable a useful ally in helping to reduce the risk of heart disease. Adequate intakes of folate in the diet appear to decrease levels of the substance in the blood called homocysteine, which, when raised, is thought to be a significant risk factor in the development of heart disease.

High Blood Cholesterol
Beets contain soluble fiber, which may help to lower low-density lipoprotein (LDL) cholesterol (see page 25). Raised levels of LDL cholesterol are linked to an increased risk of heart disease. The carotenoids and flavonoids in beets may also work to prevent LDL cholesterol and artery walls from being damaged and oxidized by free radicals, which can result in heart attacks or strokes.

Muscle Depletion
Beets have a glycemic index, or GI (see page 18) of 64, so it is rapidly digested by the body and the blood sugar level rises quite quickly after consumption. This is the kind of food that athletes need to consume immediately after strenuous exercise in order to ensure that the energy reserves in their muscles are replenished as efficiently as possible. Pickled beets, and beets eaten in the form of soup are as effective as roasted or boiled beets.

CAUTION
Beet greens contain oxalic acid, which interferes with the absorption of calcium if taken in excess, and can cause kidney stones.

SEE ALSO FATS, PAGE 22; HEART DISEASE, PAGE 152; HIGH CHOLESTEROL, PAGE 154; WOMEN & NUTRITION, PAGE 140

LEGUMES

Legumes are the fruits and seeds of leguminous plants, and develop inside pods. Those that mature and dry on the plant include broad beans, chickpeas, kidney beans, lentils, soybeans, and white beans. Immature legumes, picked prior to maturation and drying, include green peas. Legumes supply an array of disease fighting phytonutrients.

KEY BENEFITS

- MAY REDUCE THE RISK OF HEART DISEASE
- HELP TO CONTROL BLOOD SUGAR LEVELS
- MAY LOWER THE RISK OF CERTAIN CANCERS
- CAN HELP TO MAINTAIN THE CORRECT LEVELS OF IRON AND CALCIUM IN THE BODY

FOOD PROFILE

★ HOW MUCH TO EAT

- 2/3 cup of red kidney beans provide about 16 percent of a woman's daily protein needs and about 14 percent of a man's daily protein needs.
- 2/3 cup of red kidney beans also supply 33 percent of an adult's daily fiber needs.
- 2/3 cup of chickpeas or haricot beans supply almost 7 percent of a woman's recommended daily calcium requirement.

📋 CHOOSING & STORING

- Buy legumes in dried, canned, or cooked forms.
- When buying dried legumes, choose those that are unbroken and of a uniform color.
- Avoid all types of dried legumes that have a sour smell.
- Store in an airtight container for no more than one year.

🍲 COOKING & EATING

- Soak all legumes, except lentils and split peas, in four times their volume of water for four hours.
- Boil, pressure-cook, or microwave legumes.

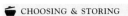

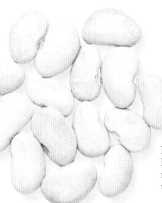

LENTILS
Magnesium, iron, zinc, and calcium are just some of the minerals contained in lentils. Red lentils also contain a small amount of carotene.

LIMA BEANS
Lima beans are believed to neutralize acidity in the stomach that arises from a meat-rich diet.

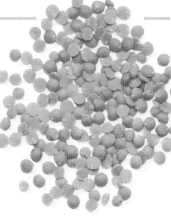

RED LENTILS

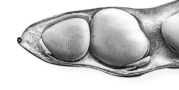

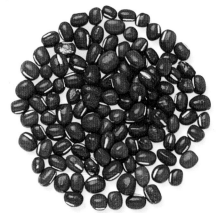

ADZUKI BEANS
Small red adzuki beans are sweeter in taste than other legumes, and are ideal served with rice. This combination supplies useful quantities of vegetable protein, along with valuable amounts of zinc.

HARICOT BEANS
A particularly good source of soluble fiber, haricot beans also contain more calcium than other legumes. Baked beans are haricot beans that have been cooked and combined with a tomato sauce.

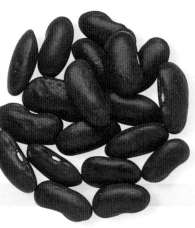
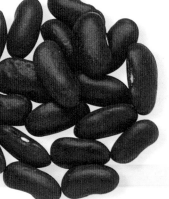

SOYBEANS
Grown in China for thousands of years, soybeans provide more protein than any other legume and have a higher fat content. They can be made into flour, then processed to form textured vegetable protein, known as TVP, which is used in vegetarian food products.

RED KIDNEY BEANS
Along with chickpeas, red kidney beans are the richest sources of protein of all the legumes.

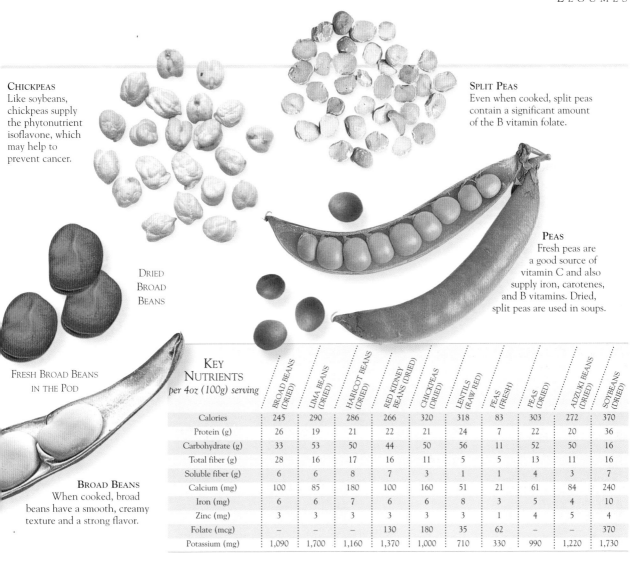

CHICKPEAS
Like soybeans, chickpeas supply the phytonutrient isoflavone, which may help to prevent cancer.

SPLIT PEAS
Even when cooked, split peas contain a significant amount of the B vitamin folate.

DRIED BROAD BEANS

PEAS
Fresh peas are a good source of vitamin C and also supply iron, carotenes, and B vitamins. Dried, split peas are used in soups.

FRESH BROAD BEANS IN THE POD

BROAD BEANS
When cooked, broad beans have a smooth, creamy texture and a strong flavor.

KEY NUTRIENTS per 4oz (100g) serving	BROAD BEANS (DRIED)	LIMA BEANS (DRIED)	HARICOT BEANS (DRIED)	RED KIDNEY BEANS (DRIED)	CHICKPEAS (DRIED)	LENTILS (RAW RED)	PEAS (FRESH)	PEAS (DRIED)	ADZUKI BEANS (DRIED)	SOYBEANS (DRIED)
Calories	245	290	286	266	320	318	83	303	272	370
Protein (g)	26	19	21	22	21	24	7	22	20	36
Carbohydrate (g)	33	53	50	44	50	56	11	52	50	16
Total fiber (g)	28	16	17	16	11	5	5	13	11	16
Soluble fiber (g)	6	6	8	7	3	1	1	4	3	7
Calcium (mg)	100	85	180	100	160	51	21	61	84	240
Iron (mg)	6	6	7	6	6	8	3	5	4	10
Zinc (mg)	3	3	3	3	3	3	1	4	5	4
Folate (mcg)	–	–	–	130	180	35	62	–	–	370
Potassium (mg)	1,090	1,700	1,160	1,370	1,000	710	330	990	1,220	1,730

HEALING PROPERTIES

🌿 TRADITIONAL USES
In Chinese medicine, legumes are believed to be good for the kidneys because of their diuretic properties. Red legumes, such as adzuki beans, red lentils, and kidney beans, are thought to influence the heart and small intestine. Yellow legumes, such as yellow peas and soybeans, are believed to help the spleen, pancreas, and stomach. White legumes, such as lima beans, assist the lungs and large intestine. Black and brown legumes, such as brown lentils, are believed to be good for the bladder. Green legumes, such as green peas, help the liver and gallbladder. An Ayurvedic dish called "kitcheri," a dish containing yellow mung beans, is thought to help irregular digestion.

✳ SPECIFIC BENEFITS
Heart Disease
Studies have revealed that when people with high levels of blood fat and cholesterol add legumes to their diet, these levels decrease. It is therefore possible that a legume rich diet could help in the battle against heart disease. The cholesterol and fat lowering effects of legumes probably come from their protein and fiber, and possibly the phytates that they contain.

Diabetes
Legumes are digested slowly. Once they have finally been broken down in the intestines, they are then gradually absorbed into the bloodstream as glucose, causing a gradual rise in blood sugar levels. This means that only small amounts of the hormone insulin need to be released to keep blood sugar levels within the normal range. For people who have non-insulin and insulin-dependent diabetes, a regular inclusion of legumes in their diets may help to improve their long-term control of blood sugar levels.

Cancer of the Colon
The insoluble fiber in legumes does not get digested in the small intestine but moves on into the large intestine, or colon, where bacteria act on it and produce short-chain fatty acids. These are thought to nourish the lining of the colon and protect it from carcinogenic invaders. Insoluble fiber adds to the physical bulk of the stools, helping them to move along more rapidly. This helps to prevent cancer causing substances from attaching themselves to the colon wall.

Anemia
A regular intake of legumes can add a significant amount of calcium and iron to the diet, especially for vegetarians. These minerals are important for building and maintaining strong bones and for the prevention of anemia.

> **CAUTION**
>
> Legumes contain proteins called lectins. If legumes are eaten undercooked, the lectins can cause vomiting and diarrhea. The lectins are destroyed by boiling the legumes fast for ten minutes.

SEE ALSO ANEMIA, PAGE 160; CANCER, PAGE 214; DIABETES, PAGE 218; HEART DISEASE, PAGE 152

SOYBEANS

T his pea-sized legume is an excellent source of protein, and therefore a useful food for vegetarians. Soybeans are also very rich in phytonutrients known as isoflavones, which are believed to account for the lower rates of breast and prostate cancers in countries where soybeans are consumed regularly. Soybeans can be yellow, black, or red, and all are high in nutrients.

> ### KEY BENEFITS
> - MAY HELP TO PREVENT BREAST CANCER
> - COULD REDUCE PROSTATE CANCER
> - LOWER LEVELS OF BLOOD CHOLESTEROL
> - MAY REDUCE THE RISK OF OSTEOPOROSIS

FOOD PROFILE

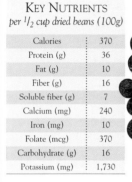

KEY NUTRIENTS
per ¹/₂ cup dried beans (100g)

Calories	370
Protein (g)	36
Fat (g)	10
Fiber (g)	16
Soluble fiber (g)	7
Calcium (mg)	240
Iron (mg)	10
Folate (mcg)	370
Carbohydrate (g)	16
Potassium (mg)	1,730

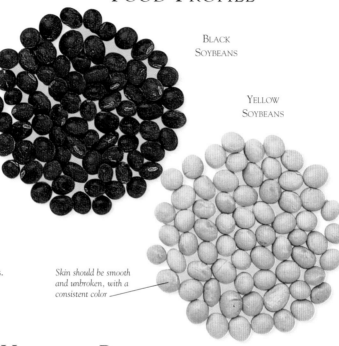

BLACK SOYBEANS

YELLOW SOYBEANS

Skin should be smooth and unbroken, with a consistent color

DISEASE FIGHTERS
Soybeans contain substances called "lignans," which have the ability to fight viruses, bacteria, and fungal infections. The lignans perform these functions in addition to their potential role in helping to prevent cancer.

★ HOW MUCH TO EAT
- A 1-cup serving of soybeans supplies about 15 percent of an adult's daily recommended intake of calcium, and provides about 25 percent of the protein needed daily. Eaten regularly, soybeans and soy products can make a significant contribution to calcium intakes and may help to maintain bone density.

CHOOSING & STORING
- Store in airtight jars in the refrigerator for up to six months to avoid rancidity.

COOKING & EATING
- Dried soybeans need to be cooked for at least three hours before eating; fresh beans can be steamed. Serve in stews and soups, or with salads. Soybeans served with rice supply all the essential amino acids.

HEALING PROPERTIES

🗹 TRADITIONAL USES
Soybeans were first described in ancient Chinese manuscripts in 2800 BC, at which time they were known as the "beef" of China. In traditional Chinese medicine, soybeans are believed to have "cooling" properties that strengthen the spleen and pancreas, cleanse the blood, and boost milk secretion in breast-feeding mothers. Rich in potassium, soybeans have also been used to relieve high blood pressure.

✠ SPECIFIC BENEFITS
Breast Cancer
The isoflavones found in soybeans and tofu called genistein and diadzein may help to inhibit the growth of cancerous breast cells. They seem to block the effect of

potentially harmful, naturally circulating estrogens in the blood. In laboratory studies, genistein has been shown to inhibit the growth of breast cancer cells.

Prostate and Other Cancers
The prostate gland has been found to contain estrogen receptors, as have the colon and uterus. In areas where soybeans and soy products are eaten regularly, reduced rates of cancers in these organs have been reported.

High Blood Cholesterol
A number of studies have revealed that 25–50g of soy protein eaten daily for four weeks can decrease low-density lipoprotein (LDL) cholesterol (*see page 25*) by as much as 10–20 percent in

people with high cholesterol. People with normal levels can also benefit. LDL cholesterol is able to damage the arteries, which may increase the risk of heart disease. It is the saponins and isoflavones in soy, especially genistein, that appear to have the LDL lowering effect. The genistein in soy may also improve the ability of the arteries to dilate, which helps to prevent blockages.

Osteoporosis
It is possible that the isoflavone diadzein in soy products could prevent decreases in bone mass in people with osteoporosis. The theory is that the isoflavone helps to reduce the amount of calcium that naturally leaches out of the bones.

OTHER FORM

Soy Products
Soybeans are used to make soy sauce and tofu (beancurd), and non-dairy milk and yogurt, which are alternatives for people who have an intolerance to dairy products. Tofu supplies both protein and calcium. It is made by soaking soybeans, then adding water to make a purée. This is strained, then the liquid boiled, to form curds.

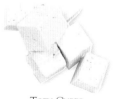

TOFU CUBES

SEE ALSO CANCER, PAGE 214; HIGH CHOLESTEROL, PAGE 154; OSTEOPOROSIS, PAGE 199

MUSHROOMS

STAR NUTRIENTS & PHYTONUTRIENTS

 K Bc Lentinan, D-fraction, Biotin

There are estimated to be more than 38,000 types of mushroom, some of which are poisonous, but most of which are edible. They fall into two types – cultivated and wild. Some mushrooms are believed to have health-giving effects, from thinning the blood to preventing tumors. Since they are low in calories, they can also be a useful ingredient in a weight-loss diet.

KEY BENEFITS

- MAY BOOST THE IMMUNE SYSTEM BY STIMULATING WHITE BLOOD CELLS
- BELIEVED TO HAVE ANTICANCER PROPERTIES
- MAY PREVENT CLOTS BY THINNING THE BLOOD

FOOD PROFILE

KEY NUTRIENTS
per 4oz (100g)

Calories	13
Protein (g)	2
Potassium (mg)	320
Copper (mg)	1
Pantothenic acid (mg)	2
Biotin (mcg)	12
Folate (mcg)	44
Iron (mg)	1
Vitamin B₃ (mg)	3
Fiber (g)	1

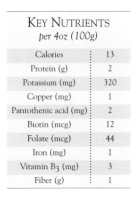

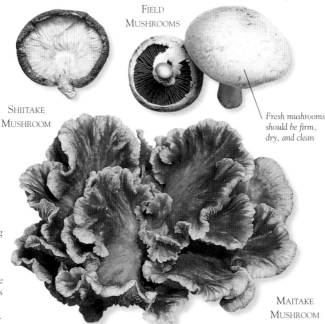

FIELD MUSHROOMS

SHIITAKE MUSHROOM

Fresh mushrooms should be firm, dry, and clean

MAITAKE MUSHROOM

A USEFUL SOURCE OF IRON
Mushrooms contain about 1mg of iron per 1¹/₂ cups. Unlike many vegetable sources of iron, mushrooms do not contain phytates, which reduce the body's ability to absorb this mineral, so the iron present in mushrooms is readily absorbed.

★ HOW MUCH TO EAT
- Five average-sized mushrooms supply about 25 percent of the recommended daily adult intake of copper. Eaten regularly, shiitake and maitake mushrooms may help to improve the function of the immune system.

CHOOSING & STORING
- Choose undamaged mushrooms with an earthy fragrance.
- Store mushrooms in a brown paper bag in the refrigerator for up to one week.

COOKING & EATING
- Gently wipe to remove dirt. Trim stems but do not peel.
- Cultivated mushrooms may be eaten raw.
- Maitake mushrooms can be obtained from Mailto, 64 Fairview Dr., East Hanover, NJ 07936 (Mailto:Fscalora@aol.com).

HEALING PROPERTIES

⬚ TRADITIONAL USES
Mushrooms have been used in traditional Eastern medicine for centuries. The shiitake is a well-known Japanese remedy for a variety of disorders. It has also been used to prevent heart disease, build resistance against viruses and disease, and treat fatigue and viral infections. In China, during the Ming dynasty, this mushroom was recorded as increasing stamina, and in the 15th century it was given to warrior priests for its energy giving properties.

⬚ SPECIFIC BENEFITS
Immune Deficiency
Members of the *Polyporaceae* family of mushrooms are unusually rich in medicinal properties. Of these, the maitake mushroom has

probably been studied the most, and it has recently been the subject of considerable research in the West. Maitake extracts have been shown to stimulate the immune system by increasing white blood cell activity. The specific extracts in these mushrooms that have been identified as being beneficial include two sugars, known as trehalose and chitin, as well as beta-1-6-D-glucans. These extracts appear to stimulate the immune system to launch attacks on invading bacteria and viruses, as well as helping it to respond if faced with a similar invader in the future. In addition to the maitake's effects on the immune system, it contains polyporenic acids, including nemotinic, acetic, and malic acids, which can

inhibit and kill microscopic organisms such as bacteria. The presence of phenolic compounds, quinones, and terpenoids in many other mushrooms have similar effects. This wide range of antibiotic substances found in mushrooms helps them to fight off the bacteria that grow in the warm, moist places where they thrive.

Cancer
Mushrooms contain the phytonutrient called lentinan. This plant chemical, along with another phytonutrient found in maitake mushrooms known as D-fraction, appears to be able to suppress tumor growth. This potential cancer fighting effect of mushrooms is an area of intensive ongoing research.

Heart Disease
Another wild mushroom, known as the wood ear mushroom, or black tree fungus, is believed to help to stop blood cells from clumping together and causing buildups on artery walls. By helping to keep the blood thin, wood ear mushrooms perform a similar role to fish oils, which are thought to help reduce the risk of heart disease by thinning the blood.

CAUTION
It is recommended that you only buy wild mushrooms from dependable retail outlets. Certain wild fungi can damage the heart, liver, and kidneys. Some can be fatal.

SEE ALSO CANCER, PAGE 214; HEART DISEASE, PAGE 152

SALAD LEAVES

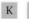 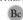

T he leaves of lettuce, young spinach, endive, chicory, and cress are used widely in salads. Many other exotic and unusual leaves, such as raddichio, arugula, and red leaf, are now readily available and are gaining in popularity. Salad leaves are low in calories and contain a surprising amount of minerals and vitamins, which all help to maintain a healthy body.

KEY BENEFITS

- GIVE SOME PROTECTION AGAINST CATARACTS
- MAY HELP TO PREVENT COLONIC CANCER, HEART DISEASE, AND SPINA BIFIDA
- HELP TO COMBAT INSOMNIA
- PROVIDE IRON AND CALCIUM FOR BONES

FOOD PROFILE

★ HOW MUCH TO EAT

- Spinach and endive are the richest suppliers of folate. A $^3/_4$-cup serving supplies 130mcg of folate. A woman who consumes 200mcg of folate daily, together with 400mcg of folic acid supplements, may reduce the risk of giving birth to a baby with spina bifida.

CHOOSING & STORING

- Avoid salad leaves that are damp or have brown edges.
- Choose lettuce and chicory that feel heavy for their size.
- Put in a refrigerator as soon as possible after purchase.

COOKING & EATING

- Wash leaves in cold water, then pat dry with a dish towel.
- Tear rather than cut leaves to minimize the loss of vitamin C.
- Use leaves raw in salads.

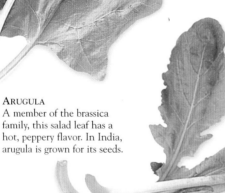

ARUGULA
A member of the brassica family, this salad leaf has a hot, peppery flavor. In India, arugula is grown for its seeds.

WATERCRESS
Fresh watercress can be used to treat lung cancer, porphyria, muscle cramps, and night blindness. (*See also page 64*)

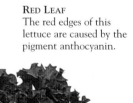

SPINACH
Known for their iron content, spinach leaves also supply calcium.

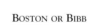

BOSTON OR BIBB LETTUCE
More beta carotene and vitamin C is found in this lettuce than in other varieties.

RED LEAF
The red edges of this lettuce are caused by the pigment anthocyanin.

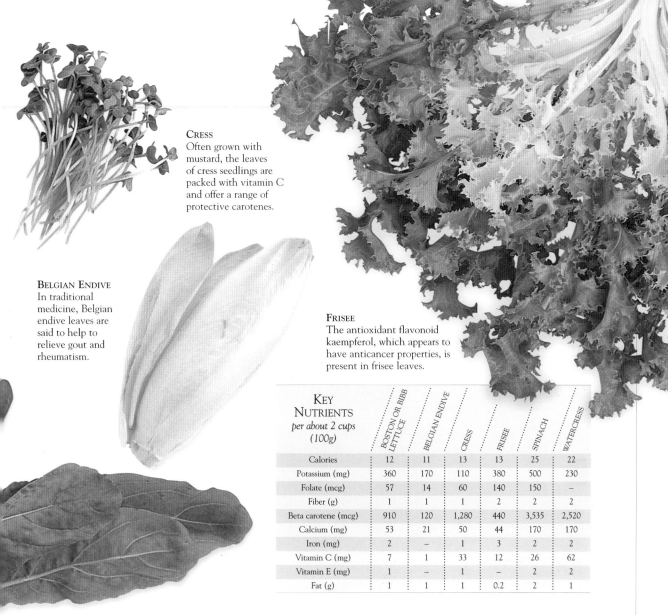

CRESS
Often grown with mustard, the leaves of cress seedlings are packed with vitamin C and offer a range of protective carotenes.

BELGIAN ENDIVE
In traditional medicine, Belgian endive leaves are said to help to relieve gout and rheumatism.

FRISEE
The antioxidant flavonoid kaempferol, which appears to have anticancer properties, is present in frisee leaves.

KEY NUTRIENTS per about 2 cups (100g)	BOSTON OR BIBB LETTUCE	BELGIAN ENDIVE	CRESS	FRISEE	SPINACH	WATERCRESS
Calories	12	11	13	13	25	22
Potassium (mg)	360	170	110	380	500	230
Folate (mcg)	57	14	60	140	150	–
Fiber (g)	1	1	1	2	2	2
Beta carotene (mcg)	910	120	1,280	440	3,535	2,520
Calcium (mg)	53	21	50	44	170	170
Iron (mg)	2	–	1	3	2	2
Vitamin C (mg)	7	1	33	12	26	62
Vitamin E (mg)	1	–	1	–	2	2
Fat (g)	1	1	1	0.2	2	1

HEALING PROPERTIES

☑ TRADITIONAL USES
The leaves of wild lettuce are used by traditional herbalists in the West as a sedative, and are prescribed for insomnia. In Chinese medicine, lettuce is used as a diuretic and to "dry out" digestive problems. It is given to start or increase a mother's milk production. Spinach strengthens the blood and cleanses it of toxins that can cause skin disease. In China, people believe that spinach helps bowel movements, the flow of urine, and relieves herpes irritations.

✠ SPECIFIC BENEFITS
Cataracts
Studies have revealed that regularly eating spinach may reduce the risk of cataracts forming. The phytonutrients lutein and zeathanxin in spinach may be responsible. Their antioxidant properties could help to protect proteins in the eye lens from becoming permanently damaged.

Cancer of the Colon
There is evidence that regularly eating salad leaves decreases the risk of colonic cancer. This is partly due to their supply of antioxidants, which may stop or deactivate the production of carcinogens, and partly due to the fiber that they provide. Fiber appears to reduce the risk of colonic cancer in several ways. It binds carcinogens and keeps them away from the colon wall. It increases stool bulk, thereby diluting potential carcinogens. It also provides food for bacteria in the colon, which then produce substances that increase the acidity. Cancers are less likely to grow in an acidic environment.

Heart Disease
Salad leaves, especially cress, frisee, spinach, and lettuce, supply good amounts of folate. Regularly eating folate-rich foods is believed to help reduce the risk of heart disease in susceptible people.

Spina Bifida
Intakes of folate and folic acid supplements can reduce the risk of spina bifida, a defect of the spinal column.

Stress and Insomnia
The white, latexy sap that oozes from lettuce stalks when they are snapped contains small amounts of a natural sedative called lactucarium. Wild lettuce is known to contain more lactucarium than cultivated varieties.

Anemia
Frisee is a particularly good source of iron, which is required by the blood for the formation of hemoglobin. Spinach also contains iron, but the presence of substances called phytates blocks some of its absorption.

Osteoporosis
Salad leaves, especially spinach, cress, and frisee, contain calcium, which the body needs for the formation of strong bones. As with iron, the absorption of calcium is slightly inhibited by phytates, but the leaves are still useful sources of calcium.

SEE ALSO ANEMIA, PAGE 160; CATARACTS, PAGE 202; CANCER, PAGE 214; HEART DISEASE, PAGE 152

WATERCRESS

 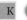

A member of the brassica family, this hot-tasting aquatic plant has been gathered and eaten as a food since ancient times, but it was not until the 19th century that people began to grow it commercially. Noted for its liver cleansing properties, watercress supplies iron, and is packed with antioxidant nutrients and phytonutrients, including plenty of vitamin C and beta carotene.

AKEY BENEFITS

- IMPROVES LIVER FUNCTION
- MAY HELP TO REDUCE MILD FLUID RETENTION THROUGH ITS DIURETIC EFFECTS
- MAY HELP TO PREVENT CANCER
- IMPROVES NIGHT BLINDNESS

FOOD PROFILE

AKEY NUTRIENTS
per 1 bunch (100g)

Calories	22
Vitamin C (mg)	62
Calcium (mg)	170
Iron (mg)	2
Potassium (mg)	230
Beta carotene (mcg)	2,520
Vitamin E (mg)	2
Nicotinic acid (mg)	1
Fiber (g)	2
Fat (g)	1

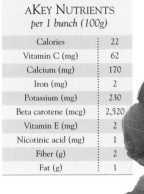

Orange color of beta carotene is masked by green chlorophyll

A NATURAL ANTIBIOTIC
The peppery taste of watercress is caused by a benzyl mustard oil, which is also present in nasturtium leaves. This oil is a powerful natural antibiotic which, unlike modern synthetic antibiotics, is not harmful to the body's intestinal flora.

★ HOW MUCH TO EAT

- A 20g bunch of watercress supplies more than 50 percent of the recommended daily intake of vitamin C.
- A 4-cup serving of watercress supplies 170mg of calcium.

CHOOSING & STORING

- Look for crisp, deep green watercress stems and firm, dark green leaves. Yellow leaves indicate aging and loss of flavor.
- Keep watercress wrapped in a paper towel and store in the refrigerator for up to five days.

COOKING & EATING

- Wash watercress thoroughly before use and shake to remove any excess water.
- Use in salads, soups, sandwiches, and for making vegetable juice.

HEALING PROPERTIES

✍ TRADITIONAL USES

According to the Greek writer Xenophon, the Persians used to eat large quantities of raw watercress when subjected to heavy physical labor. In medieval Europe, herbalists recommended its blood cleansing and restorative properties, and its stimulating effect on the spleen, liver, and gallbladder. A natural diuretic, watercress remains a chief ingredient in cleansing therapies in which the mustardlike oils are thought to purify the blood.

✜ SPECIFIC BENEFITS

Lung Cancer
In tests on smokers, one substance in tobacco smoke that causes lung cancer, called NNK (nicotine-derived nitrosaminoketone), was partly detoxified by eating 2 cups of watercress three times a day. It is the isothiocyanate in watercress that appears to have this effect. This is probably also capable of working on other enzymes that detoxify cancer-causing substances. A 2-cup serving of watercress supplies 5–10mg of this protective substance. Watercress also boasts a large range of antioxidant phytonutrients that seem to play a role in reducing the risk of cancers. A number of studies reveal that those populations that regularly consume cruciferous vegetables such as watercress appear to have lower rates of cancers of the colon, rectum, and thyroid than those that do not. In laboratory tests, the isothiocyanates in watercress inhibit other enzymes involved in causing DNA damage and cancer. Eating watercress regularly may reduce the risk of cancer.

Porphyria
People who suffer from the sun-sensitive condition porphyria have, in tests, shown a threefold increase in their tolerance of sunlight when taking large amounts of beta carotene. Watercress is rich in beta carotene. The vitamin C also present is likely to improve the body's ability to absorb beta carotene.

Muscle Cramps
Watercress is one of the richest vegetable sources of calcium. A good source of this mineral is very important for strong bones and teeth and healthy muscles, nerves, and blood. Watercress also supplies the mineral iron. The beta carotene and vitamin C that are present in watercress help the body to absorb it.

Night Blindness
Eating watercress can help to improve night blindness. The beta carotene in its leaves is needed for the formation of visual purple, the pigment in the retina of the eye that helps us to see in the dark.

CAUTION

Wild watercress grows mainly in polluted waters and may carry liver flukes. Only buy commercially produced watercress that has been grown on filtered, shallow, gravel bottom beds.

SEE ALSO CANCER, PAGE 214; MUSCLE CRAMPS, PAGE 196; PLANT NUTRIENTS, PAGE 34

TOMATOES

STAR NUTRIENTS & PHYTONUTRIENTS

C E   Lycopene, Beta carotene

One of the most popular vegetables in the world, the tomato is actually a fruit. Eaten raw, cooked, sun-dried, and canned, tomatoes are used in an array of products, including juices, soups, sauces, ketchups, chutneys, purées, and pastes. They supply potassium, vitamin C, and fiber, and are among the richest natural food sources of the antioxidant pigment lycopene.

KEY BENEFITS

- LINKED WITH LOWERING THE RISK OF PROSTATE CANCER AND OTHER TYPES OF CANCER
- MAY HELP TO REDUCE HEART DISEASE
- ASSOCIATED WITH IMPROVED MENTAL AND PHYSICAL CAPACITY IN OLD AGE

FOOD PROFILE

KEY NUTRIENTS
per ½ cup (100g)

Calories	17
Protein (g)	1
Fat (g)	0.3
Fiber (g)	1
Potassium (mg)	250
Beta carotene (mcg)	620
Beta cryptoxanthin (mcg)	35
Vitamin C (mg)	17
Vitamin E (mg)	1
Folate (mcg)	17

LONG-LIFE VEGETABLE
The taste that makes tomatoes so delicious relies on the interaction of sugars, malic and citric acids, and a number of other substances. Scientists have recently created tomato plants that yield tomatoes with improved shelf life and higher amounts of lycopene.

SALAD TOMATOES

CHERRY TOMATOES

BEEFSTEAK TOMATO

★ HOW MUCH TO EAT

- One tomato weighing about 3oz supplies 36 percent of the recommended adult daily intake of vitamin C. Canned tomatoes contain slightly less vitamin C than fresh ones. Tomatoes are rich in lycopene. Eaten regularly, they may reduce the risk of heart disease.

CHOOSING & STORING

- Avoid light, puffy looking tomatoes, as they are not tasty.
- Store at room temperature, out of direct sunlight.

COOKING & EATING

- For the best flavor, eat tomatoes raw. Add to salads or grill, bake, or microwave, and make into soups, pastes, and purées. Cooking does not destroy lycopene, so all forms are a useful source of this antioxidant.

HEALING PROPERTIES

✎ TRADITIONAL USES
Tomatoes have been used for a long time in Eastern medicine to cleanse the liver and are said to have "cooling" properties. These, combined with their sweet-and-sour flavor, are thought to build the "yin" fluids in the body, which relieve dryness and thirst. An increased intake of tomatoes is also thought to be a tonic for the stomach and digestion, and they are said to alkalize the blood and help treat rheumatism and gout.

❖ SPECIFIC BENEFITS
Prostate Cancer
Research in the US has looked into the relationship between prostate cancer and the consumption of various fruits and vegetables. Out of the 46 types of fruit and vegetable studied, tomatoes, and their derivatives, such as tomato sauce, were significantly associated with a reduction in the risk of prostate cancer. Men who ate ten servings of these foods each week had a significantly lower rate of prostate cancer than those who ate one-and-one-half servings. It was the powerful antioxidant called lycopene in the tomatoes that was believed to offer this protective effect. Lycopene is one of the most efficient carotenoids when it comes to "mopping up" cancer-causing free radicals in the body.

Other Cancers
Research in Italy has revealed that when people ate seven or more servings of tomatoes a week, a 60 percent lower risk of cancers of the mouth, esophagus, stomach, colon, and rectum was observed. Tomatoes contain the substances p-coumaric acid and chlorogenic acid, which are thought to prevent the formation of potentially cancer-causing substances called nitrosamines.

Heart Disease
Research carried out in Europe has discovered that men who had the highest levels of lycopene in their fat stores were half as likely to have a heart attack as men with low lycopene reserves. The lycopene in tomatoes appears to protect against heart disease by deactivating free radicals that damage low-density lipoprotein (LDL) cholesterol (*see page 25*).

Damaged LDL cholesterol appears to block blood flow, which can eventually lead to heart attacks.

Aging
Scientists at the University of Kentucky believe that the consumption of tomatoes, and therefore the intake of the antioxidant pigment lycopene, more than protects against heart disease and cancers. They studied 88 women over the age of 75 and found that those with lower lycopene levels were less able to attend to their needs than those with higher levels of lycopene. The researchers attribute these startling findings to lycopene's anti-oxidant ability to prevent free radicals from damaging joints, muscles, and even brain cells.

SEE ALSO CANCER, PAGE 214; FATS, PAGE 22; HEART DISEASE, PAGE 152; THE ELDERLY & NUTRITION, PAGE 144

GARLIC

STAR NUTRIENTS & PHYTONUTRIENTS

K Zn Fe Se Bc Allicin

The medicinal benefits of garlic have been recorded since ancient times. Archaeological evidence suggests that garlic has been cultivated in Central Asia from at least 3000 BC. A member of the onion family, garlic has been used to treat bronchitis, colds, whooping cough, and influenza. Modern research has identified its uses in tackling the widespread phenomena of heart disease.

KEY BENEFITS
- MAY HELP TO REDUCE CHOLESTEROL AND BLOOD FATS
- ANTIBACTERIAL AND ANTIFUNGAL PROPERTIES
- APPEARS TO COMBAT VIRAL CONDITIONS
- COULD PROTECT AGAINST STOMACH CANCER

FOOD PROFILE

KEY NUTRIENTS
per 1 large head (100g)

Calories	98
Protein (g)	8
Carbohydrate (g)	16
Potassium (mg)	620
Zinc (mg)	1
Calcium (mg)	19
Selenium (mcg)	2
Iron (mg)	2
Sodium (mg)	4
Magnesium (mg)	25

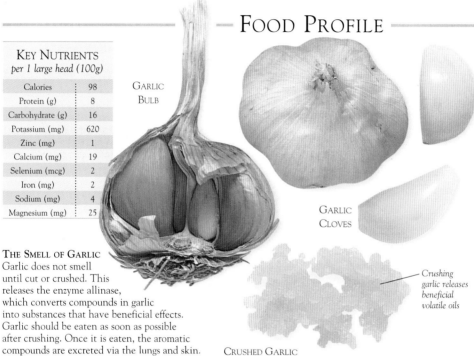

GARLIC BULB

GARLIC CLOVES

Crushing garlic releases beneficial volatile oils

CRUSHED GARLIC

THE SMELL OF GARLIC
Garlic does not smell until cut or crushed. This releases the enzyme allinase, which converts compounds in garlic into substances that have beneficial effects. Garlic should be eaten as soon as possible after crushing. Once it is eaten, the aromatic compounds are excreted via the lungs and skin.

★ HOW MUCH TO EAT
- An average serving of garlic is less than $1/2$ an ounce. The quantity of nutrients supplied is low compared to the daily recommended intakes. However, every clove is full of sulfurous compounds that fight infections. Several servings a week may reduce the risk of heart disease.

CHOOSING & STORING
- Choose plump, unbruised bulbs that are neither soft and soggy, nor starting to dry. Avoid torn skins and bulbs with sprouts.
- Keep for several weeks in a dry place where air can circulate, away from other vegetables.

COOKING & EATING
- Add crushed garlic toward the end of cooking to avoid singeing. Whole cloves can be boiled for two minutes, peeled, and then used in casseroles.

HEALING PROPERTIES

✍ TRADITIONAL USES
In ancient Rome, Pliny named 61 ailments cured by garlic. The British herbalist Culpeper believed it was a remedy for all diseases. Garlic is well known for its ability to promote circulation and inhibit colds. Poultices of chopped garlic were used in folk medicine to draw out the swelling from boils. Garlic's antibacterial effects are also well documented. In World War I surgeons used garlic juice to stop wounds from becoming septic.

✜ SPECIFIC BENEFITS
High Cholesterol
Garlic may reduce levels of low-density lipoprotein (LDL) cholesterol (*see page 25*), increase levels of high-density lipoprotein (HDL) cholesterol, and decrease blood fats. The allicin and other compounds appear to bring about this effect. Studies have found an association between low blood fats and regular garlic consumption. Regularly adding fresh garlic to cooking may therefore help to decrease the risk of heart disease.

Blood Clots
Ajone, one of the volatile substances that is produced when garlic is crushed, appears to reduce the formation of blood clots. This potentially makes garlic a useful treatment for those with heart disease. Research has shown that the clotting mechanisms reduce significantly when people are given daily supplements of garlic for one month.

High Blood Pressure
Powdered garlic (equal to 2.5g of fresh garlic) has been shown to lower blood pressure. Eating fresh garlic may also help this condition.

Food Poisoning
Garlic has been shown to fight many of the bacteria that cause food poisoning, including *Salmonella*.

Fungal Infections
Garlic has antifungal capabilities and is reported to be more effective than drugs against fungal infections such as yeast infections.

Viral Infections
Research shows that garlic is able to fight parainfluenza type 3, herpes simplex type 1, and influenza B viruses.

Stomach Cancer
Evidence from studies around the world suggest that diets high in garlic decrease the risk of stomach cancer. This is thought to be due to allicin compounds that may prevent cancerous changes from occurring in the stomach wall. Garlic's antibacterial effect is also important; it can help act against *Helicobacter pylori*, the bacteria that causes stomach ulcers, which in turn can become cancerous.

CAUTION
Doses of garlic should not be given as a remedy to those on anticoagulant therapy, or to pregnant women, as they may cause contractions. Garlic may also interfere with diabetic drugs.

SEE ALSO CANCER, PAGE 214; HIGH CHOLESTEROL, PAGE 154; HIGH BLOOD PRESSURE, PAGE 155; INFECTIONS, PAGE 212

ONIONS

 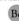 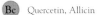
Related to garlic, the onion family includes chives, shallots, and leeks. Onions have been used in cooking and for their medicinal properties for thousands of years. Traditionally used as a home remedy for coughs and colds, these vegetables are consumed worldwide. Recent discoveries relating to the onion family and its antioxidant effects make this a particularly interesting vegetable.

KEY BENEFITS

- MAY HELP TO PREVENT CANCER AND CIRCULATORY DISORDERS
- MAY HELP TO PREVENT HEART DISEASE
- ASSOCIATED WITH A REDUCED RISK OF BLADDER CANCER IN SMOKERS

FOOD PROFILE

KEY NUTRIENTS per ⅔–1 cup (100g)	ONIONS	SPRING ONIONS
Calories	36	23
Fiber (g)	1	2
Fat (g)	–	0.5
Potassium (mg)	160	260
Vitamin C (mg)	5	26
Calcium (mg)	25	39
Folate (mcg)	17	54
Biotin (mcg)	1	–
Vitamin B₆ (mg)	0.2	0.1
Vitamin E (mg)	0.3	–

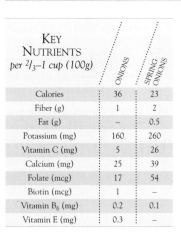

SCALLIONS

PEELING ONIONS
Preparing onions makes many people cry. This unusual effect is due to a series of complicated processes in which the sulfurous compounds in onions are converted into a substance called propanethial S-oxide, which stimulates the tear glands.

PEELED ONION

BROWN ONION

★ HOW MUCH TO EAT

- An average-sized onion weighs about 90g and provides about 5 percent of an adult's daily potassium needs. It is also a rich source of quercetin. Eaten three to four times a week, onions may help to reduce the risk of heart disease.

CHOOSING & STORING

- Onions should be firm and free from sprouts, with a thin skin that is not cracked. Avoid strong-smelling onions.
- Store in a dry place.

COOKING & EATING

- Eat raw, baked, boiled, braised, sautéed, roasted, casseroled, stir-fried, and in soups. Fresh, raw onion is more beneficial to health than cooked onion.

HEALING PROPERTIES

✔ TRADITIONAL USES

Onions are a traditional folk remedy for coughs, colds, and bronchitis. Simmering an onion in water with a little honey, then eating the onion, and repeating this every four hours is a well established remedy for coughs. Bronchial inflammations were also treated by pressing onions on to the chest. Fresh slices of onion were placed on insect bites to reduce the swelling. Onion tea is said by herbalists to act as a sedative.

✦ SPECIFIC BENEFITS

Cancer and Circulatory Disorders
Quercetin is a phytonutrient present in onions which, like vitamins E and C, is a strong antioxidant. It appears to be able to "mop up" potentially harmful free radicals in the body which, if left intact, may spark cancerous changes and diseases such as atherosclerosis. Although present in apples and tea, research has shown that the absorption of quercetin from onions may be 32 percent more efficient and quicker than from these other sources. Quercetin absorbed from onions was found to remain in the body for approximately 24 hours. It has therefore been speculated that a regular intake of onions in the diet could lead to a buildup of quercetin in blood plasma. The presence of querticin could make a significant contribution to antioxidant defences in the blood and help to protect against several different kinds of disease.

Heart Disease
Women in particular benefit from high intakes of quercetin when it comes to preventing heart disease. A Finnish study of flavonoids over a 26-year period revealed that people with higher intakes of flavonoids had significantly less chance of dying from heart disease than those with lower intakes. The main sources of flavonoids in this study were onions and apples, which are both very rich in quercetin. This substance is believed to reduce the risk of heart disease by preventing low-density lipoprotein (LDL) cholesterol (see page 25) from being damaged by free radicals. Quercetin is thought to help by inhibiting the formation of blood clots. The intake of quercetin in onions is very important in the prevention of heart disease when other vegetables and fruits that supply useful antioxidants, such as vitamins C and E, are in short supply.

Bladder Cancer in Smokers
Tobacco smoking is one of the major causes of bladder cancer in humans. It is believed that flavonoids such as the quercetin present in onions are converted into substances that protect the bladder lining from carcinogens. The substances seem to alter the rates at which the cancer forming substances are absorbed, by reacting with, or binding to, toxins. Regular intakes of onions may form part of a strategy in the prevention of cancer.

SEE ALSO CANCER, PAGE 214; COLDS AND INFLUENZA, PAGE 184; HEART DISEASE, PAGE 152

CHILIES & PEPPERS

I n Central and South America, chilies and peppers (capsicum) were eaten as long ago as 7000 BC and cultivated from about 5000 BC. They have been a part of the region's diet ever since. Christopher Columbus introduced the plants to Europe, and their use quickly spread throughout the world. Known for their "hot" flavor, these foods are rich in carotenoids and vitamin C.

KEY BENEFITS

- MAY PROTECT AGAINST STOMACH ULCERS AND CANCEROUS CHANGES WITHIN THE BODY
- FIGHT INFECTIOUS DISEASES
- ACT AS NATURAL PAINKILLERS
- MAY HELP TO FIGHT THE COMMON COLD

FOOD PROFILE

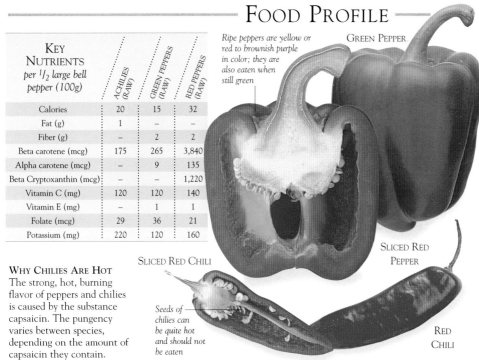

Ripe peppers are yellow or red to brownish purple in color; they are also eaten when still green

GREEN PEPPER

SLICED RED PEPPER

SLICED RED CHILI

Seeds of chilies can be quite hot and should not be eaten

RED CHILI

KEY NUTRIENTS per ¹/₂ large bell pepper (100g)	CHILIES (RAW)	GREEN PEPPERS (RAW)	RED PEPPERS (RAW)
Calories	20	15	32
Fat (g)	1	–	–
Fiber (g)	–	2	2
Beta carotene (mcg)	175	265	3,840
Alpha carotene (mcg)	–	9	135
Beta Cryptoxanthin (mcg)	–	–	1,220
Vitamin C (mg)	120	120	140
Vitamin E (mg)	–	1	1
Folate (mcg)	29	36	21
Potassium (mg)	220	120	160

WHY CHILIES ARE HOT
The strong, hot, burning flavor of peppers and chilies is caused by the substance capsaicin. The pungency varies between species, depending on the amount of capsaicin they contain.

★ HOW MUCH TO EAT

- A medium-sized pepper weighing approximately 5oz provides more than three times the recommended adult daily intake of vitamin C.

🥣 CHOOSING & STORING

- Buy well shaped, firm, thick peppers that have a bright, shiny color. Keep in the refrigerator for up to 12 days.

🍲 COOKING & EATING

- Remove the stalk and seeds from peppers before using. Slice the flesh and use it in cooked dishes or raw in salads. Peppers can also be stuffed and baked.
- Use small amounts of fresh chilies to add flavor and heat to casseroles and other dishes.
- Add the powder of different species, such as paprika, cayenne, and pimento, to different recipes.

HEALING PROPERTIES

🔖 TRADITIONAL USES

Chilies have long been used in herbalism in the West. The chili is a potent stimulant thought to help increase blood flow, tone the nervous system, stimulate appetite, relieve indigestion, and encourage sweating. Its antibacterial properties have made it a popular treatment for colds and throat problems. Many Chinese herbalists recommend that women eat hot dishes in the week prior to menstruation to ease period pains. The Mayna Jivaro people of Peru apply chilies directly to their teeth for toothache. Chili poultices and ointments have been used in the East and in the West to relieve arthritis, rheumatism, and varicose veins, and to remove warts.

✢ SPECIFIC BENEFITS

Stomach Ulcers
In Singapore and Malaysia, Chinese people are more prone to stomach ulcers than Malayan and Indian peoples, who eat more chilies than the Chinese. The apparent protective effect of chilies may be due to capsaicin increasing blood flow to the stomach lining, and also the amount of protective mucus produced by the stomach wall. In studies, scientists have found that ¹/₂ oz of chilies eaten 30 minutes before a 600mg dose of aspirin results in less damage to the stomach and duodenum than would normally be caused by the drug. In other studies, the long-term use of chilies decreased damage to the stomach lining by alcohol.

Infectious Diseases
Chilies stimulate stomach acids, which help to kill bacteria, and a diet that is rich in chilies has been used successfully to fight infectious diseases such as cholera and dysentery. Tests using an extract of capsaicin suggest that this plant chemical may enhance parts of the immune system, thereby helping to fight infections.

Cancer
Experiments have shown that capsaicin seems to be able to detoxify a wide range of chemical carcinogens which, if left free to roam the body, could set up mutations that lead to cancers. Scientists suggest that chilies in the diet could help in the management of cancer.

Pain
Modern research shows that the repeated application of capsaicin desensitizes nerves and controls pain. Capsaicin does this by overstimulating the pain receptors in the skin, making them insensitive to other causes of pain.

Colds
Peppers are a rich source of vitamin C. Their regular inclusion in the diet could reduce the severity and duration of cold symptoms.

CAUTION

Do not touch the eyes or any cuts after handling fresh chilies. Avoid using cayenne remedies, such as infusions and gargles, when pregnant or breastfeeding.

SEE ALSO CANCER, PAGE 214; COLDS & INFLUENZA, PAGE 184; INFECTIONS, PAGE 212; PEPTIC ULCERS, PAGE 171

SPROUTING VEGETABLES

STAR NUTRIENTS & PHYTONUTRIENTS

  C E Carotenes, Genistein, Daidzein

A sprouting seed is said to represent the point of greatest vitality in the life cycle of a plant because vitamin and enzyme content increases dramatically during the sprouting process. The seeds of many plants can be eaten when they are sprouting. They are known as bean or grain sprouts and include alfalfa beans, mung beans, lentils, wheat, barley, corn, and oats.

KEY BENEFITS

- USEFUL IN LOW-CALORIE DIETS
- MAY PROTECT AGAINST HEART DISEASE
- MAY HELP TO LOWER CHOLESTEROL
- POSSIBLY HAVE CANCER FIGHTING PROPERTIES

FOOD PROFILE

KEY NUTRIENTS

There has been little analysis of the nutrient content of these vegetables, except for mung beans and alfalfa. These both contain some protein, and small amounts of iron, zinc, carotenes, folate, and vitamin C.

HOME SPROUTING
Soak one part seeds in at least three parts water in a wide mouthed jar for up to 12 hours. After soaking, drain the seeds, keep them warm, and rinse them twice a day. They will sprout within three to five days, depending on the variety. Eat as soon as possible after sprouting.

MUNG BEANS

SPROUTING ALFALFA

ALFALFA SEEDS

WHEAT GRAINS

SPROUTING MUNG BEANS

SPROUTING WHEAT GRAINS

★ HOW MUCH TO EAT
- 1 cup of fresh alfalfa sprouts supply approximately 6 percent of an adult woman's daily requirement of iron.
- A 1-cup serving of mung bean sprouts provides more than 15 percent of the daily folate requirement for adults.

CHOOSING & STORING
- When buying sprouted seeds, look for those that are springy with a fresh smell.
- Avoid slimy, wet sprouts.

COOKING & EATING
- Rinse fresh sprouts in cold water, drain, and use them raw in sandwiches and salads.
- Sprouts can be added to dips, burgers, and even ice cream to give extra texture and variety.

HEALING PROPERTIES

TRADITIONAL USES
The sprouting process makes the nutrients in seeds and grains easy to digest. This is because, as the sprouts grow, enzymes partly break down the starch, protein, and fat present in seeds into sugars, amino acids, and fatty acids. This beneficial effect is particularly recognized by doctors in the East, who often prescribe sprouting vegetables as remedies for swellings and lumps, depression, and stress that are caused by a disorder of the liver. Sprouting alfalfa seeds are the most commonly prescribed. They are thought to improve the appetite and increase urinary output, making them good for cleansing the body and for helping to alleviate water retention. Sprouting

vegetables are used in the East to treat gastric ulcers and to cure people of addictions.

SPECIFIC BENEFITS
Weight Problems
Sprouting seeds are filling but low in calories and are therefore a useful food for people who are trying to reduce their calorie intake. Like other low-calorie vegetable foods, sprouts contain a range of vitamins and minerals, including vitamin C and the B group, as well as iron and calcium.

Degenerative Diseases
Sprouts are a source of the antioxidant vitamins C and E and the phytonutrients coumarins, anthocyanidins, xanthophyll, and lutein, which have antioxidant

properties. These vitamins and phytonutrients apparently seem to help fight various substances that can cause heart disease and certain cancers in the body.

High Cholesterol
Alfalfa stems and leaves contain chemicals called saponins, which have been reported to decrease cholesterol, reduce the amount of cholesterol absorbed from the intestines, and help to prevent a form of arteriosclerosis (the hardening and thickening of artery walls) called atherosclerosis. A study on a small number of people with high cholesterol levels revealed that the addition of alfalfa seeds to their diets helped to normalize cholesterol levels.

Cancer
Alfalfa seeds contain the isoflavonoids known as daidzein and genistein, also found in soybeans. These antioxidants are known to have similar properties to the hormone estrogen in the body. Once in the body, they can mimic estrogen and block its receptor sites in the breasts. They may therefore be able to help prevent breast cancer. They are also thought to lower the incidence of cancer of the prostate gland. Genistein is known to help stop the proliferation of cells and reduce the formation of blood vessels to new cancer cells. It is thought that this may be the reason that genistein seems to be able to prevent the formation of cancers within the body.

SEE ALSO CANCER, PAGE 214; HEART DISEASE, PAGE 152; HIGH CHOLESTEROL, PAGE 154; OBESITY, PAGE 178

SEAWEEDS

| Ca | K | Fe | Iodine, Carotenes |

Seaweeds have been a part of human diets for many thousands of years. There is evidence from burial sites that seaweeds were eaten in the Stone Age, and they are mentioned in ancient Chinese and Japanese medical texts. Low in fat, seaweeds supply a range of minerals, including potassium, iodine, calcium, magnesium, and iron, as well as fiber.

KEY BENEFITS

- MAY PROTECT AGAINST CERTAIN CANCERS
- USEFUL SOURCE OF IRON AND CALCIUM, PARTICULARLY FOR VEGETARIANS
- FILLING ADDITION TO MEALS, AND THEREFORE USEFUL IN WEIGHT-LOSS DIETS

FOOD PROFILE

★ HOW MUCH TO EAT

- About 1¹/₂ cups (50g) dried wakame supplies 8 percent of an adult's daily calcium requirement.
- Eating a small amount of seaweed weekly, up to ³/₄ cup (25g), helps to keep up iodine levels in the body. Seaweeds contain more iodine than fish.

CHOOSING & STORING

- Seaweeds are usually sold dried in various forms, such as sheets, flakes, granules, or powders.
- Buy from reputable health food stores or supermarkets.
- Store seaweed in airtight containers in a cool, dry place.

COOKING & EATING

- Fresh seaweed should be eaten soon after it is bought.
- The salty taste makes seaweeds ideal for sprinkling over foods or adding to soups and stews.
- Use seaweed sheets to wrap around rice cakes as a snack, or to make sushi.

DULSE
The flat, smooth leaves of dulse have a red and blue pigmentation. Fresh dulse can be used like spinach as a vegetable, or dried and toasted over a low flame and eaten like chips.

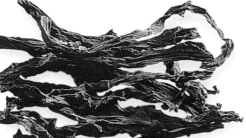
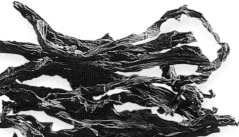

WAKAME
A deep green, curly leaved seaweed, wakame is regarded by the Japanese as good for the complexion. The hard central spine of wakame needs to be removed after softening in cold water because it does not soften in cooking.

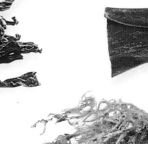

NORI
Particularly rich in iron and potassium, nori ranges from bright green to purple in color. The high iodine content helps to maintain good hearing.

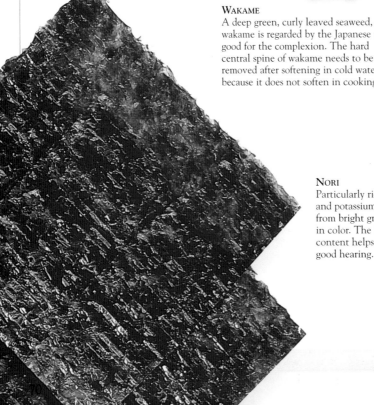
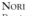

IRISH MOSS
Reddish purple to reddish green in color, raw Irish moss is an excellent source of iron. It is used in the food industry as a source of gelatinous carrageenans which set foods.

KEY NUTRIENTS per 2–3 cups (100g)	KOMBU (DRIED)	NORI (DRIED)	WAKAME (DRIED)	IRISH MOSS (RAW)	AGAR (SOAKED)	AGAR (DRIED)
Calories	43	136	71	8	2	16
Protein (g)	7	31	12	2	0.2	1.3
Fat (g)	2	2	2	0.2	0.1	1.2
Fiber (g)	59	44	47	12	15	81
Potassium (mg)	450	2,840	220	63	20	110
Calcium (mg)	900	430	660	72	110	760
Iron (mg)	13	20	12	9	4	21
Iodine (mcg)	440	1,470	16,830	–	–	–
Carotene (mcg)	340	14,910	515	–	–	–
Vitamin B_{12} (mcg)	3	28	3	–	–	–

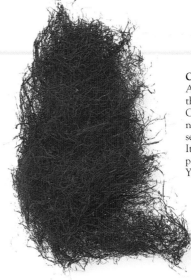

CHINESE BLACK MOSS
A hairlike seaweed with thin black strands, Chinese black moss needs to be soaked several times before use. It is often cooked with pork for Chinese New Year celebrations.

KOMBU
Exceptionally rich in calcium, kombu is a wide, ribbonlike sea plant. Good for making stock, kombu contains glutamic acid, which tenderizes legumes and enhances flavor.

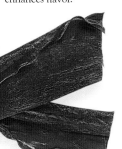

RED AGAR

WHITE AGAR

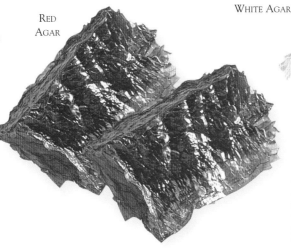

AGAR
A complex carbohydrate obtained from some seaweeds, agar is mainly used as a food thickener. It is available in threads or as a powder. Agar is flavor-free and is often described as the vegetarian gelatin.

HEALING PROPERTIES

☑ TRADITIONAL USES
In the East, some types of seaweeds are recommended in weight-loss programs, and are said to have a role to play in improving water metabolism, cleaning up the lymphatic system, and alkalizing the blood. Many practitioners prescribe seaweeds to help the thyroid gland to function properly. Other uses include the treatment of swellings, nodules, lumps, goiter, and skin diseases. According to ancient Chinese texts, "there is no swelling that is not relieved by seaweed." Kombu is used for its apparent anticoagulant effect on the blood. It is said to relieve hormonal imbalances and is used particularly for the treatment of goiter, high blood pressure, prostate problems, anemia, and swallowing difficulties. Nori is recommended in Chinese medicine for goiter, rickets, and difficulty in urinating. Wakame is given to new mothers to purify their blood, and to those with weak hair and skin. Irish moss is rich in carrageenan, which is used in Chinese medicine to treat peptic and duodenal ulcers, combat arteriosclerosis, and reduce levels of cholesterol. Dulse has been found to have antiviral properties and is also believed to help prevent motion sickness.

❖ SPECIFIC BENEFITS
In the West, seaweeds have undergone little medical research to prove their benefits in either preventing or treating diseases. However, the extracts of certain kinds of seaweed are now being investigated for their possible healing properties.

Cancer
An extract from the edible red alga Asakusa-nori (*Porphyra tenera*) has been shown, in Japanese research, to stop mutation of certain cancerous cells. The pigments in some seaweeds may be responsible for the protective action that these plants have.

Anemia
In vegetarians and those who eat little or no red meat and fish, seaweed can help to replenish or maintain body stores of iron. The regular inclusion of seaweeds in the diet, especially of vegetarians, could help to fight anemia.

Brittle Bones
Seaweeds are an excellent source of calcium, which the body absorbs well from these foods. It is then transported to and deposited in the bones.

Weight Problems
Seaweeds add physical bulk to meals yet are low in calories and fat. The gel-like makeup of these plants, and their high fiber content, make them filling and therefore a useful part of a weight loss diet.

CAUTION

Certain areas of ocean are polluted with heavy metals. Buy seaweeds from reputable companies that source their products from clean sea regions to avoid products containing poisons.

SEE ALSO ANEMIA, PAGE 160; CANCER, PAGE 214; OBESITY, PAGE 178

FRUITS

FRUITS CONTAIN LITTLE or no protein or fat, with most of their energy coming from carbohydrates. The carbohydrates in fruits is usually in the form of the fruit sugars fructose and glucose, although some underripe fruits, such as bananas, also supply starch. The sugars in fruits give them their sweetness, while a variety of organic acids, such as citric or malic acid, provide a refreshing edge. As fruits ripen, the concentration of sugars rises, while that of acids falls. Fruits supply vitamin C, some B vitamins, and good amounts of potassium and fiber, along with protective phytonutrients. There is a growing body of compelling evidence to suggest that a good intake of fruits can fortify the body against a variety of degenerative diseases.

FRUIT FIBERS

The fibrous content of fruits plays a key role in determining their texture. The crispness of certain apples, the softer consistency of a pear, and the pithy structure of oranges are the result of their fiber content. The small amounts of insoluble fiber in fruits help to bulk up the stools and speed their passage through the large intestine, while soluble fibers, such as pectin, appear to maintain blood sugar and cholesterol levels.

FRUIT SUGARS

Fructose is about one and a half times sweeter than sucrose (table sugar). It is said that the innate human preference for sweet foods came from an early discovery that sweet fruits were safer than other plant foods, and were less likely to contain the naturally occurring alkaloids and toxins often associated with a bitter taste. Fructose intolerance is an inherited condition in which the metabolism of fructose is affected. Symptoms such as diarrhea and liver and kidney problems can occur if those affected eat fruits. The condition responds well to the exclusion of fruits and other sources of fructose from the diet. Supplements will usually be necessary to ensure that good intakes of vitamin C are maintained. Sadly, not all the phytonutrients found in fruits can be so easily replaced.

THE PROTECTIVE POWERS OF FRUITS

All fruits are literally bursting with an array of phytonurients. In red, yellow, and orange fruits, these are present in the form of carotenoids, which appear to have far-reaching protective effects in all body systems. Carotenoids occur as alpha carotene and beta carotene in oranges, bananas, berries, grapes,

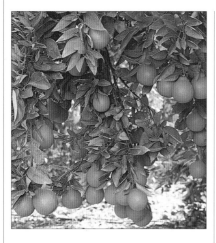

FRUIT FARMING

Today's sophisticated systems of farming, storage, and transportation ensure that a wide variety of fruits from every climatic region can be enjoyed virtually all year round. There is now an increasing demand for organically produced fruits that are grown without artificial fertilizers. This method favors crop rotation and natural fertilizers. Organically farmed fruits often look less perfect than those produced by modern, quality-controlled methods.

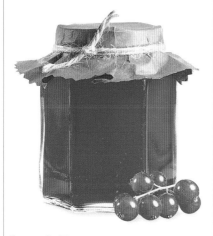

JAMS & PRESERVES

Fruits contain sugar and a natural setting agent, pectin, and can be boiled with additional sugar to make jams, preserves, and marmalades. Although these are made with whole or cut fruits, the fruits are boiled, which is thought to destroy some vitamins and minerals. In addition, jam is 60 percent sugar, which may cause tooth decay and obesity. Acid fruits make the best preserves. Barely ripe fruits are preferred for jam-making because it is at this stage that the pectin content is highest. Pectin is also made commercially and used as a setting agent in jellies and ice cream.

blackcurrants, mangoes, papayas, watermelons, and star fruits, while beta cryptoxanthin is found in mangoes, peaches, papayas, and oranges. Lutein is present in bananas, oranges, berries, and grapes, and lycopene occurs in watermelons. Phytoene is present in mangoes, and papayas, and phytofluene in apricots and peaches. Along with vitamin C, all of these plant nutrients have antioxidant properties that appear to help protect against blocked arteries, and encourage the replication of normal cells. Flavonoids such as quercetin and rutin, found in apples, grapes, and citrus fruits, appear to prevent cancer-forming substances from causing damage in the body, reduce the risk of malignant changes to cells, and help to keep the skin's structural component collagen firm and strong. Apples, grapes, and strawberries contain another type of phytonutrient – ellagic acid – that seems to be able to neutralize today's sources of pollution, such as cigarette smoke. Berries are rich in lignans, substances that cause estrogen-like activities in the body, which in turn are able to fight cancerous changes, especially in the breast and colon, and are also thought to play a part in reducing the risk of heart disease.

WHOLE FRUITS

It is possible to extract substances from fruits and package them in supplement form. For some people there may be compelling reasons for enhancing the diet with extra quantities of nutrients in this way. Supplements are not, however, a substitute for whole fruits, which contain a wide mix of vitamins, minerals, fiber, and phytonutrients. It is thought that these act in synergy once consumed, helping to improve each other's absorption and function in the body. It is recommended that five servings of fruits or vegetables be consumed daily. Eating excessive quantities of certain fruits may, however, lead to diarrhea. Some fruits contain derivatives of hydroxyphenylistan, which stimulates the muscles of the large intestine and increases the speed at which stools are moved through and out of the body.

STORAGE & PREPARATION

Citrus fruits, berries, and other kinds of fruits add color, flavor, texture, and natural sweetness to the diet, in the form of both sweet and salty dishes. Most fruits benefit from cool storage to preserve their nutrients and maintain their texture. All fruits should be washed before they are consumed and, where possible, eaten raw and with the skin intact.

MAIN FRUIT GROUPS

A fruit is the part of a plant that contains and protects the seeds. Sweet, juicy fruits are edible, but some fruits are inedible and can even be poisonous. Below is a list of the main fruit groups.

• **BERRIES** include raspberries, cranberries, melons, gooseberries, kiwis, avocados, grapes, and red currants.

• **CITRUS FRUITS** include oranges, lemons, limes, tangarines, kumquats, uglis, clementines, and grapefruits.

• **DRIED AND SEMIDRIED ("READY-TO-EAT") FRUITS** include raisins, currants, and dates. Various succulent fruits can also be eaten in a dried form, for example, apricots, bananas, figs, and sundried tomatoes.

• **FRUIT WITH PITS** include peaches, cherries, apricots, blackberries, nectarines, plums, cherries, mangoes, coconuts, and prunes.

• **FALSE FRUITS** include rowan berries, apples, figs, strawberries, and breadfruits.

• **FRUIT-VEGETABLES** include green, yellow, red, cherry, and plum tomatoes; eggplants; cucumbers; gherkins; red, yellow and green peppers; and rhubarb.

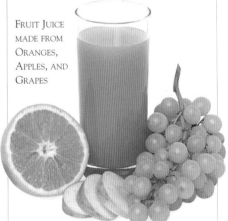

FRUIT JUICE MADE FROM ORANGES, APPLES, AND GRAPES

FRUIT JUICES

Fresh fruit juices, drinks made from blended fruits, and fruit teas count toward the daily recommended intake of five servings, or 14oz (400g) (raw weight), of fresh fruits and vegetables. Fruit teas may lose some value if the temperature of the water is high. Fresh, unsweetened fruit juices are the healthiest and, diluted with water, make a refreshing and healthy drink. An even healthier option would be to juice fresh fruit at home, thereby ensuring that no sugar or preservatives are added. This is an effective way of increasing daily consumption of water and fruit.

APPLES

 K C Quercetin, Soluble fiber, Cellulose

The old saying "an apple a day keeps the doctor away" may be very well founded. As research continues to discover the significance of phytonutrients, it is becoming apparent that apples may indeed play an important role in our long-term well-being, not just because of the vitamins, minerals, and fiber that apples supply, but also due to the additional antioxidants that they contain.

KEY BENEFITS

- HELP TO REDUCE THE RISK OF HEART DISEASE
- REGULAR INTAKE MAY HELP TO REDUCE HIGH LEVELS OF BLOOD CHOLESTEROL
- GOOD FOOD FOR PEOPLE WITH DIABETES

FOOD PROFILE

KEY NUTRIENTS
per 1 small apple (100g)

Calories	47
Protein (g)	0.4
Fat (g)	0.1
Carbohydrate (g)	12
Fiber (g)	2
Soluble fiber (g)	1
Insoluble fiber (g)	0.4
Cellulose (g)	0.6
Potassium (mg)	120
Vitamin E (mg)	1
Vitamin C (mg)	6

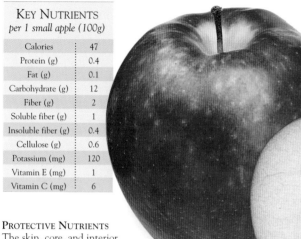

RED DELICIOUS APPLE

Skin is rich in soluble fiber pectin, an anticholesterol agent

GRANNY SMITH APPLE

PROTECTIVE NUTRIENTS
The skin, core, and interior membranes of apples are stockpiled with phytonutrients that are believed to protect the fruit from ultraviolet light, insects, fungi, viruses, and bacteria, and to act as plant hormone and enzyme controllers.

★ HOW MUCH TO EAT

- An average-sized eating apple weighs about 4oz (112g) and provides 10 percent of the recommended daily intake of vitamin C. It is also rich in soluble fiber. Regular consumption may help to lower cholesterol levels.

🛍 CHOOSING & STORING

- Apples are available all year round but Fall is the best time to buy the new season's fruit. Select firm apples with bright, undamaged skins.
- Store apples for up to 14 days in the refrigerator.

🍳 COOKING & EATING

- Wash and dry. Eat whole, slice into fruit salads, or serve with cheese. Core, leave whole, and bake or microwave. Stew, or make into crumbles and pies.

HEALING PROPERTIES

✍ TRADITIONAL USES
Apples are well known for cleansing the system. Ripe apples have been used for their laxative properties since Roman times. In 1653, the British herbalist Culpeper described apple syrup as "a good cordial in faintings, palpitations, and melancholy." In Chinese medicine, apples are thought to reduce "heat" and have a "cooling effect" on the lungs. The malic and tartaric acid in apples seems to inhibit the growth of disease producing bacteria in the digestive tract.

❖ SPECIFIC BENEFITS
Heart Disease
A growing number of studies has shown that foods with high levels of quercetin, such as apples, improve the

antioxidant activity of the blood and reduce the susceptibility of low-density lipoprotein (LDL) cholesterol (*see page 25*) to damage. Studies have shown that people with a high quercetin intake have a lower than normal risk of heart disease and stroke. These observations were explained by the anti-atherosclerotic and anti-thrombotic effects of the quercetin in apples.

Cancer
Experimental studies of samples of human tumor cells suggest that in relatively high doses quercetin can halt certain cancers. Population studies around the world do not as yet, however, indicate that diets rich in quercetin generally protect against

cancer. Meanwhile, some studies have shown that quercetin could be particularly beneficial to smokers. Tobacco carcinogens are known to damage the cells of the bladder wall, where they set up cancerous growths. It has been discovered that smokers who eat more flavonoids, including the quercetin found in apples, were partially protected from bladder wall damage caused by tobacco.

High Cholesterol
Apples contain the fiber known as pectin in good amounts. Pectin is a soluble fiber, which means that it becomes sticky and viscous when wet. Several controlled studies have shown that adding pectin to the diet leads to a modest lowering of

cholesterol levels. This may be because the pectin in apples binds to bile acids, which helps to lower levels of cholesterol in the blood. Eating apples regularly can help those with high cholesterol.

Diabetes
The pectin in apples can help to keep blood sugar levels stable. The natural sugars in apples are digested and absorbed slowly. This is probably partly due to the effect of the pectin, which forms a gel in the digestive tract. The slow rise in blood sugar levels caused by apples means that they have a low glycemic index, or GI (*see page 18*). This makes them particularly useful for those with diabetes.

SEE ALSO CANCER, PAGE 214; DIABETES, PAGE 218; HIGH CHOLESTEROL, PAGE 154

PEARS

STAR NUTRIENTS & PHYTONUTRIENTS

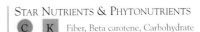

C **K** Fiber, Beta carotene, Carbohydrate

Available all year round, the pear continues to ripen once picked. Thought to have originated in western Asia, the fruit was introduced to Europe by the ancient Greeks. Digested slowly by the body, pears are particularly good for keeping hunger at bay. The most popular cultivated varieties include the Bartlet, Bosc, Anjou, and Comice.

KEY BENEFITS

- A GOOD FOOD FOR PEOPLE WITH DIABETES
- USEFUL IN WEIGHT-LOSS EATING PLANS
- REGULAR INTAKE CAN HELP TO KEEP CHOLESTEROL LEVELS STABLE

FOOD PROFILE

KEY NUTRIENTS
per ½ large pear (100g)

Calories	40
Protein (g)	0.3
Carbohydrate (g)	10
Fructose (g)	7
Fat (g)	0.1
Fiber (g)	2
Potassium (mg)	150
Vitamin C (mg)	6
Beta carotene (mcg)	18

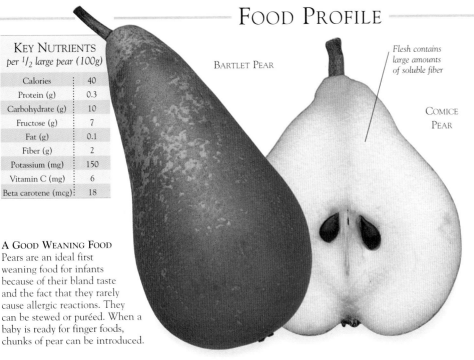

BARTLET PEAR

Flesh contains large amounts of soluble fiber

COMICE PEAR

A GOOD WEANING FOOD
Pears are an ideal first weaning food for infants because of their bland taste and the fact that they rarely cause allergic reactions. They can be stewed or puréed. When a baby is ready for finger foods, chunks of pear can be introduced.

★ HOW MUCH TO EAT
- One Bartlet pear supplies 15 percent of an adult's daily requirement of fiber. Much of this is soluble, which helps to reduce cholesterol levels and maintain blood sugar levels. Eating pears regularly may be useful for people with diabetes.

🥄 CHOOSING & STORING
- Choose well shaped, plump, firm pears with undamaged skins.
- Avoid pears with dull skins and spots near the base. These marks indicate a mealy flesh.
- Store pears for several days in the refrigerator.

🍳 COOKING & EATING
- Wash pears and eat raw, or add to fruit salads. Alternatively, poach whole in wine, or purée and make into a sorbet. Use in crumbles, pies, tarts, and cakes.

HEALING PROPERTIES

📖 TRADITIONAL USES
In Chinese medicine, pears are said to have "a cooling nature." They are believed to be useful for treating the lungs to eliminate "heat" and excess mucus and to soothe coughs. Pears are also recommended for moistening the lungs and throat, and for improving general dryness in the chest area. In folk medicine, pears have been used by diabetics, and to help relieve problems such as constipation and gallbladder inflammation and obstruction. Pears are believed to be useful in treating injuries to the skin.

✖ SPECIFIC BENEFITS
Diabetes
Pears have a low glycemic index, or GI (see page 18), so they are suitable for people

with diabetes. This is because pears do not contribute to big increases in blood sugar levels after they are eaten. The slow rate at which the fruit sugars are absorbed means that pears do not require large releases of insulin by the body for their digestion. Pears are therefore of benefit to those with diabetes, as they help to maintain good blood sugar control. As a result, people with both insulin-dependent and non-insulin dependent diabetes can cope with pears in their diet.

Weight Problems
Pears cause a very gradual rise in blood sugar. This prevents peaks and troughs in blood sugar levels, which may cause a sudden desire to overeat. Foods with a low GI can be

very helpful in weight-loss schemes, where one of the main problems is avoiding hunger. Fresh, raw pears have a GI of 36, one of the lowest of all fruits. The good fiber content of pears also helps to prevent overeating by keeping the stomach feeling full for a longer period of time.

High Cholesterol
Pears contain plenty of soluble fiber, which has been shown to help regulate cholesterol levels in the blood. They are therefore a useful snack and dessert food for people who have high cholesterol levels.

Food Allergies
Pears rarely cause allergic reactions. As such, pears are frequently an important part of exclusion diets (see page

245), which are advised for people who are trying to detect a food to which they are allergic.

Energy Depletion
The carbohydrates in pears are released slowly in the body, which makes them an ideal snack food for those undertaking physical activity. For best effect, they should be eaten in the two to four hour period leading up to exercise and during the recovery period between workouts.

Brain Power
Some research in the US suggests that pears, which are thought to contain the trace mineral boron, may help to improve electrical activity in the brain and therefore boost mental performance.

SEE ALSO DIABETES, PAGE 218; FOOD ALLERGIES, PAGE 210; HIGH CHOLESTEROL, PAGE 154; OBESITY, PAGE 178

APRICOTS

Documented as far back as 2000 BC in Chinese writings, the apricot originated in Eastern Asia, spread to Europe via the Arabs, and was introduced to the Mediterranean by the Romans. The sweet taste of this fruit comes from the high proportion of sucrose carbohydrate that it contains. Its yellow to orange flesh and skin are due to the antioxidant pigment beta carotene.

KEY BENEFITS

- MAY HELP TO PREVENT CANCER
- COULD HELP TO LOWER HIGH BLOOD PRESSURE
- HELP TO PREVENT NIGHT BLINDNESS
- USEFUL IN WEIGHT-LOSS EATING PLANS

FOOD PROFILE

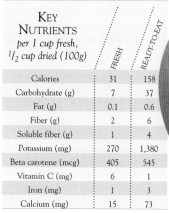

KEY NUTRIENTS per 1 cup fresh, 1/2 cup dried (100g)	FRESH	READY-TO-EAT
Calories	31	158
Carbohydrate (g)	7	37
Fat (g)	0.1	0.6
Fiber (g)	2	6
Soluble fiber (g)	1	4
Potassium (mg)	270	1,380
Beta carotene (mcg)	405	545
Vitamin C (mg)	6	1
Iron (mg)	1	3
Calcium (mg)	15	73

FRESH, DRIED, OR READY-TO-EAT? Whether fresh, "ready-to-eat," or dried, apricots are sweet and nutritious. Dark-colored, fresh apricots supply the antioxidant beta carotene, and dried apricots are a particularly rich source of potassium.

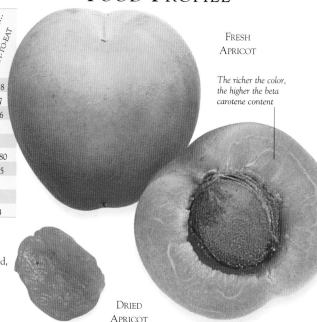

FRESH APRICOT

The richer the color, the higher the beta carotene content

DRIED APRICOT

★ HOW MUCH TO EAT

- Six average sized, "ready-to-eat" apricots provide about 13 percent of women's recommended daily intake of iron. Regular consumption of apricots may help to reduce the risk of anemia.

CHOOSING & STORING

- Look for soft, plump fruits, rather than firm, yellow ones. When buying dried apricots, avoid brightly colored ones, since these are preserved with sulfur dioxide.
- Ripen in a paper bag at room temperature. Store in a plastic bag in the refrigerator and eat within a few days.

COOKING & EATING

- Wash and eat raw, or poach or stew, then use in sorbets, tarts, jams, or chutney.

HEALING PROPERTIES

✍ TRADITIONAL USES

Recognized in traditional Chinese medicine for their copper content, apricots are used in China today to treat anemia. They are also used to "moisten the lungs" because they are said to increase the "yin" fluids in the body. For this reason, apricots may be given to treat dry lung conditions such as asthma, as well as to relieve thirst and dry throats.

▦ SPECIFIC BENEFITS

Stomach and Lung Cancers
Apricots are a useful source of beta carotene. Through studying the relationship between beta carotene and stomach cancer, a World Cancer Research Fund report concluded in 1998 that a high intake of carotenoids could

possibly reduce the risk of this disease. The protection against cancer is likely to be due to beta carotene's ability to "mop up" the substances that are responsible for sparking cancerous changes in cells.

The World Cancer Research Fund report of 1998 also concluded that carotenes probably offer protection against lung cancer in both smokers and nonsmokers, and in men and women alike. Regularly including apricots in the diet helps to boost carotene intakes.

High Blood Pressure
"Ready-to-eat" apricots are a particularly rich source of potassium, supplying 1.4g per 4oz serving. Including between 2.5 and 3.9g of extra potassium in the diet every

day has been shown to lower blood pressure in people with both normal and high levels.

Depression in the Elderly
Puréed apricots make an excellent dessert for elderly people who are suffering from mental depression and confusion due to a lack of potassium in the diet.

Night Blindness
A lack of carotene-rich foods can lead to poor night vision, especially in the elderly, who often eat few fresh fruits and vegetables. Apricots are a good source of carotene.

Energy Depletion
Fresh apricots are digested slowly, releasing a gentle stream of sugar into the blood. People who exercise regularly

need this kind of slow releasing fuel several hours before, and again between exercising sessions, to replace energy in the muscles.

Weight Problems
Fresh apricots taste sweet, yet provide relatively few calories. They are also rich in fiber and release a slow burning form of sugar into the bloodstream. It is easy to see why apricots make an excellent, low-calorie snack food for dieters.

CAUTION

Never eat apricot kernels. They contain a substance called amygdalin that releases cyanide into the body. If left untreated, this can cause respiratory failure, paralysis, or even death.

SEE ALSO CANCER, PAGE 214; DEPRESSION, PAGE 233; FATIGUE, PAGE 235; HIGH BLOOD PRESSURE, PAGE 155

PEACHES

Like other orange-colored fruits, peaches get their pigmentation from a variety of antioxidant carotenes. Originating in the mountains of Tibet and China, peaches were first cultivated in about 2000 BC. By 300 BC they had reached Greece, and by the first century AD the Romans, and soon the rest of Europe, were enjoying and benefiting nutritionally from this delicious fruit.

KEY BENEFITS
- MAY HELP TO LOWER BLOOD PRESSURE
- MAY HELP TO PREVENT CANCER
- COULD HELP TO IMPROVE MALE FERTILITY
- HELP TO COMBAT GUM DISEASE

FOOD PROFILE

KEY NUTRIENTS per ½ peach (100g)	FRESH	DRIED
Calories	33	219
Carbohydrate (g)	8.0	53
Potassium (mg)	160.0	1,100
Vitamin C (mg)	31.0	–
Fiber (g)	1.0	7
Soluble fiber (g)	1	4
Carotene (mcg)	58	445
Calcium (mg)	7	36
Sodium (mg)	1.0	6
Fat (g)	0.1	1

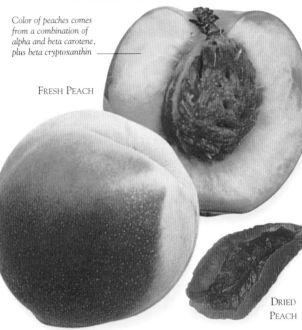

Color of peaches comes from a combination of alpha and beta carotene, plus beta cryptoxanthin

FRESH PEACH

DRIED PEACH

PEACH PITS
Peaches can be classified according to how easily the pit is removed. A "freestone" peach has an easily detachable pit and soft flesh. A "clingstone" peach has firm flesh and a firmly attached pit.

★ HOW MUCH TO EAT
- A large 5oz peach provides eight per cent of the daily adult fiber requirement. Most of this is soluble fiber, which helps to keep cholesterol levels down. Regular consumption may help reduce the risk of heart disease.

CHOOSING & STORING
- Look for a pale yellow to golden yellow skin with a red blush. The flesh should yield slightly when pressed gently.
- Store at room temperature, or place in the refrigerator for a few days.

COOKING & EATING
- Eat raw, whole or sliced, or add to fruit salads. To cook peaches, stew, poach, or bake them.

HEALING PROPERTIES

TRADITIONAL USES
According to Chinese medicine, the softness of this fruit makes it ideal for treating acute inflammation of the stomach. The fruit should be cooked, then puréed. Dry coughs and dry conditions of the lungs are also treated with peaches. Eaten regularly, they are thought to "moisten the lungs" and intestines.
Applying a poultice of fresh peach to the face is said to improve the complexion. The ground peach kernel is used to strengthen the circulation and is thought to reduce tumors and uterine fibroids.

SPECIFIC BENEFITS
High Blood Pressure
High blood pressure is often symptom-free, and it can go undiagnosed. Eventually it may lead to both heart disease and strokes. Losing excess weight and increasing the amount of potassium consumed in the diet can help to reduce high blood pressure. Consuming fresh peaches regularly adds significant amounts of potassium to the diet. When peaches are out of season, dried ones can be eaten.

Cancer & Heart Disease
The presence of antioxidant carotenes, flavonoids, and vitamin C in peaches means that this fruit may play an important role in combatting degenerative diseases such as heart disease and certain types of cancer. Consumed regularly, the nutrients in this fruit may intervene at various stages in the development of disease.

Male Infertility
Studies indicate that men with fertility problems can possibly be helped by increasing their intake of vitamin C to 500mg twice a day in supplement form. In tests on the general quality of sperm, there was an improvement in just one week in the number of sperm present, their mobility, and lifespan. The amount of sperm "clumping" rather than swimming freely, was reduced from 37 to 14 percent, and after four weeks to only 11 percent. Diets that include regular intakes of fruits rich in vitamin C, such as peaches, can help to boost levels of vitamin C in the body. This is particularly important for smokers, in whom attack from free radicals increases dramatically if vitamin C intakes are low. Sperm count improves when vitamin C intakes are boosted to 250mg a day, an amount that can easily be obtained from fruits such as peaches. Sperm counts in male smokers can be improved by as much as 24 percent and sperm mobility by 18 percent if 250mg of vitamin C is consumed daily.

Gum Disease
One of the first signs of vitamin C deficiency is loosening of the teeth and bleeding gums. Evidence suggests that gum disease is three and a half times more common than normal in people with low levels of vitamin C in their blood. A medium peach supplies about 34mg of this vitamin.

SEE ALSO CANCER, PAGE 214; GUM DISEASE, PAGE 206; HIGH BLOOD PRESSURE, PAGE 155; INFERTILITY IN MEN, PAGE 227

PINEAPPLES

STAR NUTRIENTS & PHYTONUTRIENTS

C K Bromelain, Fiber, P-coumaric acid

The medicinal properties of pineapples were recognized and exploited by native South Americans, who were the first people to cultivate them. The juicy, yellow, fragrant fruit is packed with protective phytonutrients and also contains the protein digesting enzyme bromelain and the antioxidant vitamin C. Pineapples can be eaten fresh or canned, and the juice makes a refreshing drink.

KEY BENEFITS

- HELP TO DISSOLVE BLOOD CLOTS THAT CAN CAUSE THROMBOSIS
- RELIEVE INDIGESTION
- MAY PREVENT CANCER
- HELP TO HEAL WOUNDS

FOOD PROFILE

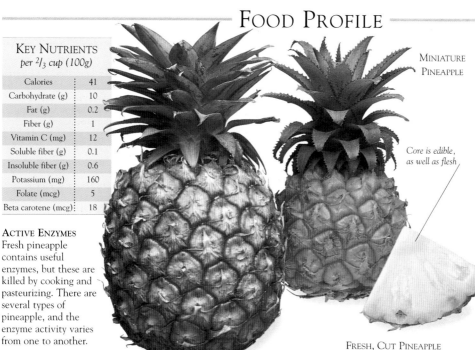

MINIATURE PINEAPPLE

Core is edible, as well as flesh

FRESH, CUT PINEAPPLE

KEY NUTRIENTS
per ²/₃ cup (100g)

Calories	41
Carbohydrate (g)	10
Fat (g)	0.2
Fiber (g)	1
Vitamin C (mg)	12
Soluble fiber (g)	0.1
Insoluble fiber (g)	0.6
Potassium (mg)	160
Folate (mcg)	5
Beta carotene (mcg)	18

ACTIVE ENZYMES
Fresh pineapple contains useful enzymes, but these are killed by cooking and pasteurizing. There are several types of pineapple, and the enzyme activity varies from one to another.

★ **HOW MUCH TO EAT**
- ¹/₂ cup of pineapple supplies over 25 percent of an adult's daily vitamin C requirement.

🍚 **CHOOSING & STORING**
- Choose a ripe pineapple because this fruit does not ripen after being picked. The pineapple should not be too green. It should be firm to the touch but should still have some "give." The base should smell sweet.
- Leave an uncut pineapple upside down (standing on its tufty top) overnight so that the sugars move through the fruit. Store at room temperature.

🍲 **COOKING & EATING**
- Eat pineapple raw, on its own, and use in salads.
- Add chunks to stir-fries or cook with seafood.

HEALING PROPERTIES

🌿 TRADITIONAL USES
Native South Americans believed that the pineapple had healing properties. They used the juice to aid digestion and to keep the skin clean. Warriors applied pineapple poultices to wounds and used the leaves as bandages. The Chinese believe the fruit to have a "neutral" nature and a sweet-and-sour flavor. These properties are thought to keep the body cool in the heat of summer. In China, the fruit is used to treat conditions such as sunburn, diarrhea, indigestion, and worms.

✴ SPECIFIC BENEFITS
Thrombosis
The enzyme bromelain, which can be found in pineapples, has been shown to be effective in treating blood clots that may lead to thrombosis. Blood clots are everyday occurrences and are needed to stop blood from leaking into organs. When they are no longer needed, they should dissolve naturally. When clots do not dissolve, they can block blood vessels and cause a heart attack or stroke. Bromelain supplements have been shown to reduce deaths in people with heart disease from an expected 20 percent to less than two percent. Bromelain appears to function by stimulating the production of plasmin, a substance in the blood that breaks down clots.

Indigestion
Bromelain extract is used in the food industry to tenderize meat. The enzyme helps to start the breakdown of the protein structures in the meat. A similar process seems to occur in the stomach if bromelain is taken either in the form of fresh pineapple, or as a supplement. This enzyme can often be particularly useful for people with bad digestion. Bromelain can be used to break down solid or semisolid masses of undigested food lodged in the stomach. Known as bezoars, these masses cause stomach pains. They can be treated by cutting them up with an endoscopic attachment, then giving the patient a drink containing bromelain. It has been shown that if a large lump of meat gets stuck in the throat, a bromelain drink, sipped at regular intervals, can help to reduce it so that it is able to be swallowed.

Cancer
Pineapples contain the phytonutrients p-coumaric and cholorgenic acid, which appear to stop nitric oxide and amines from combining in the stomach and creating the cancer causing substances called nitrosamines.

Wounds
Bromelain is used in medicine to impregnate specially formulated bandages, along with antibiotic drugs.

CAUTION

People who have a history of stomach ulcers should avoid eating pineapples, especially unripe ones, because they have a high acid content. The acid in the fruit can also damage the teeth.

SEE ALSO CANCER, PAGE 214; HEARTBURN, PAGE 170; THROMBOSIS, PAGE 157

PRUNES

A prune is a dried plum, usually the d'Agen sugar plum, that has been processed without removing the pit. Taken to medieval Europe from the Middle East by the Crusaders, almost 70 percent of the world's prunes now come from California. Prunes are rich in fiber and known for their laxative properties. They supply a good range of vitamins and minerals.

KEY BENEFITS

- HELP TO TREAT AND PREVENT CONSTIPATION
- MAY HELP TO PREVENT IRON DEFICIENCY
- CAN HELP TO REDUCE FAT IN BAKED GOODS
- MAY HELP TO TREAT HIGH BLOOD PRESSURE

FOOD PROFILE

KEY NUTRIENTS per 2/3 cup dried (100g)	PRUNES	READY-TO-EAT PRUNES	CANNED IN JUICE
Calories	160	141	79
Fat (g)	0.5	0.4	0.2
Carbohydrate (g)	38	34	20
Fiber (g)	7	6	2
Soluble fiber (g)	4	4	1.5
Potassium (mg)	860	760	340
Iron (mg)	3	3	2
Calcium (mg)	38	34	26
Beta carotene (mcg)	155	140	140
Selenium (mcg)	3	3	–

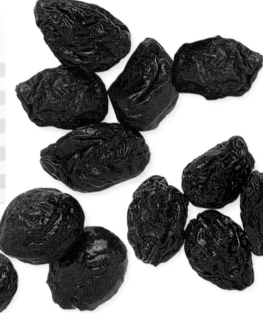

WRINKLED RICHES
It takes about 8 lbs of fresh plums to make 2 1/4 lbs of prunes. Carotenes in the fruits' purple outer skins survive the drying process, which means that prunes can add valuable antioxidants to the diet.

★ HOW MUCH TO EAT

- A 1/2-cup serving of "ready-to-eat" prunes supplies 28 percent of an adult's daily fiber needs.
- The same serving provides 15 percent of a woman's daily iron requirement.

CHOOSING & STORING

- Buy "ready-to-eat" prunes in cans or sealed packets.
- Keep sealed prunes for up to six months, and canned prunes for up to a year.

COOKING & EATING

- For winter fruit salads, soak prunes with other dried fruits.
- Use in stuffing for pork and game, or add to pork and rabbit casseroles or stews.
- Serve stewed on breakfast cereals and in cakes.
- Prune purée can be used as a fat substitute in some baked foods, such as brownies and carrot cake.

HEALING PROPERTIES

📖 TRADITIONAL USES

In Chinese medicine, prune juice is recommended as a useful morning elixir for refreshing and detoxifying the body after sleeping. Prune juice is best drunk slightly warmed and, if taken cold, should not be colder than body temperature. In Japan, eating prunes is traditionally considered to bestow great natural beauty. In the West, prunes and prune juice have been recommended as a cure for constipation for centuries.

✦ SPECIFIC BENEFITS

Constipation
Both fresh and dried prunes help to relieve and prevent constipation by speeding up the rate at which stools pass through the colon, or large intestine. Prunes work in two ways. First, they provide fiber as a food for bacteria found in the colon. The bacteria ferment the fiber and, in the process, increase the bulk of the stools. The muscular walls of the colon, therefore, have more material to work on, which increases the strength and speed of their contractions so that they can push waste through the body more quickly. Second, prunes and prune juice contain derivatives of a substance called hydroxyphenylisatin, which directly stimulates the smooth muscle of the colon wall. This stimulation sets off increased activity in the colon, which again helps to speed up the movement of the stools. A typical 1/2-cup serving of prunes contains 10g of the substance sorbitol, a type of sugar that has a laxative effect on the colon.

Iron Deficiency
Vegetarians and people who eat very little red meat risk taking in inadequate amounts of iron and running down their body's reserves of this mineral. A lack of iron can eventually lead to anemia, the symptoms of which include severe fatigue and difficulty in concentrating. Prunes are a good source of "non-hem" iron (*see page 160*), supplying 3mg of iron per 1/2-cup serving.

Weight Problems
Cooks have long known that, in times of fat shortages, margarine or butter can be substituted by a similar weight of prune purée in soft, chewy, baked recipes, such as muffins, brownies, and carrot cake. The prune purée adds bulk and substance to the recipe, and does not have the fat content of butter or margarine. It is therefore useful for people on low fat diets who wish to eat a sweet treat that has a fraction of the fat of traditional products. It is possible to buy ready-made prune purée.

High Blood Pressure
Prunes are an excellent source of potassium and can help people to reach target intakes of 3,500mg of this mineral daily. An adequate daily intake of potassium in the diet helps to maintain a good balance of fluid in the body and to regulate blood pressure levels.

SEE ALSO CONSTIPATION, PAGE 175; HIGH BLOOD PRESSURE, PAGE 155; MINERALS, PAGE 30; OBESITY, PAGE 178

FIGS

Among the oldest recorded crops, fig remains have been found at historic sites dating back as far as 7800 BC. Figs have been used for their mild laxative effects for centuries. Their nutritional value depends on whether they are fresh, dried, or in the popular, partly dried, "ready-to-eat" form. Dried and "ready-to-eat" figs are a very good source of iron and potassium.

KEY BENEFITS

- RELIEVE MILD CONSTIPATION AND PROMOTE REGULAR BOWEL HABITS
- MAY REDUCE ANEMIA
- MAY PLAY A ROLE IN PREVENTING OSTEOPOROSIS

FOOD PROFILE

KEY NUTRIENTS per ¹/₂ cup dried (100g)	FRESH	DRIED	READY-TO-EAT
Calories	43	227	209
Fat (g)	0.3	2	2
Fiber (g)	2	8	7
Potassium (mg)	200	970	890
Calcium (mg)	38	250	230
Iron (mg)	0.3	4	4
Zinc (mg)	0.3	0.7	0.6
Carotenes (mcg)	150	64	59
Folate (mcg)	–	9	8
Vitamin C (mg)	2	1	1

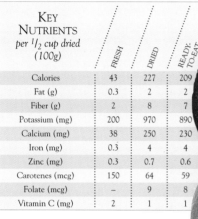

A NATURAL LAXATIVE
The laxative effect of figs is said to be due to the substance known as "mucin." This is also believed to give figs a soothing and gently cleansing effect in the intestines, and to help to prevent hemorrhoids. Syrup of figs has a more potent laxative effect than the fresh or dried fruit.

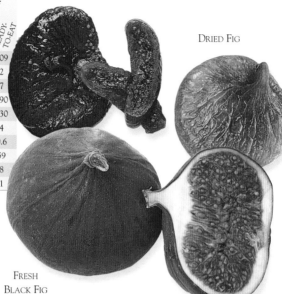

DRIED FIG

FRESH BLACK FIG

★ HOW MUCH TO EAT

- Two fresh figs weighing 4oz are a useful source of fiber, supplying 7 percent of the recommended daily intake. Dried and "ready-to-eat" figs are rich in calcium. Three dried figs provide 21 percent of a woman's recommended daily intake of calcium.

🍲 CHOOSING & STORING

- Fresh figs should be soft, plump, and sweet-smelling, with an undamaged skin. Store in the refrigerator for a few days.
- Buy dried figs from a reputable source and store for up to one month in an airtight container.

🍳 COOKING & EATING

- Wash and dry fresh figs and serve with fromage frais, cheese, or ham. Poach, caramelize, or use to make fig tart or ice cream.
- Dried and "ready-to-eat" figs can be stewed or eaten as snacks.

HEALING PROPERTIES

✍ TRADITIONAL USES

In traditional Chinese medicine, figs are thought to help eliminate toxins and are used to treat boils. The fig is considered to be one of the most alkaline fruits, and it therefore helps to balance acidic conditions that occur from over consumption of meat and refined foods. For asthma and sore throats, Chinese medicine suggests eating fig soup. Fresh figs can be rubbed onto the gums to relieve toothache, and the milky latex inside figs is recommended for warts. In Western herbalism, a concoction of figs is given for colds and to dislodge mucus in the respiratory tract. Syrup of figs is recommended for poor bowel movements and to prevent constipation.

✸ SPECIFIC BENEFITS

Constipation
While there has been little clinical research on the role that figs play in relieving constipation, it is generally accepted that they increase the peristaltic movements in the large intestine, which encourage the contents to move out of the body rapidly. Doctors often suggest figs and syrup of figs for people with constipation. Figs are especially useful for young children, who usually require only a very mild laxative.

Anemia
Both dried and "ready-to-eat" figs supply iron. Adequate iron intakes are vital for the production of hemoglobin in the blood. Women in the West often have poor or nonexistent iron reserves which, at times of extra demand, such as during menstruation and pregnancy, can lead to anemia. The iron in figs is "non-hem" iron (see page 160), which is less well absorbed than iron from meat. It is therefore advisable to eat figs with a source of vitamin C, such as orange juice, to enhance the absorption of iron. Dried and "ready-to-eat" figs make a good snack and they are also useful for teenage girls who have become vegetarians, as a way of increasing their iron intake.

Osteoporosis
Dried and "ready-to-eat" figs are an excellent, nondairy source of the bone building mineral calcium. They are useful for teenage girls who have become vegans and wish to avoid dairy products. Calcium is very important for healthy bone growth in children and teenagers. If the calcium intakes are poor during peak growing periods in young people, maximum bone mass will not be achieved. If the body's calcium reserves do not reach their peak during growth, there may be a greater than normal risk of bone fractures and osteoporosis in later life.

CAUTION

Fresh figs contain a milky, latex-like substance that can cause mouth and skin eruptions in certain susceptible people. These people should avoid eating figs in their raw state.

SEE ALSO ANEMIA, PAGE 160; CONSTIPATION, PAGE 175; OSTEOPOROSIS, PAGE 199

GRAPES

STAR NUTRIENTS & PHYTONUTRIENTS	
K	Ellagic acid, Anthocyanidins, Fiber, Flavonoids

Long valued in hot climates as a refreshing, energy boosting food, grapes were traditionally used to treat conditions such as arthritis and rheumatism, and for their diuretic effects. Grapes are said to cleanse, strengthen, and rejuvenate the body. They supply a range of phytonutrients, plenty of potassium, and relatively large amounts of sugar.

KEY BENEFITS

- MAY PLAY A ROLE IN FIGHTING CARCINOGENS
- HELP TO IMPROVE SYMPTOMS OF ARTHRITIS
- MAY HELP URINARY DISORDERS
- COULD LOWER RAISED BLOOD PRESSURE

FOOD PROFILE

KEY NUTRIENTS per 4oz (100g)	GRAPES	RAISINS
Calories	60	272
Carbohydrate (g)	16	69
Glucose (g)	8	34.5
Fructose (g)	8	34.8
Potassium (mg)	210	1020
Fiber (g)	1	2
Soluble fiber (g)	0.4	1
Vitamin C (mg)	3	1
Carotenes (mcg)	17	12

HIGH-ENERGY FOOD
The sweetness of grapes comes from their high sugar content. About 15–25 percent of their calories comes from glucose and fructose. Grapes are a low glycemic index (GI) food (see page 18), since they raise blood sugars slowly.

Reddish-purple color comes from antioxidant pigment anthocyanidins

BLACK GRAPES

GREEN GRAPES

RAISINS

★ HOW MUCH TO EAT

- A small bunch of grapes supplies vitamins and minerals and is a rich source of antioxidant phytonutrients such as ellagic acid. Regular consumption several times a week may help to reduce the risk of cancer caused by pollution.

CHOOSING & STORING

- Select grapes with firm stalks and plump, undamaged fruits.
  - Look for an amber tinge on green grapes and a dark tone on red grapes.
  - Store in the refrigerator for several days.

COOKING & EATING

- Wash, rinse, then pat dry. Serve alone, with cheese, or as a garnish for fish or meat dishes.
- If cooking grapes, they should be skinned and deseeded first.

HEALING PROPERTIES

✔ TRADITIONAL USES

According to traditional Chinese medicine, the grape is said to contain salts that purify the blood and cleanse the glands and organs. Chinese doctors advise a ten day grape cure to cleanse the body, in which only grapes and grape juice are consumed. Grapes are also believed to increase "qi" energy and strengthen bones and sinews. Grapes have been used in the West to help relieve arthritis and rheumatism, water retention, and to treat painful urination. About 1¼ cups of grapes a day is traditionally recommended for long-term urinary problems, and 2½ cups a day for acute problems. Grape juice is said to have positive effects on disorders such as hepatitis and jaundice.

✚ SPECIFIC BENEFITS

Cancer
Grapes contain the phytonutrient ellagic acid which, under laboratory conditions, appears to help neutralize cancer causing substances before they cause mutations. Ellagic acid is thought to fight off carcinogens caused by pollution, barbecued meats, and tobacco smoke.

Rheumatoid Arthritis
Rich in several antioxidant flavonoids, grapes may play a role in treating arthritis. They seem to stop or hinder the action of certain enzymes that can otherwise damage the substances that produce cartilage and bone in the joints.

High Blood Pressure
Grapes are rich in potassium, which may help to lower high blood pressure. Intakes of 2.5–3.9g a day have been found to lower blood pressure in men. It has been estimated that regular daily intakes of 2.3–3.1g of potassium could result in a 25 percent reduction in deaths related to high blood pressure.

Mental Confusion
A lack of potassium can lead to mental confusion and depression. The elderly, who tend to consume low amounts of fruits and vegetables, are particularly at risk. Eating grapes is a simple, palatable way in which to increase intakes of potassium.

OTHER FORM

Red Wine
Wine produced from red grapes contains antioxidants that are thought to reduce the risk of heart disease. Low to moderate consumption (one or two glasses) of wine a day may therefore be beneficial to the heart.

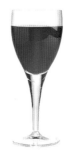

GLASS OF RED WINE

SEE ALSO CANCER, PAGE 214; HIGH BLOOD PRESSURE, PAGE 155; KIDNEY DISORDERS, PAGE 192; RHEUMATOID ARTHRITIS, PAGE 197

BERRIES

This large group of cultivated and wild fruits includes blueberries, gooseberries, strawberries, raspberries, mulberries, cranberries, and red currants. All of them are bursting with water-soluble plant chemicals known as bioflavonoids. These powerful antioxidants may be responsible for many of the berries' health-giving properties, and they also contribute to their wide array of colors.

STAR NUTRIENTS & PHYTONUTRIENTS

  C **K** **Bc** Anthocyanidins, Fiber

KEY BENEFITS

- MAY HELP TO PREVENT VARICOSE VEINS
- MAY EASE RHEUMATOID ARTHRITIS
- CAN BE PART OF A WEIGHT-LOSS DIET
- MAY HELP TO REDUCE THE RISK OF CANCERS

FOOD PROFILE

★ HOW MUCH TO EAT

- An average ³/₄-cup serving of whole strawberries supplies 62 percent of an adult's daily vitamin C requirement.
- ²/₃ cup of raspberries provide 15 percent of an adult's daily folate requirement.
- 1¹/₄ cups of cranberry juice, taken daily, is believed to help to reduce the risk of developing urinary infections.
- 1 cup of black currants supply 200mg of vitamin C, which is five times the recommended daily intake.

CHOOSING & STORING

- Buy plump, brightly colored fruits that are free from brown or soft patches and mold.
- Store in a refrigerator.

COOKING & EATING

- Wash all berries before eating.
- Most berries are best eaten raw.
- Use in jams, pies, fruit crumbles, and sorbets or use to make fruit juices.

BLACKBERRIES

Blackberries contain at least twice as much vitamin E as most common berries, and supply more folate.

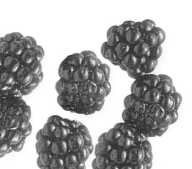

STRAWBERRIES

Strawberry juice is said to have antibacterial properties. Women through the ages have also used the crushed wild fruits to make freckles fade.

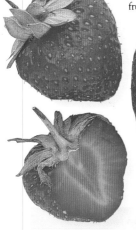
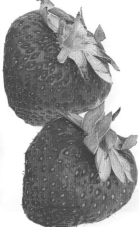

CRANBERRIES

The tart flavor makes raw cranberries unpalatable to most people. Juice can be made by crushing the berries and mixing the pulp with sugar and water. (See also page 85)

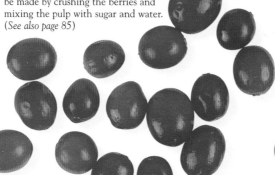

RED CURRANTS

These berries contain less citric acid than blackcurrants yet have similar amounts of sugar, so they taste sweeter.

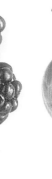
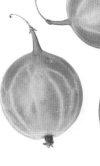
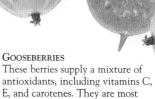

GOOSEBERRIES

These berries supply a mixture of antioxidants, including vitamins C, E, and carotenes. They are most palatable when cooked.

BLACK CURRANTS

The intense color of black currants is due to bioflavonoids, which are the antioxidant pigments present in purple and blue berries.

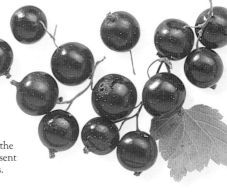

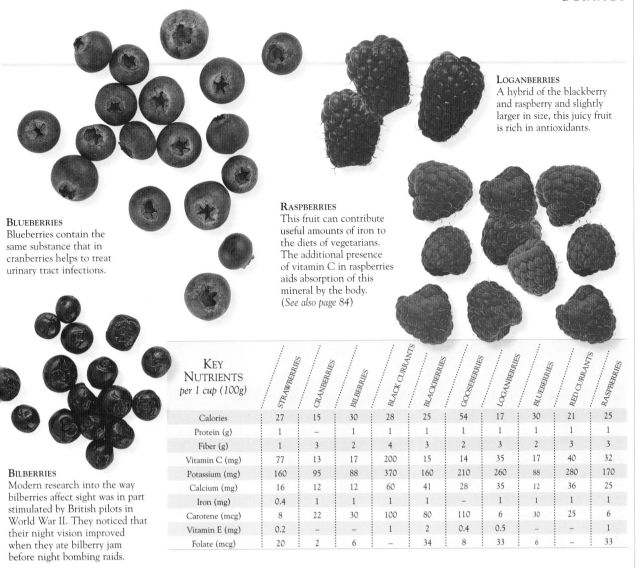

LOGANBERRIES
A hybrid of the blackberry and raspberry and slightly larger in size, this juicy fruit is rich in antioxidants.

RASPBERRIES
This fruit can contribute useful amounts of iron to the diets of vegetarians. The additional presence of vitamin C in raspberries aids absorption of this mineral by the body. (*See also page 84*)

BLUEBERRIES
Blueberries contain the same substance that in cranberries helps to treat urinary tract infections.

BILBERRIES
Modern research into the way bilberries affect sight was in part stimulated by British pilots in World War II. They noticed that their night vision improved when they ate bilberry jam before night bombing raids.

KEY NUTRIENTS per 1 cup (100g)	STRAWBERRIES	CRANBERRIES	BILBERRIES	BLACK CURRANTS	BLACKBERRIES	GOOSEBERRIES	LOGANBERRIES	BLUEBERRIES	RED CURRANTS	RASPBERRIES
Calories	27	15	30	28	25	54	17	30	21	25
Protein (g)	1	–	1	1	1	1	1	1	1	1
Fiber (g)	1	3	2	4	3	2	3	2	3	3
Vitamin C (mg)	77	13	17	200	15	14	35	17	40	32
Potassium (mg)	160	95	88	370	160	210	260	88	280	170
Calcium (mg)	16	12	12	60	41	28	35	12	36	25
Iron (mg)	0.4	1	1	1	1	–	1	1	1	1
Carotene (mcg)	8	22	30	100	80	110	6	30	25	6
Vitamin E (mg)	0.2	–	–	1	2	0.4	0.5	–	–	1
Folate (mcg)	20	2	6	–	34	8	33	6	–	33

HEALING PROPERTIES

☑ TRADITIONAL USES
Raspberry leaves are used in traditional herbal medicine to strengthen the uterus and to stop heavy menstrual flow. The antibacterial properties of strawberry juice have been used by herbalists in the West to protect against typhoid epidemics. Strawberries have also been prescribed by herbalists as a liver tonic. Cranberry and raspberry juice are used in the West to treat urinary tract infections. In Chinese medicine, doctors use strawberries to correct disorders of the spleen and pancreas, to "moisten the lungs," and to treat sore throats. In China, mulberries are said to help slow down prematurely graying hair, and to prevent insomnia, constipation, and stiff joints.

▦ SPECIFIC BENEFITS
Varicose Veins
Bioflavonoids, particularly anthocyanidins, are found in bilberries and other red, blue, and purple berries. These substances may have a role to play in preventing varicose veins and broken veins and capillaries, and in strengthening artery walls. They seem to prevent the destruction of the protein collagen, which is responsible for maintaining the structure of skin and blood vessels.

Rheumatoid Arthritis
Studies carried out over many weeks on people with rheumatoid arthritis revealed that the oil from black currant seeds could be a potential treatment for the disease. The oil contains the essential fatty acids, gammalinolenic acid (GLA) and alphalinolenic acid (ALA), which appear to "dampen down" inflammatory responses in the body. Treatment with 10.5g of black currant oil a day for six months showed a modest but significant reduction in pain.

Weight Problems
Berries contain only between 15 and 30 calories per 1-cup serving, so it is possible to eat a large amount of these fruits in a calorie-controlled diet. Berries cause a slow increase in blood sugar, which helps to promote a feeling of fullness and does not lead to a large release of insulin. Insulin is the hormone produced to control blood sugar levels and encourage the retention of excess sugar as fat.

Cancer of the Colon
Berries supply fiber, which bulks up the stools and makes them move faster through the colon. This may reduce the risk of colonic cancer.

Stomach Cancer
Strawberries contain the plant chemicals p-coumaric acid and chlorogenic acid. These appear to prevent carcinogens known as nitrosamines from forming in the stomach, and may reduce the risk of cancer.

> **CAUTION**
>
> Drinking high doses of raspberry leaf infusions should be avoided during early pregnancy since they can stimulate contractions of the uterus.

SEE ALSO CANCER, PAGE 214; CATARACTS, PAGE 202; COLDS AND INFLUENZA, PAGE 184

RASPBERRIES

STAR NUTRIENTS & PHYTONUTRIENTS

 Quercetin, Lutein, Myricetin, Ellagic acid

Described as the king of berries, the raspberry was first cultivated about 500 years ago. Wild varieties still grow in Europe and Western Asia. Both the raspberry and its leaves have formed an important part of home cures for centuries, and they are well known for their healing properties. Recent research suggests that this delicious fruit also has a role to play in cancer prevention.

KEY BENEFITS

- MAY HELP TO PREVENT TOBACCO AND ENVIRONMENTALLY INDUCED CANCERS
- PREPARE THE BODY FOR CHILDBIRTH
- BOOST THE BODY'S ANTIOXIDANT LEVELS

FOOD PROFILE

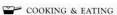

KEY NUTRIENTS
per 1/2 cup (100g)

Calories	25
Protein (g)	1
Fiber (g)	3
Calcium (mg)	25
Potassium (mg)	170
Magnesium (mg)	19
Vitamin C (mg)	32
Folate (mcg)	33
Vitamin E (mg)	1
Iron (mg)	1

RASPBERRY LEAVES

FRESH RASPBERRIES

CLEANSING BERRIES
An infusion of raspberry leaves is a cleansing diuretic and helps to treat rheumatic problems. It is also given to men who have prostate problems.

★ **HOW MUCH TO EAT**

- A 1/2-cup serving of fresh raspberries provides 16 percent of the day's folate intake for men and women. A similar portion of raspberries also supplies 80 percent of the daily recommended vitamin C requirements.

🥣 **CHOOSING & STORING**

- Buy plump, brightly colored fruit with no brown patches.
- Store raspberries covered, in the refrigerator, for as little time as possible before eating.

🍲 **COOKING & EATING**

- Wash gently, then pat dry. Eat whole within 24 hours of purchase, or use in fruit tarts, sorbets, and soufflés.

HEALING PROPERTIES

📋 **TRADITIONAL USES**
In Chinese medicine, raspberries are traditionally used to benefit the liver and kidneys and help them to cleanse the blood of toxins. Raspberries are particularly beneficial for excessive and frequent urination, especially at night. Women with irregular menstrual cycles are recommended to eat raspberries on a regular basis, and they have also been used in the East to treat anemia and to encourage labor during childbirth. In Chinese herbalism, the dried, unripe fruit is used to treat impotence and premature ejaculation in men. Ripe raspberries are also said to benefit the eyesight. The unripe raspberry is said to have estrogenlike effects on the female sex organs. Western herbalism uses the whole raspberry to help ease

indigestion and rheumatism, while the juice is given for sore throats and coughs.

✳️ **SPECIFIC BENEFITS**
Cancer
Raspberries contain the phytonutrient called ellagic acid, which appears to be particularly efficient at fighting pollutants derived from cigarette smoke, processed foods, and barbecued meats. Ellagic acid seems to neutralize the cancer causing substances before they can invade healthy cells. In laboratory experiments, ellagic acid has been found to inhibit the development of lung cancer.

Childbirth
Both traditional medicine and modern research acknowledge the stimulating effect of the raspberry leaf on the uterus. An infusion of raspberry

leaves sets up rhythms in the smooth muscle lining of the uterus in pregnant women. This is caused by a number of stimulants in raspberries.

Viral Infections
Raspberries contain tannic acid, which is believed to be responsible for the antiviral activity that scientists have noted in various extracts from the raspberry fruit.

Heart Disease
Raspberries are bursting with a wide variety of antioxidant substances. In addition to vitamins C and E, these red berries also supply the plant chemicals quercetin, lutein, myricetin, and ellagic acid. All of these phytonutrients have strongly antioxidant effects on the body and appear to play a role in the prevention of heart disease and certain types of cancer.

Weight Problems
Raspberries are low in calories, and are an ideal food for dieters who are on a calorie-reduced eating plan. The idea of this form of diet is to increase the volume of food consumed while simultaneously reducing the total number of calories. In a typical 1/2-cup serving of fresh raspberries, water constitutes 87g, making them particularly suitable for this diet. The sweetest of all the berries, raspberries also add a welcome flavor and texture to any low-fat diet.

CAUTION

Raspberry leaf infusions can be taken by women to ease childbirth. However, high doses should be avoided during early pregnancy since they can stimulate the uterus.

SEE ALSO CANCER, PAGE 214; HEART DISEASE, PAGE 152; INFECTIONS, PAGE 212; WOMEN & NUTRITION, PAGE 140

CRANBERRIES

The cranberry is one of only three fruits native to North America. Used by Native Americans long before the 1620 landings of the European pilgrims, cranberries grow in bogs or marshes. The fruit supplies fiber and vitamin C, but the main health benefit comes from the phytonutrients that appear to maintain the health of, and fight diseases in, the urinary tract.

KEY BENEFITS

- HELP FIGHT URINARY TRACT INFECTIONS
- NATURALLY ANTIBACTERIAL
- MAY HELP THOSE WITH URINARY STONES
- MAY HELP THOSE WITH KIDNEY STONES

FOOD PROFILE

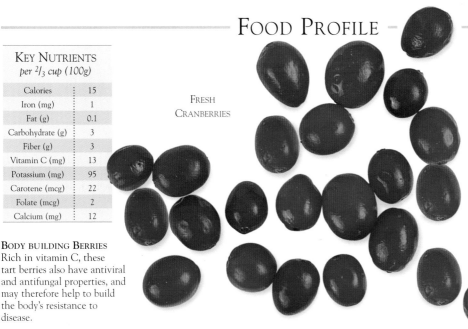

FRESH CRANBERRIES

KEY NUTRIENTS
per 2/3 cup (100g)

Calories	15
Iron (mg)	1
Fat (g)	0.1
Carbohydrate (g)	3
Fiber (g)	3
Vitamin C (mg)	13
Potassium (mg)	95
Carotene (mcg)	22
Folate (mcg)	2
Calcium (mg)	12

BODY BUILDING BERRIES
Rich in vitamin C, these tart berries also have antiviral and antifungal properties, and may therefore help to build the body's resistance to disease.

★ HOW MUCH TO EAT

- Cranberries are often consumed as juice. An average 1/4 cup taken daily is believed to reduce the risk of urinary infections.

🍲 CHOOSING & STORING

- Drinking cranberry juice is the easiest way to benefit from the therapeutic properties of this fruit. Choose a well-known brand and refrigerate after opening.
- Store berries, jellies, and purées according to pack instructions.

🥘 COOKING & EATING

- The juice should be drunk cold. It can be used in jellies, sorbets, and ice-pops.
- Use cranberry jelly with turkey and in sandwiches.

HEALING PROPERTIES

✍ TRADITIONAL USES

Crushed cranberries and cranberry juice were used by Native Americans to treat and prevent urinary tract infections long before the discovery of antibiotics. It is said that Native Americans introduced the European settlers to these berries as a treatment for scurvy. In the West, the first recorded use of cranberries by doctors to treat infections of the urinary tract was in 1923. They believed that cranberries made the urine so acidic that bacteria could not multiply. A later theory was that it was the benzoic acid in cranberry juice that helped to prevent infections. Both theories have now been dismissed. It is, as yet, a mystery phytonutrient that seems capable of preventing bacteria from setting up an infection in the urinary tract.

❖ SPECIFIC BENEFITS

Cystitis
The bacterium known as *Escherichia coli* accounts for 85 percent of all urinary tract infections. One of the most common of these infections is cystitis, which is especially prevalent in women. Scientists are now recommending the traditional use of cranberries and cranberry juice to deal with such infections. The presence of benzoic acid in cranberries has been thought to play a role in their therapeutic and protective effects. However, new research is showing that the effect is possibly due to the presence of a "polymeric compound" in cranberries, of unknown nature. This unidentified compound helps to prevent *Escherichia coli* from sticking to the walls of the bladder and urinary tract, and thereby acts to prevent bacteria from

multiplying and setting up an infection. The same effect is exhibited by blueberries and blueberry juice. Eating these berries and drinking these fruit juices regularly may help to reduce the incidence of urinary infections and the use of antibiotics to treat them.

Bacterial Infections
Cranberries have been found to have an "antiadherence" effect on several types of bacteria that are found in the urine and stools. This means that the cranberries can help to flush the bacteria out of the body. One study was able to show that cranberry juice had a limited capacity to clear infected urine of bacteria. In another study, people were given a combination of orange juice, vitamin C, and cranberry juice, which was found to make their urine more acidic. This could prove

to be a way of treating and preventing long-term urinary tract infections. Although cranberries are not a complete substitute for antibiotics, these fruits and their juice may enhance the effect of drugs that are used to treat such conditions.

Urinary Stones
Regular intake of cranberry juice to acidify urine is thought to be useful in the treatment of bad-smelling urine and urinary stones in people with urostomies (artificial urine drainage).

CAUTION

Drinking more than 4 cups of cranberry juice a day can cause diarrhea in some people and may result in uric acid stones in others. It may therefore be best to restrict intake to 1 cup twice a day.

SEE ALSO CYSTITIS, PAGE 190; INFECTIONS, PAGE 212

CITRUS FRUITS

STAR NUTRIENTS & PHYTONUTRIENTS

C   Bc   K   Lycopene, Fiber

The evergreen shrubs or trees on which citrus fruits grow can reach up to 32 feet or more in height. They grow best in subtropical, Mediterranean-type climates. Citrus fruits are well known for being high in vitamin C, which is essential for good health. Scientists have discovered that they are also packed with a wide variety of phytonutrients and different kinds of dietary fiber.

KEY BENEFITS

- MAY HELP TO PREVENT CANCERS OF THE STOMACH AND COLON
- HIGH INTAKES MAY REDUCE RISK OF CATARACTS
- HELP THE BODY TO ABSORB IRON AND REDUCE THE RISK OF ANEMIA

FOOD PROFILE

★ HOW MUCH TO EAT

- A medium sized 5$^{1}/_{2}$oz grapefruit supplies about 10 percent of an adult's recommended daily intake of the mineral potassium.
- One orange supplies more than 90 percent of an adult's daily vitamin C requirement. Blood oranges contain the antioxidant pigment beta carotene.

🥢 CHOOSING & STORING

- Look for evenly colored fruits without brown or soft patches.
- Choose fruits that have the brightest-colored skin.
- Store at room temperature.

🍳 COOKING & EATING

- Eat raw, squeeze to make juice, or divide into segments and add to vegetable and fruit salads.
- Use in marmalades, chutneys, sorbets, jellies, and mousses.

KUMQUATS
These citrus fruits have a tender skin that can be eaten with the flesh, making them a particularly good source of protective phytonutrients.

ORANGES
Unusually for fruit, oranges provide a source of the B vitamin folate, which may help to reduce the risk of heart disease and spina bifida in babies. (*See also* page 88)

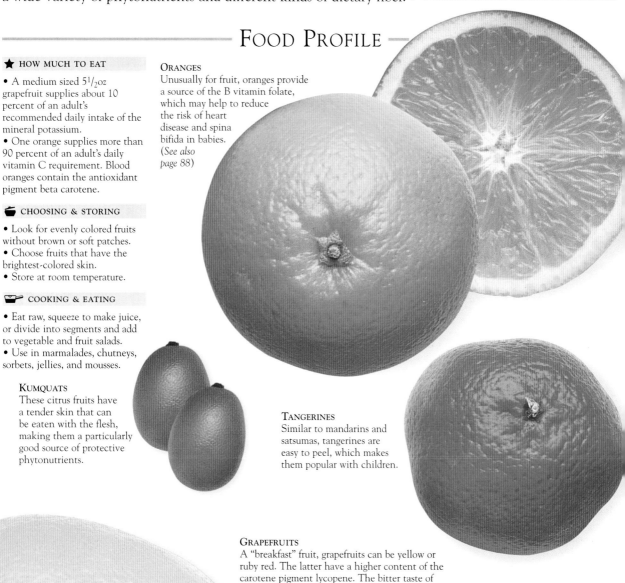

TANGERINES
Similar to mandarins and satsumas, tangerines are easy to peel, which makes them popular with children.

GRAPEFRUITS
A "breakfast" fruit, grapefruits can be yellow or ruby red. The latter have a higher content of the carotene pigment lycopene. The bitter taste of grapefruits comes from the substance naringin.

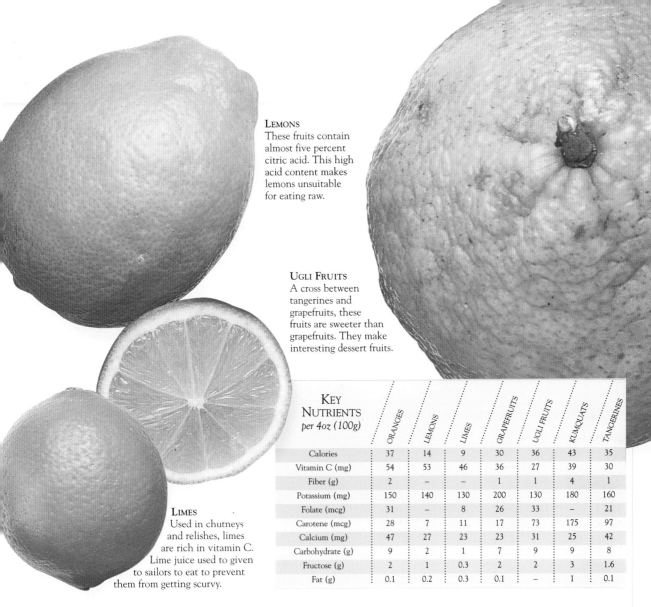

LEMONS
These fruits contain almost five percent citric acid. This high acid content makes lemons unsuitable for eating raw.

UGLI FRUITS
A cross between tangerines and grapefruits, these fruits are sweeter than grapefruits. They make interesting dessert fruits.

LIMES
Used in chutneys and relishes, limes are rich in vitamin C. Lime juice used to given to sailors to eat to prevent them from getting scurvy.

KEY NUTRIENTS per 4oz (100g)	ORANGES	LEMONS	LIMES	GRAPEFRUITS	UGLI FRUITS	KUMQUATS	TANGERINES
Calories	37	14	9	30	36	43	35
Vitamin C (mg)	54	53	46	36	27	39	30
Fiber (g)	2	–	–	1	1	4	1
Potassium (mg)	150	140	130	200	130	180	160
Folate (mcg)	31	–	8	26	33	–	21
Carotene (mcg)	28	7	11	17	73	175	97
Calcium (mg)	47	27	23	23	31	25	42
Carbohydrate (g)	9	2	1	7	9	9	8
Fructose (g)	2	1	0.3	2	2	3	1.6
Fat (g)	0.1	0.2	0.3	0.1	–	1	0.1

HEALING PROPERTIES

☑ TRADITIONAL USES
Grapefruits are used in Chinese medicine to help digestion and stop belching. They are also prescribed to help overcome the effects of drinking too much alcohol. The juice and pulp are used to make a tea that is given to people with a fever. The skin is thought to regulate the spleen and pancreas and thus help to relieve a buildup of gas in the digestive system. In the East, extract of grapefruit seeds is said to be a strong natural antibiotic. Lemons and limes are often used to treat dysentery, colds, influenza, and coughs, and infestations of parasites. They are prescribed to encourage bile formation, to cleanse and improve blood circulation, and to calm the nerves.

❖ SPECIFIC BENEFITS
Stomach Cancer
Studies have revealed that those who regularly eat citrus fruits have up to 60 percent less risk of developing stomach cancer than people who do not. It is likely that the vitamin C in the fruits blocks the formation of cancer causing substances in the stomach. It may also help to prevent gastritis (an irritation of the stomach lining), which may lead to cancers forming in the cells of the stomach lining.

Cancer of the Colon
The fiber in the pith of citrus fruits is insoluble. It therefore helps to increase stool weight and the speed at which stools are passed. This may reduce the risk of colonic cancer.

Cataracts
The lens of the human eye naturally contains a high level of vitamin C. It has been shown that people who consume less than 125mg of vitamin C a day have a fourfold increase in the risk of developing cataracts compared with those who consume more than 500mg a day. It seems likely therefore that the inclusion of citrus fruits in the diet could help to boost lens protection.

Anemia
Vitamin C helps the body to absorb iron in the diet. It is particularly important for vegetarians to consume plenty of vitamin C rich foods, such as citrus fruits, to decrease the risk of iron deficiency, which can lead to anemia.

OTHER FORM
Marmalade
Probably invented in France in 1692 by a nobleman's chef, this fruit spread is made like jam. Oranges are used, and also limes, grapefruits, and lemons. Marmalade contains the fruits' skins, and therefore has more phytonutrients than if just the flesh were used.

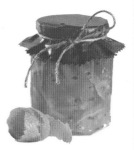

ORANGE MARMALADE

SEE ALSO ANEMIA, PAGE 160; CANCER, PAGE 214; CATARACTS, PAGE 202

ORANGES

 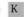

Believed to have evolved in China and Southeast Asia, oranges have long been used in traditional Chinese medicine. They are now grown widely around the world and are the most popular citrus fruits. Sweet oranges include the valencia, red-fleshed blood oranges, and the navel orange. Seville oranges are too bitter to eat raw, but are used for making marmalade.

KEY BENEFITS

- MAY HELP TO FIGHT HEART DISEASE
- HELP MAINTAIN VITAMIN C LEVELS IN SMOKERS
- FIGHT THE COMMON COLD
- MAY PROTECT AGAINST CANCERS

FOOD PROFILE

KEY NUTRIENTS
per ¹/₂ orange (100g)

Calories	37
Vitamin C (mg)	54
Fiber (g)	2
Folate (mcg)	31
Potassium (mg)	150
Carbohydrate (g)	9
Fructose (g)	2
Fat (mg)	0.1
Carotenes (mcg)	28
Calcium (mg)	47

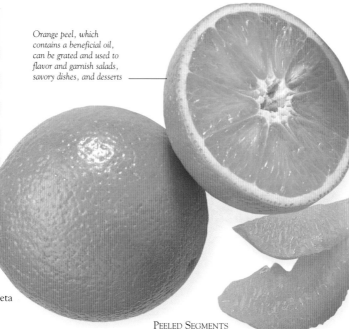

Orange peel, which contains a beneficial oil, can be grated and used to flavor and garnish salads, savory dishes, and desserts

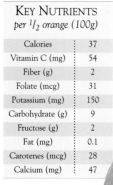

PEELED SEGMENTS

PROTECTIVE PROPERTIES
As well as having a high vitamin C content, oranges supply a range of protective, antioxidant phytonutrients including alpha and beta carotene, beta cryptoxanthin, and lutein.

★ HOW MUCH TO EAT
- An average-sized 6oz orange supplies 15 percent of an adult's recommended daily folate intake, and 90 percent of the daily recommended intake of vitamin C.

CHOOSING & STORING
- Choose thin-skinned oranges that are heavy for their size.
- Avoid fruits with soft areas, which indicate decay.
- Reject fruits with shriveled skin, which suggests aging.

COOKING & EATING
- Peel and eat the segments, or cut an orange into quarters.
- Add to fruit and green salads.
- Serve with duck, veal, chicken, and ham dishes.
- Use in milk shakes, sorbets, fruit salads, and to fill pancakes.
- Use seville oranges to make homemade marmalade.

HEALING PROPERTIES

☑ TRADITIONAL USES
Oranges are used in Chinese medicine to stimulate the digestive system and treat constipation. They are thought to combat dysentery, indigestion, and excessive mucus buildup. Believed to "move stagnation," oranges are also used to make a cooling expectorant for coughs. They are given for stress and sleeplessness, and to calm nerves. Oranges have long been recognized for their ability to fight scurvy and keep gums strong.

✠ SPECIFIC BENEFITS
Cholesterol Damage
Studies of populations around the world show that diets rich in vitamin C help to protect against heart disease. Vitamin C may work with vitamin E to prevent damage to LDL cholesterol (*see page 25*) by free radicals. Damaged LDL cholesterol can block arteries, leading to heart disease.

Vitamin C Deficiency
The official recommended daily intake of vitamin C is 60mg. Nutritionists that subscribe to the "Optimum Nutrition" school (*see page 13*) recommend intakes of 400mg for those aged between 25 and 50 and 800mg for those over 50. Oranges and orange juice can make useful contributions to these daily requirements of vitamin C.

Common Cold
Good intakes of vitamin C appear to help reduce the severity of cold symptoms and decrease their duration.

Cancer
Oranges and orange juice are rich in the phytonutrient hesperitin. In laboratory experiments, extracts of hesperitin were found to inhibit breast cancer cell growth and tumor formation. Hesperidin (a form of hesperitin) was found to help to prevent mouth cancers. The skins of oranges contain the phytonutrients nobiletin and tangeretin, which may stop invasion by cancerous cells. Orange juice is rich in phytonutrients called limonoids, which may also have anticancer properties.

Spina Bifida
Oranges contain folate, which, if taken with folic acid supplements, may help to prevent spina bifida in babies.

OTHER FORM

Orange Juice
This fruit juice can be canned, bottled, frozen, or freshly squeezed. A typical 1-cup glass of juice supplies almost 80mg of vitamin C and 40mg of folate. When counting daily fruit and vegetable intakes, a glass of orange juice counts as one "serving."

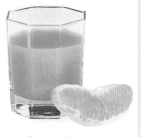

FRESHLY SQUEEZED ORANGE JUICE

SEE ALSO CANCER, PAGE 214; COLDS & INFLUENZA, PAGE 184; HEART DISEASE, PAGE 152; HIGH CHOLESTEROL, PAGE 154

PAPAYAS (PAW-PAWS)

The papaya plant probably originated in southern Mexico. It is a treelike herb that grows up to 32 feet high, and the fruits are now widely available. Papayas are particularly rich in vitamin C and are also a useful source of antioxidants and fiber. They have a low acidity and therefore lack the tartness of many fruits, making them palatable to young children.

KEY BENEFITS
- MAY HELP TO PREVENT CANCER
- MAINTAIN VITAMIN C LEVELS IN SMOKERS
- MAY HELP TO IMPROVE MALE FERTILITY
- REJUVENATE WHITE BLOOD CELLS IN THE ELDERLY

FOOD PROFILE

KEY NUTRIENTS
per 3/4 cup (100g)

Calories	36
Vitamin C (mg)	60
Carotenes (mcg)	810
Fiber (g)	2
Potassium (mg)	200
Sodium (mg)	5
Glucose (mg)	3
Fructose (mg)	3
Sucrose (mg)	3
Iron (mg)	1

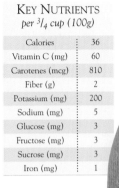

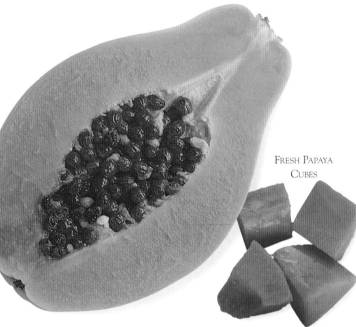

FRESH PAPAYA CUBES

MEAT TENDERIZER
The enzyme papain, which is known to break down protein, is contained in papaya fruits and leaves. In traditional Mexican cooking, the leaves are wrapped around meat to tenderize it and make it more digestible.

★ **HOW MUCH TO EAT**
- 1 cup of papaya provides 140 percent of the daily adult requirement of vitamin C.

CHOOSING & STORING
- Select sweet-smelling fruits with firm, even, yellow skins.
- Keep unripe fruits at room temperature until soft to the touch, which indicates ripeness.
- Store ripe fruits for up to two weeks in the refrigerator.

COOKING & EATING
- Cut in half lengthwise, scoop out the seeds, sprinkle with lime juice, and remove the flesh from the skin.
- Peel, seed, slice, and use in fruit salads, sorbets, and ice cream; or serve with chicken, pork, or scallops.
- Crush the seeds and use them in salad dressings.

HEALING PROPERTIES

🌿 TRADITIONAL USES
In Chinese medicine, papayas have traditionally been given to those who find it difficult to digest protein rich foods. They are also thought to help clean the teeth by breaking down trapped deposits. The fruits can be used to treat intestinal worms; they can be pickled in cider vinegar and eaten with the pickling liquid; alternatively, the seeds can be soaked in water to make a tea. Ripe papayas are often given to relieve dysentery, rheumatism, and the over-production of mucus.

✴ SPECIFIC BENEFITS
Cancer
The World Cancer Research Fund's report of 1997 on diet and cancer revealed that regular dietary intakes of vitamin C and carotenoids probably protect against lung cancer and possibly against cervical, colonic, pancreatic, breast, and bladder cancers. They can reduce the activity of potentially harmful free radicals, which could spark or promote cancerous changes within various cells and organs of the body. The papaya is a rich source of vitamin C and also contains a range of carotenes.

Vitamin C Deficiency
Cigarettes contain an abundance of oxidants, which stretch the antioxidant defense systems of the body. Smoking therefore speeds up the rate at which the body uses up vitamin C. Smokers need 120mg of vitamin C a day to achieve the same levels of the vitamin in the blood as nonsmokers. One papaya provides virtually all of this requirement. Optimum Nutritionists (see page 13) suggest taking upwards of 400mg of vitamin C per day.

Male Infertility
Vitamin C is essential for the proper formation of semen and sperm. Damage to genetic material has been shown to increase dramatically in men who have a low intake of vitamin C. This damage is repaired within a month of increasing their intake of this important nutrient. Tests have shown that men who are infertile due to sperm clumping can reduce the problem by increasing their intakes of vitamin C to 500mg a day. Sperm quality, quantity, mobility, and lifespan will also improve with increased daily intakes of vitamin C.

Aging
Vitamin C may lessen the risk of cataracts, strengthen capillaries, and reduce the risk of heart disease. Some researchers believe that it may help to delay aging by rejuvenating the white blood cells. Papaya is an ideal food for the elderly because it is palatable and easy to digest.

CAUTION
Do not use papaya in jellies or any recipes that need to set, because the papain enzyme will destroy the protein cross links in gelatin and eggs, preventing them from setting.

SEE ALSO CANCER, PAGE 214; INFERTILITY IN MEN, PAGE 227; THE ELDERLY & NUTRITION, PAGE 144

BANANAS

One of the oldest cultivated plants in the world, the banana is thought to have evolved from a wild species. Actually a treelike plant, the banana can reach up to 6–29 feet in height. A good source of fiber, potassium, and magnesium, bananas are mentioned in ancient writings as far back as 600 BC, which highlights the importance of this fruit over the centuries.

KEY BENEFITS

- CONVENIENT LOW-FAT ENERGY SOURCE
- HELP TO MAINTAIN BLOOD SUGAR LEVELS
- MAY IMPROVE MENTAL CONFUSION
- PLAY A ROLE IN REDUCING BLOOD PRESSURE
- PROTECT AGAINST HEART DISEASE

FOOD PROFILE

KEY NUTRIENTS
per 1 banana (100g)

Calories	95
Carbohydrate (g)	23
Fiber (g)	1
Potassium (mg)	400
Vitamin C (mg)	11
Magnesium (mg)	34
Copper (mg)	0.1
Folate (mcg)	14
Vitamin B$_6$ (mg)	0.3
Fat (g)	0.3

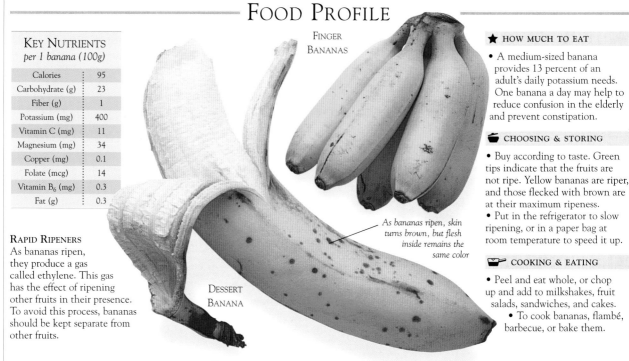

FINGER BANANAS

As bananas ripen, skin turns brown, but flesh inside remains the same color

DESSERT BANANA

RAPID RIPENERS
As bananas ripen, they produce a gas called ethylene. This gas has the effect of ripening other fruits in their presence. To avoid this process, bananas should be kept separate from other fruits.

★ **HOW MUCH TO EAT**
- A medium-sized banana provides 13 percent of an adult's daily potassium needs. One banana a day may help to reduce confusion in the elderly and prevent constipation.

📖 **CHOOSING & STORING**
- Buy according to taste. Green tips indicate that the fruits are not ripe. Yellow bananas are riper, and those flecked with brown are at their maximum ripeness.
- Put in the refrigerator to slow ripening, or in a paper bag at room temperature to speed it up.

🍴 **COOKING & EATING**
- Peel and eat whole, or chop up and add to milkshakes, fruit salads, sandwiches, and cakes.
- To cook bananas, flambé, barbecue, or bake them.

HEALING PROPERTIES

📗 **TRADITIONAL USES**
In traditional Chinese medicine, bananas are used to lubricate the intestines and lungs and to treat constipation and ulcers. Bananas are recommended for dry coughs in the form of a thick soup. Underripe bananas are said to have astringent properties, and are recommended steamed to treat diarrhea.

🔳 **SPECIFIC BENEFITS**
Quick-energy Boost
A very ripe banana that is speckled with many black patches and spots contains about 23g of sugar and 2g of starch. The sugars are rapidly digested and absorbed across the intestinal wall and into the bloodstream. This makes bananas a perfect snack following exercise, when a

rapid sugar burst is required within an hour of the activity to give the muscles the best chance of refueling and replenishing their stores of carbohydrate (glycogen). Due to this rapid absorption of sugar, ripe bananas have a high glycemic index, or GI (*see page 18*). Ripe bananas, are not, however, recommended for people with diabetes, or for dieters. Bananas that are mostly yellow have a medium glycemic index.

Diabetes
Underripe bananas can be useful for those who need to maintain steady blood sugar levels, such as people with diabetes. A banana that is mainly green with small areas of yellow skin contains 2g of

sugar and 23g of starch. The starch is known as a "resistant starch" because it is not well-digested in the small intestine. It passes on to the colon, where it is metabolized then absorbed into the bloodstream and used as energy. This slow breakdown of the carbohydrate in underripe bananas results in gently raised blood sugar levels.

Confusion in the Elderly
A lack of potassium can result in depression and confusion. Elderly people are particularly vulnerable, since they tend to eat few fresh fruits and vegetables. Ripe bananas, which are high in potassium, are easy to chew and digest. One ripe banana supplies about 13 percent of the daily requirement of potassium.

High Blood Pressure
Bananas are low in salt and high in potassium, which means that they are an ideal food source for people with high blood pressure. The potassium present in bananas appears to help lower blood pressure in several ways. It seems to encourage the body to excrete salt, and also appears to dilate the blood vessels, increasing their width and reducing the pressure of the blood flow.

Heart Disease
The potassium in bananas may be able to protect the heart, not only by reducing blood pressure, but also by inhibiting the activity of potentially harmful free radicals and by preventing the formation of blood clots.

SEE ALSO DIABETES, PAGE 218; HEART DISEASE, PAGE 152; HIGH BLOOD PRESSURE, PAGE 155

MANGOES

STAR NUTRIENTS & PHYTONUTRIENTS

   C E K Beta carotene, Fiber

One of the earliest known tropical fruits, the mango originated in the foothills of the Himalayas in India and Burma. Cultivated for more than 4,000 years, it is now grown in both tropical and subtropical areas of the world. Increasingly popular in the West, mangoes are highly nutritious, supplying good amounts of vitamin C, carotenes, fiber, and easily digested carbohydrate.

KEY BENEFITS

- MAY HELP TO CONTROL BLOOD PRESSURE
- MAY HELP TO PREVENT ANEMIA
- COULD PLAY A ROLE IN PREVENTING CERVICAL CANCER
- MAY STRENGTHEN THE IMMUNE SYSTEM

FOOD PROFILE

KEY NUTRIENTS
per ³/₄ cup (100g)

Calories	57
Potassium (mg)	180
Vitamin C (mg)	37
Beta carotene (mcg)	2,000
Vitamin E (mg)	1
Fiber (mg)	3
Soluble fiber (g)	0.5
Insoluble fiber (g)	1.6
Iron (mg)	1
Vitamin B₃ (mg)	1

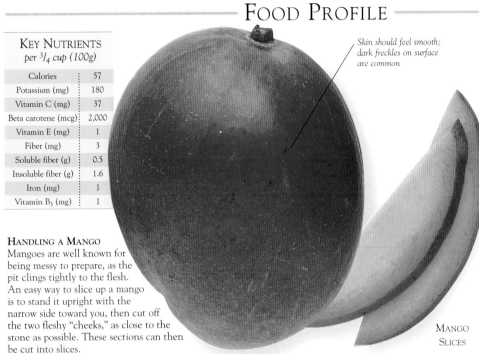

Skin should feel smooth; dark freckles on surface are common

MANGO SLICES

HANDLING A MANGO
Mangoes are well known for being messy to prepare, as the pit clings tightly to the flesh. An easy way to slice up a mango is to stand it upright with the narrow side toward you, then cut off the two fleshy "cheeks," as close to the stone as possible. These sections can then be cut into slices.

★ HOW MUCH TO EAT
- A whole mango, weighing about 1¼lbs, supplies 11 percent of an adult's daily potassium requirements. Eaten on a regular basis, mangoes may help to reduce blood pressure.

🥣 CHOOSING & STORING
- Look for a smooth skin with areas of deep green, yellow, and red. The skin should yield slightly when pressed.
- Underripe green mangoes ripen at room temperature in a few days. Ripe fruits stay fresh for two weeks in the refrigerator.

🍲 COOKING & EATING
- Peel off the skin and eat like a banana. Alternatively, slice mangoes and sprinkle with lime juice. Use in fish dishes, milk shakes, sorbets, and ice creams.

HEALING PROPERTIES

✒ TRADITIONAL USES
According to Chinese medicine, mangoes are said to "dry up" conditions such as excessive sweating and diarrhea. They are also said to counteract the effects of rich, oily foods, by helping to break down fats and protein. Chinese doctors believe that mangoes help to join the heart and mind and settle disjointed thoughts.

❖ SPECIFIC BENEFITS
High Blood Pressure
Mangoes are a good source of potassium, which is a key mineral for people with high blood pressure. Following scientific studies, it has been calculated that intakes of 2,300–3,100mg of potassium a day could lower blood pressure; it is estimated that this could lead to a 25 percent reduction in deaths related to high blood pressure (hypertension).

Anemia
The risk of anemia in vegetarians is high, particularly in women in the West, who often have depleted iron reserves. It is essential that plant sources of iron are consumed with nutrients that enhance iron absorption. Vitamin C and beta carotene, both present in mangoes, do just that. While vitamin C's ability to improve iron absorption is well known, recent research has revealed that beta carotene has a similar function. Beta carotene is thought to work by forming a complex substance with iron that keeps the iron soluble in the intestines and makes it difficult for plant chemicals such as phytates to block its absorption.

Cervical Cancer
Mangoes contain the antioxidant known as beta cryptoxanthin. A study of more than 15,000 women over 15 years has shown that high levels of beta cryptoxanthin in the blood were associated with a significant reduction in the risk of cervical cancer. Women may wish to improve their dietary intake of beta cryptoxanthin from sources such as mangoes to protect against this type of cancer.

Infections and Tumors
A diet high in foods that are rich in beta carotene may help to strengthen the immune system, especially in the elderly. Research has shown that certain types of immune cell become more active when beta carotene supplements are taken. Mangoes, which are rich in this antioxidant pigment, may help to improve the activity of these natural "killer" cells against viruses and tumors. Eaten regularly, mangoes may help to reduce the risk of both viral infections and tumor growth.

CAUTION
Mango skin contains a substance to which some people are highly allergic. Contact with the skin can cause an almost instant rash. People who are affected can still eat the sweet flesh.

SEE ALSO ANEMIA, PAGE 160; CANCER, PAGE 214; HIGH BLOOD PRESSURE, PAGE 155

CEREALS & GRAINS

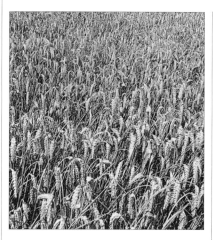

CEREALS ARE MEMBERS OF the grass family. The grain, or kernel, is found at the top of the stem and is the fruit of the plant. It consists of an outer husk (bran), a starchy inner part (endosperm), and a nutritious seed (germ). Cereal foods provide about 30 percent of the total calories eaten in the West, but this figure rises dramatically in parts of rural Asia and Africa, where cereals supply between as much as 70 and 80 percent of calorific requirements.

STAPLE CEREALS

Various cereals are the staple foods in different countries around the world. Wheat makes the most significant contribution to diets in many European countries, while rice is the most important grain consumed in the Far East, and corn is the main staple cereal of Africa and Central America. These global differences are due mostly to the climatic conditions that determine which cereal thrives in a particular region. Wheat, barley, and oats grow best in temperate zones, whereas rice, corn, and millet thrive in tropical and subtropical regions.

NUTRITIONAL PROFILES

Grains are major suppliers of carbohydrates, mostly in the form of starch, in the human diet. They also provide both soluble and insoluble fiber, and make large contributions of protein. The protein content of cereals varies between grains, with oats and wheat providing 11g and 13g per 3oz (100g), and rice and millet supplying about 6g each per 3oz (100g). Grains naturally provide a range of minerals, such as calcium, iron, and zinc, although the presence of certain fibrous compounds, known as phytates, can reduce the body's ability to absorb the minerals. Grains contain many B group vitamins, and the germ supplies vitamin E.

FORTIFICATION OF CEREALS

The milling of a cereal grain involves the removal of the bran. A cereal that is finely milled is stripped down to the endosperm. Less refined cereals contain some of the outer layers of the grain, while 100 percent whole-grain cereals leave the germ and outer layers. As these layers are stripped away, so too are vitamins, minerals, fiber, and phytonutrients. In some countries, the calcium, iron, and vitamins B_1 and B_3 (niacin) lost through milling wheat to produce white flour are, by law, put back into bread flour. Wholewheat bread provides more folate and vitamin E than white bread, and twice as much fiber.

HOW MUCH TO EAT?

It is recommended that about a third of food intake should be in the form of bread, other cereals, and potatoes. This means that some grains should be included in most meals, preferably prepared and served with as little fat as possible. The guidelines for healthy eating suggest between six and 14 servings a day. Two tablespoons of boiled rice, one slice of bread or toast, and three tablespoons of breakfast cereal each count as one serving. Grains have only been cultivated for the last 10,000 years, and some scientists believe that humans are not yet fully able to tolerate them. Health problems, such as an allergic reaction to gluten, may occur as a result of excessive grain consumption.

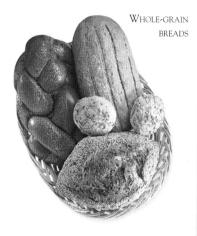

WHOLE-GRAIN BREADS

WHOLE-GRAIN FOODS

Whole foods, such as whole grains, nuts, lentils, beans, seeds, fresh fruits, and vegetables, are excellent sources of carbohydrates, which break down into essential blood sugars. Whole grains are generally more nutritious than refined versions. When increasing consumption of high-fiber, whole-grain cereals, it is important to ensure good fluid intakes. Increasing fiber in the diet should be accompanied by six to eight glasses of fluid a day to prevent hard, dry stools.

CEREALS & DISEASE

Cereals provide the body with a powerful mixture of protective substances, including fiber, antioxidant vitamins and minerals, and phytonutrients. It is considered likely that these are involved in the prevention of some cancers and heart disease. Wheat gluten is, however, one of the most common food allergens. Gluten can irritate the walls of the small intestine, and should be avoided by those who are sensitive to this protein. Foods that may contain gluten include cookies, breads, cereals, cakes, pastries, and pasta. Rye, buckwheat, quinoa, and corn can be used as gluten-free alternatives in some dishes.

CANCER & HEART DISEASE

The European Cancer Prevention Group believes that the consumption of a diet rich in high-fiber cereals is associated with a reduced risk of cancer of the colon and rectum. This protection is likely to come from the ability of the insoluble fiber in wholegrains to increase the weight of the stools, and speed their passage through the colon. In addition, bulky, loose stools help to dilute the colon contents, including potential carcinogens, making them less of a threat to the surrounding colon wall. Evidence also suggests that a high-fiber cereal diet may protect against the risk of breast cancer. Swiftly moving, bulky stools allow less time for the absorption of estrogens in the colon, and so reduce the body's overall estrogen pool. Reduced circulation of estrogen is thought to reduce the risk of breast cells dividing abnormally to produce tumors. Whole-grain wheat products also supply lignans, and rye, oats, and wheat supply acid lactones. Both are plant estrogens. These appear to latch onto estrogen receptors in breast tissue (as well as receptors in the ovaries and endometrium, and in the prostate gland in men), thereby blocking human estrogen and reducing its potential to make these cells divide abnormally. The lignans in whole-grain cereals also have antioxidant and anti-inflammatory properties that appear, along with vitamin E, to protect against heart disease. Soluble fibers, found in oats particularly, are capable of reducing low-density lipoprotein (LDL) cholesterol (*see page 25*), which may help to reduce the risk of blocked arteries. The bulking up of the stools can help to reduce the risk of constipation, which is thought to reduce the risk of a variety of other problems, such as varicose veins, heartburn, and irritable bowel syndrome.

MAIN CEREAL GROUPS

There are a number of categories of cereals and grains, and many uses for these versatile foods. Below are some examples of each.

• **WHEAT** is the most popular cereal, but in some regions wheats are low in selenium, which may have caused a reduction in intakes of this mineral.

• **RICE** is the second most important cereal in the human diet. Polished white rice loses both vitamin B and fiber.

• **MAIZE** is popular as the vegetable corn, which is harvested early before the grain has matured.

• **RYE** is a popular grain used in the production of crispbreads and rye breads.

• **BARLEY** is grown mainly for the production of malt for brewing beer or fermenting whiskey. Much of the world's production is used for animal feed.

• **OATS** contain a soluble fiber known to help reduce cholesterol levels. They are mainly used in the human diet as rolled oats for making cooked cereal.

• **MILLET** is ground into flour to make unleavened bread or cooked cereal, and may also be toasted prior to cooking.

• **SORGHUM** can be fermented to make beer, but is mostly ground into flour and used for cooked cereal, chapatis, and tortillas.

• **QUINOA** is used in breakfast cereals, cookies, and other foods, and is a good alternative to grain containing gluten, such as wheat, oats, rye, and barley. Quinoa provides calcium and iron.

• **BUCKWHEAT** flour is made from buckwheat and is suitable for pancakes, cookies, pasta, and breads.

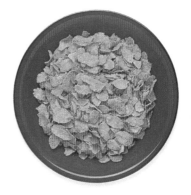

BREAKFAST CEREALS

Most processed cereals contain fast-releasing sugars and have added sugar. Oats, sugar-free cornflakes, or millet flakes are a healthier alternative to most standard cereals. Some cereals contain added vitamins and minerals.

RICE

 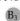

Originating in Asia, rice was the staple food of China by 2800 BC, and soon after assumed a similar role in India. Its nutritional value depends on the extent of the milling process. When just the husk is removed, the bran remains attached to the grain. This is brown rice, which is high in fiber. White rice is produced by milling to remove the pericarp, testa, and germ.

> ### KEY BENEFITS
> - PROVIDES ENERGY FAST
> - MAY HELP REDUCE THE RISK OF COLON CANCER
> - HELPS TO MAINTAIN THE NERVOUS SYSTEM
> - MAY REDUCE BLOOD PRESSURE AND CHOLESTEROL LEVELS

FOOD PROFILE

KEY NUTRIENTS per ½–⅓ cup (100g)	BROWN RICE (COOKED)	WHITE RICE (COOKED)
Calories	141	138
Protein (g)	3	3
Fat (g)	1	1
Carbohydrate (g)	32	31
Fiber (g)	1	0.1
Potassium (mg)	99	54
Magnesium (mg)	43	11
Phosphorus (mg)	120	54
Vitamin B₁ (mg)	0.14	–
Vitamin B₃ (mg)	1.3	1

NUTRITIONAL VALUE
Parboiling rice helps the B vitamins to migrate from the outer layers of the bran into the grains, where they are trapped. The value of parboiling rice was first recognized in Malaya, where Chinese immigrants, who ate raw rice, had the B vitamin deficiency beriberi, and Indians, who ate parboiled rice, did not.

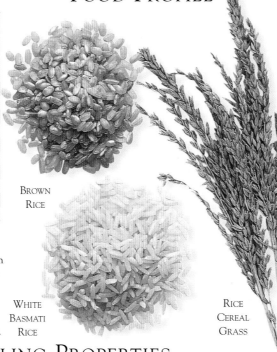

BROWN RICE

WHITE BASMATI RICE

RICE CEREAL GRASS

★ HOW MUCH TO EAT
- 1⅔ cup of cooked brown rice provides 11 percent of an adult's daily fiber requirement.

🍲 CHOOSING & STORING
- Rice should be bought from a reputable outlet. Many forms of rice are now available, including instant, canned, and raw rice.
- Store rice in a cool, dry place in a sealed container, away from pests, until required.

🍚 COOKING & EATING
- Rice can be boiled, steamed, oven-cooked, or fried.
- Brown rice requires a longer cooking time than white rice because the water and heat have to penetrate the layers of bran.
- The uses for rice in cooking are numerous. Common dishes include risotto, paella, kedgeree, and rice pudding.

HEALING PROPERTIES

✍ TRADITIONAL USES
In Chinese medicine, rice is used to treat problems of the nervous system, such as depression. It is also given to soothe the stomach and is recommended for diarrhea. Basmati rice is considered particularly light and easy to digest. Sprouted rice is used in Chinese medicine to improve appetite and poor digestion.

✳ SPECIFIC BENEFITS
Energy Deficiency
The body can digest and absorb the carbohydrate in rice relatively quickly. Rice is therefore a useful food to eat in order to refuel the muscles with energy after physical activity. Brown rice also supplies magnesium, which is required for muscle tone and protein synthesis.

Cancer of the Colon
Brown rice may decrease the risk of colonic cancer. This is partly because the rice bran helps to bulk up the stools and speed up the muscular contractions of the intestinal wall. Carcinogens in the stools have less time to stick to the colon wall, where they can trigger cancerous changes.

Nervous and Metabolic Health
The B vitamins found in brown rice are able to help keep the nervous system in good condition and to aid the conversion of blood sugar into cellular energy.

High Blood Pressure
Brown rice provides a particularly good supply of potassium, which is needed for maintaining water balance and keeping blood pressure down. It contains virtually no sodium, which has the opposite effect. People with high blood pressure can include rice (without salt) in their diets.

High Cholesterol
Oil made from the bran of rice contains a number of substances that together are described as "oryzanol." Oryzanol reduces cholesterol absorption and synthesis.

Celiac Disease
Rice does not contain the protein gluten. For this reason, it is acceptable in a gluten-free diet for those with celiac disease. Rice rarely causes allergic reactions and is often used as a staple food in diagnostic elimination diets.

OTHER FORM
Rice Cakes
Puffed rice is used to make rice cakes, which are a useful low-fat, high-carbohydrate snack for those on weight-loss diets. Rice cakes can be used in place of breads for people who are allergic to wheat. They are available salted and unsalted.

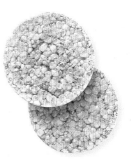

UNSALTED RICE CAKES

SEE ALSO ALLERGIES, PAGE 210; CANCER, PAGE 214; HIGH CHOLESTEROL, PAGE 154; HIGH BLOOD PRESSURE, PAGE 155

OATS

This cereal has been cultivated since 1000 BC, and is now an important crop in Europe. Oat grains can be rolled, flaked, or made into oatmeal or flour for porridge and bread. They contain more protein than other cereals, and are well-known for lowering cholesterol. Oat and oat bran are two of the least processed foods. They are additive and preservative free, and 100 percent natural.

> **KEY BENEFITS**
> - HELP TO LOWER BLOOD CHOLESTEROL
> - USEFUL IN WEIGHT-REDUCING DIETS BECAUSE THEY SATISFY APPETITE
> - SUITABLE FOR PEOPLE WITH DIABETES TO INCLUDE IN THEIR DIETS

FOOD PROFILE

KEY NUTRIENTS per 1 heaping cup (100g)	ROLLED OATS (COOKED IN WATER)	OATMEAL (RAW)
Calories	49	375
Protein (g)	2	11
Fat (g)	1	9
Carbohydrate (g)	9	66
Fiber (g)	1	7
Soluble fiber (g)	0.5	4
Insoluble fiber (g)	0.3	2
Iron (mg)	1	4
Zinc (mg)	0.4	3
Vitamin E (mg)	0.2	2

MILLED OATS
Oatmeal is finely milled oat grains. It contains vitamin E and fat. To stop the fat from turning rancid, oatmeal must be heat-treated. This prevents lipase enzymes from attacking the fatty acids, creating a bitter flavor.

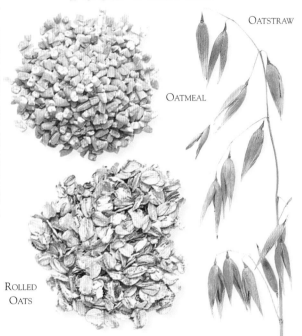

OATSTRAW

OATMEAL

ROLLED OATS

★ **HOW MUCH TO EAT**
- 1 cup of oatmeal supplies about 40 percent of an adult's daily iron requirements.

🥡 **CHOOSING & STORING**
- Oatmeal should have a creamy appearance flecked with brown.
- It must have a sweet, "nutty" aroma and, if tasted dry, should be free from any bitter flavor.

🍳 **COOKING & EATING**
- Oatmeal can be made into porridge with hot water or milk, or used in cakes, pies, fruit crumbles, and cookies.
- Instant oatmeal can be eaten mixed with cold milk.
- Oat bran, made from the coarse husks of the oat grain, can be added to stews and casseroles. Oat bran is one of the richest sources of soluble fiber.

HEALING PROPERTIES

📋 **TRADITIONAL USES**
Herbalists in the West use oatmeal externally for skin problems because it has a high silica content. The whole plant, oatstraw, is used to make tinctures and decoctions which are given to treat insomnia, anxiety, and depression. These tinctures and decoctions promote sweating, so they are useful additions to remedies for colds and chills. In the East and West, rolled oats are eaten for their antidepressant qualities. They contain saponins, alkaloids, and B vitamins, which help to lift mood. In the West, oat bran is used as a treatment for heart disease. Chinese medicine also recommends oat water as an internal antiseptic.

✳ **SPECIFIC BENEFITS**
High Cholesterol
Adding oats to the daily diet may help to reduce cholesterol. Eating $1/3$–$1/2$ cup of oatmeal daily, in combination with a low fat diet, can reduce high cholesterol levels by nine percent. It is estimated that every one percent reduction in cholesterol yields a two percent reduction in the risk of heart disease.

Weight Problems
The inclusion in the diet of high-fiber, high-carbohydrate cereals such as oats assists in weight loss and maintenance because the cereals can displace fatty, high-calorie foods in the diet. Oats take a long time to eat, especially when raw in muesli, and this brings about the feeling of being full. They also slow the emptying of the stomach. Oats take a long time to digest, resulting in a steady release of sugar into the bloodstream and a decreased release of insulin. Insulin encourages the storage of excess sugar as fat. Foods that are rich in carbohydrates, such as oats, are also believed to stimulate those centers in the brain that trigger the message to stop eating.

Diabetes
People with diabetes should keep their blood sugar levels as close to normal as possible. Large intakes of some carbohydrates cause rapid increases in blood sugar. Oats are digested slowly, however, and provide a suitable carbohydrate in diabetic diets.

OTHER FORM

Oatmeal
This is made from finely ground oats, and is used to make porridge, bread, cookies, and oatcakes. The characteristic taste of oatmeal comes partly from the steam treatment applied to the oats before they are ground. Oatmeal provides useful amounts of iron and is best eaten with foods that are rich in vitamin C.

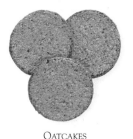

OATCAKES

SEE ALSO DIABETES, PAGE 218; HIGH CHOLESTEROL, PAGE 154; OBESITY, PAGE 178

CORN

STAR NUTRIENTS & PHYTONUTRIENTS

| K | P | Carbohydrate, Niacin, Fiber |

A lso known as sweetcorn, Indian corn, or maize, corn is native to the American continents, where people began to cultivate it by about 5000 BC. It was a particularly important food crop for the Incas, Aztecs, and Mayan peoples. Corn was introduced to Europe in the 1700s. It is a rich source of carbohydrates and supplies good amounts of vitamin B_1.

KEY BENEFITS

- MAY LOWER THE RISK OF SPINA BIFIDA IN BABIES
- CAN HELP TO PREVENT HEART DISEASE
- USEFUL IN WEIGHT-LOSS DIETS
- MAY REDUCE CANCER OF THE COLON

FOOD PROFILE

KEY NUTRIENTS per 2/3 cup (100g)	CORN KERNELS (CANNED)
Calories	122
Protein (g)	3
Fat (g)	1
Carbohydrate (g)	27
Fiber (g)	1
Potassium (mg)	220
Magnesium (mg)	23
Phosphorus (mg)	79
Vitamin B_3 (mg)	2
Folate (mg)	8

MAKING NIACIN AVAILABLE
The body is unable to absorb the B vitamin niacin from corn unless it is cooked in an alkaline solution, such as lime water. For populations that rely on corn as a staple food, this is essential because other sources of niacin are scarce.

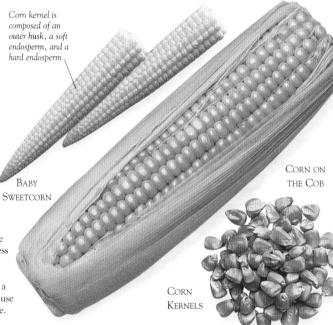

Corn kernel is composed of an outer husk, a soft endosperm, and a hard endosperm

BABY SWEETCORN

CORN ON THE COB

CORN KERNELS

★ HOW MUCH TO EAT

- A 1/3-cup serving of the cereal cornflakes with added folic acid and milk supplies 55 percent of the daily recommended amount of this essential B vitamin.
- Corn kernels and corn on the cob both contribute useful amounts of fiber.

CHOOSING & STORING

- Choose corn on the cobs with firm, juicy kernels and dark silks that are damp to the touch.
- Wrap in damp paper and store for one day in the refrigerator.

COOKING & EATING

- Remove silks from corn on the cobs. Boil, roast, or barbecue the cobs whole.
- Cornflakes are best eaten with fresh, cold milk.

HEALING PROPERTIES

✑ TRADITIONAL USES
In the East corn is believed to nourish the heart, regulate digestion, and also act as a diuretic. Corn silks can be infused to make a tea thought to be a diuretic and good for high blood pressure, water retention, gallstones, kidney stones, or urinary infections. Doctors in the East use a tea made from dried kernels in order to strengthen the kidneys. Blue corn, grown in the US, tones the kidneys.

✜ SPECIFIC BENEFITS
Spina Bifida
Cornflakes with added folic acid can supply more than 100mg of the B vitamin per 30g serving. Fortified foods and folic acid supplements may help lower the risk of spina bifida in unborn babies.

Heart Disease
Good daily intakes of folate and folic acid can lower the level of homocysteine in the blood. It is believed that a high level of this substance can damage artery walls by injuring the blood vessel lining and accelerating scar tissue buildup, leading to blood clots and heart disease.

Weight Problems
Research shows that the more fat people eat, the more likely they are to put on weight. It has also been found that those who eat the most fat eat the least amount of starchy and sugary foods, and those who eat more starch and sugar eat less fat. This is known as the sugar fat seesaw. Fat has twice the number of calories of sugar and starch, so people

trying to lose weight should eat more sugar and starch. Studies show that 2/3 cup of a cereal, such as cornflakes, eaten every day, with low-fat milk, can tip the seesaw.

Cancer of the Colon
Diets that are rich in starch may prevent cancer of the colon, or large intestine. Not all the starch from cereals, such as corn, is digested and therefore absorbed in the small intestine. Some reaches the colon where the bacteria naturally present use it to produce short-chain fatty acids (SCFAs). These SCFAs appear to increase the acidity in the colon, control cell division, and help to repair damaged DNA which might otherwise result in tumors.

OTHER FORM

Popcorn
When heated, some types of corn kernel pop open to reveal a light, puffy center. Corn can be popped in the microwave, or in a covered pan with some oil. Nutritional values vary depending on the cooking method, the type of oil used, and the flavorings that are added to the popped corn.

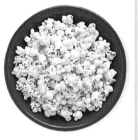

PLAIN POPCORN

SEE ALSO CANCER, PAGE 214; DIGESTIVE SYSTEM, PAGE 168; HEART DISEASE, PAGE 152; OBESITY, PAGE 178

WHEAT

STAR NUTRIENTS & PHYTONUTRIENTS

K Carbohydrate, Fiber, Phytosterols, Protein

Although its origins are the subject of some debate, it is likely that wheat was first cultivated from wild species in south-west Asia in about 8000 BC. It is now one of the world's most important plant foods. Of the two varieties of wheat, hard wheats, used in bread and pasta, have the most protein; soft wheats, used in cakes and biscuits, supply carbohydrate, vitamins, and minerals.

KEY BENEFITS

- MAY HELP TO PREVENT CANCER OF THE COLON
- MAY LOWER THE RISK OF BREAST CANCER
- MAY HELP TO PREVENT AND CURE THE BLOCKAGE OF ARTERIES, LOWERING THE RISK OF HEART DISEASE

FOOD PROFILE

KEY NUTRIENTS per 4oz (100g)	WHOLEMEAL WHEAT	WHEATGERM
Calories	310	302
Carbohydrate (g)	64	45
Protein (g)	13	27
Fat (g)	2	9
Fiber (g)	9	16
Selenium (mcg)	53	3
Iron (mg)	4	9
Calcium (mg)	38	55
Vitamin B_1 (mg)	0.5	2
Vitamin E (mg)	1.4	22

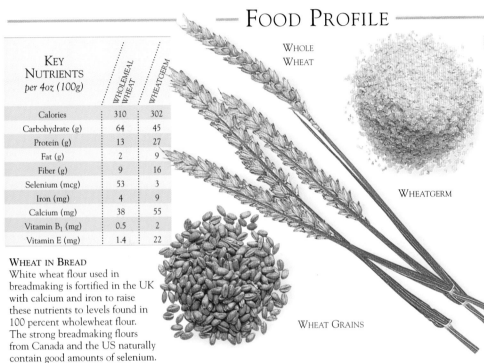

WHOLE WHEAT

WHEATGERM

WHEAT GRAINS

WHEAT IN BREAD
White wheat flour used in breadmaking is fortified in the UK with calcium and iron to raise these nutrients to levels found in 100 percent wholewheat flour. The strong breadmaking flours from Canada and the US naturally contain good amounts of selenium.

★ HOW MUCH TO EAT

- 1 cup of wholewheat flour supplies 50 percent of an adult's recommended daily intake of fiber.
- A heaping tablespoon of wheatgerm supplies an adult's daily vitamin E requirements.

🍲 CHOOSING & STORING

- Wheat is usually bought as pre-milled flour. Buy small quantities and use as soon as possible.
- Store flour in clean, airtight containers in a cool, dry place.

🍳 COOKING & EATING

- Flour is used to make bread, cakes, cookies, pastries, and pasta.
- Soaked cracked wheat grains can be added to bread dough.
- 100 percent wholewheat based breakfast cereals are best eaten with cold milk.

HEALING PROPERTIES

📋 TRADITIONAL USES

In the East, wheat is often recommended as a toner for the kidneys. It is also believed to nourish the mind, helping people to remain calm and focused, especially if they have insomnia, are irritable, or are going through menopause. Wheat is also used for treating palpitations. It is mildly astringent and is said to help cure bedwetting in children as well as diarrhea and sweating.

❖ SPECIFIC BENEFITS

Cancer of the Colon
Studies suggest that 100 percent wholewheat products in the diet protect against cancer of the colon. Wheat bran is rich in insoluble fiber, which remains intact and undigested until it reaches the colon. It bulks up the stools and increases the speed at which they pass through the colon. This gives carcinogens less time to latch on to the colon wall and set up cancerous changes. Wheat bran is "digested" by bacteria in the colon, producing short chain fatty acids (SCFAs).

Breast Cancer
One hundred percent wholewheat products may help to reduce the risk of breast cancer, partly due to the fact that they contain plant estrogens, substances that can mimic the hormone estrogen. Phytosterols latch onto estrogen receptors in breast tissue, blocking human estrogen, which may trigger breast cancer, thus lowering the risk of cancerous

changes in breast cells. Wholewheat products also have an ability to interfere with the internal cycling of estrogen. They increase the speed of the movement of stools through the intestine, which gives circulating estrogen less time to be reabsorbed into the blood across the colon wall.

Blocked Arteries
Inclusion of wheatgerm in the diet may improve the long-term intake of vitamin E and help to stop the oxidation of low-density lipoprotein (LDL) cholesterol (see page 25). Once oxidized, this type of cholesterol can narrow and block arteries, causing heart disease. High intakes of vitamin E may help to reverse blockage of arteries as well as

OTHER FORM

Pasta
Various kinds of pasta are made from wheat flour or semolina plus water, and occasionally eggs. They may be fresh or dried, wholemeal or white, depending on the flour used. Pasta is a good source of carbohydrate, B vitamins, and in the case of wholewheat pasta, insoluble fiber.

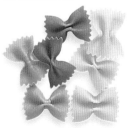

PASTA BOWS

SEE ALSO CANCER, PAGE 214; ; HIGH BLOOD CHOLESTEROL, PAGE 154; WOMEN'S HEALTH, PAGE 220

BREADS

The first "flat" breads appear to have been made in the Middle East about 9,000 years ago from crudely ground wheat and barley. The ancient Egyptians are believed to have found ways to make the raised, or leavened, breads that we eat today. Breads are a major energy source in many countries, and all types are highly nutritious, providing protein, iron, calcium, and B vitamins.

KEY BENEFITS

- SUPPLY EASILY ABSORBABLE ENERGY
- MAY HELP TO REDUCE THE RISK OF COLONIC CANCER
- MAY HELP TO REDUCE THE RISK OF OSTEOPOROSIS, ANEMIA, AND INFERTILITY

FOOD PROFILE

★ HOW MUCH TO EAT

- Two thick slices of wholewheat bread a day provide 12 percent of the 25g of fiber required daily by adults. Including bread in the diet on a regular basis may help to boost bone density and reduce the risk of osteoporosis.

🍚 CHOOSING & STORING

- Bread should be as fresh as possible when bought.
- Store in a bread bin or freeze and use as needed.

🍲 COOKING & EATING

- Eat fresh bread as the main starch component of a meal to accompany casseroles and other main courses.
- Eat toasted or untoasted, spread with a little butter and a sweet or savory topping or filling.
- Use to make bread-and-butter pudding, bread pudding, or breadcrumbs.

FOCACCIA
An increasingly popular, Mediterranean-style bread, focaccia is brushed with olive oil and sprinkled with salt. It is therefore slightly higher in calories than standard white bread.

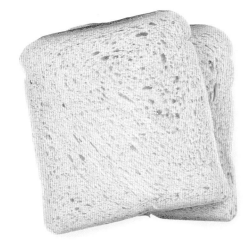

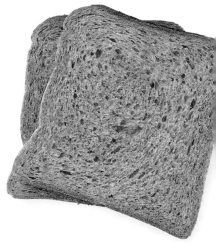

WHITE BREAD
White bread making flour is made from wheat grain that has had the fibrous husk, or endosperm, removed. In certain countries, including the US, many of the nutrients are lost during the milling process, and the calcium, iron, thiamin and niacin have to be replaced by law.

WHOLEWHEAT BREAD
Made from 100 percent wheat grain flour, wholewheat bread contains twice as much insoluble fiber as white bread, which helps to bulk up the stools. Inclusion of the germ means it also has extra vitamin E and twice the folate.

HEALING PROPERTIES

📑 TRADITIONAL USES
Bread has been a major source of sustenance in all its forms throughout history. At the end of the 1800s in the West, eating wholewheat bread was prescribed as a natural method of colonic irrigation.

✖ SPECIFIC BENEFITS
Energy Depletion
Bread contains little fat and is rich in carbohydrate, making it relatively low in calories compared to many baked

goods. White and wholemeal bread are rapidly digested and absorbed, which makes them ideal for people needing a burst of energy after exercise. The B vitamins in bread help the energy to be fully utilized by the body's cells.

Cancer of the Colon
The wheat bran present in wholewheat bread bulks up the stools and speeds their passage through the colon, thereby possibly helping to

remove some potentially carcinogenic substances before they can set up cancers in the colon. White bread supplies small amounts of fiber. All types of bread provide starch. Some starch is left undigested and is used in the colon by bacteria, which metabolize the starch to make short-chain fatty acids. These become an energy source for the body. Their presence helps to create a hostile environment for cancer forming substances.

Osteoporosis
White bread provides calcium which is well absorbed by the body because the calcium blocking phytates have been removed in the milling process. White bread is a good source of calcium for those who consume few dairy products, and also for children. A poor intake of calcium during the crucial phase of growth in childhood can increase the risk of osteoporisis in later life.

SEE ALSO ANEMIA, PAGE 160; CONSTIPATION, PAGE 175; HEART DISEASE, PAGE 152; INFERTILITY IN MEN, PAGE 227

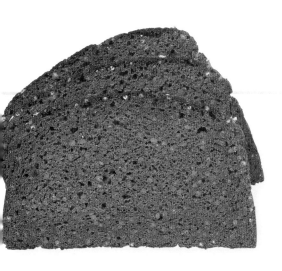

RYE BREAD

A staple in Germany and Russia, this bread is made from a high proportion of rye flour and supplies good amounts of thiamin and iron. Dark rye bread contains twice the fiber of the light version. Pumpernickel bread is made from dark rye flour, rye meal, and cracked rye grains.

SLICED BROWN BREAD

Bread that has the B vitamin folic acid added raises intakes of this essential B nutrient to approximately 100mcg per serving. All bread making flour in the US has added folic acid. In the UK and other countries in the West the addition of folic acid is voluntary.

NAAN BREAD

This traditional Indian bread is made with white flour and a little yeast, rolled into flat teardrop shapes, then baked in a hot tandoori oven. Naan is brushed with clarified butter prior to serving and can have as much as 79g of fat per portion.

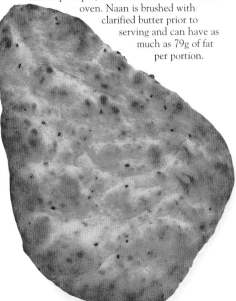

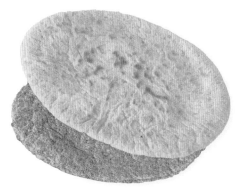

PITA BREAD

This flat bread is similar to breads made in ancient times. Pita bread provides useful amounts of iron and vitamins B_1 and niacin.

KEY NUTRIENTS per 4–5 slices (100g)	WHOLEWHEAT BREAD	BROWN BREAD	WHITE BREAD	PITA BREAD	RYE BREAD	NAAN BREAD	FOCACCIA
Calories	215	218	235	265	219	336	278
Protein (g)	9	9	8	9	8	9	7
Fat (g)	3	2	2	1	2	13	10
Carbohydrate (g)	42	44	49	58	46	50	40
Fiber (g)	6	4	2	2	4	2	2
Soluble fiber (g)	2	1	1	–	2	1	–
Insoluble fiber (g)	3	2	0.5	–	1.8	1	–
Calcium (mg)	54	100	110	91	80	160	–
Iron (mg)	3	2	2	2	3	1	–
Zinc (mg)	2	1	1	1	1	1	–

Anemia

The addition of iron to white bread makes it a useful source of this essential mineral, particularly for vegetarians, who risk low intakes of easily absorbable iron. The lack of phytates in white bread makes it easier for the body to absorb the iron across the intestinal wall and into the bloodstream, where it is used to make hemoglobin. Hemoglobin carries oxygen to all the cells in the body.

Infertility in Men

Selenium is a strong antioxidant that is able to fend off free radical attacks that could otherwise lead to heart disease. In addition, selenium is essential for male fertility. North American hard wheats are grown in selenium-rich soils, but bread made from soft European wheat, which is artificially strengthened with gluten, has led to decreased intakes of selenium in the UK.

Spine and Heart Problems

Wholewheat bread and breads that are fortified with folic acid contribute to the average daily intake of this important B vitamin. Good intakes of folic acid by pregnant women have been shown to help protect unborn babies from spina bifida. Folic acid encourages the complete fusion of the spinal cord within the first weeks of pregnancy. Folic acid also seems to lowers harmfully high levels of homocysteine, which is considered as much of a risk in the development of heart disease as high cholesterol and high blood pressure.

CAUTION

Wheat grains used in bread-making contain the protein gluten. People with celiac disease are intolerant to gluten, which interferes with digestion and absorption. The cause is still unknown.

SEE ALSO MINERALS, PAGE 30; OSTEOPOROSIS, PAGE 199; VITAMINS, PAGE 26

NUTS

There is evidence that nut trees were being grown as a source of human food as long ago as 10,000 BC, making them one of the earliest crops to have been cultivated. Approximately 25 kinds of nut are grown today as food crops around the world. They add a huge array of nutrients to people's diets, ranging from protein to iron, zinc, calcium, and potassium, and many trace elements.

KEY BENEFITS

- HELP TO BOOST THE IMMUNE SYSTEM
- LOWER CHOLESTEROL LEVELS
- MAY HELP TO REDUCE THE RISK OF HEART DISEASE AND OTHER DISEASES OF AGING
- HELP TO PREVENT OSTEOPOROSIS

FOOD PROFILE

★ HOW MUCH TO EAT

- Six fresh Brazil nuts provide 408 percent of a man's daily selenium requirement.
- A $^1/_2$-cup serving of cashew nuts provides 17 percent of an adult's daily iron requirement. Twenty fresh cashews provide 11 percent of a adult's daily zinc requirement.
- $^1/_2$ cup of almonds supply about 13 percent of a teenage girl's calcium requirement.

🥣 CHOOSING & STORING

- Always check the "use-by" date on nuts and avoid buying any nuts in their shell that seem light in weight for their size.
- Nuts in their shell should not rattle when shaken, as this indicates aging and dryness.
- Avoid buying nuts that smell musty or rancid.

🍳 COOKING & EATING

- Nuts make the perfect snack and can be eaten roasted or raw.
- Grate and chop nuts and use in savory and sweet dishes.

COCONUTS

Unlike other nuts, much of the fat of the coconut is saturated. Flaked coconut is prepared by shredding and drying the nut's endosperm. Coconut milk in the center of the nut contains vitamin C.

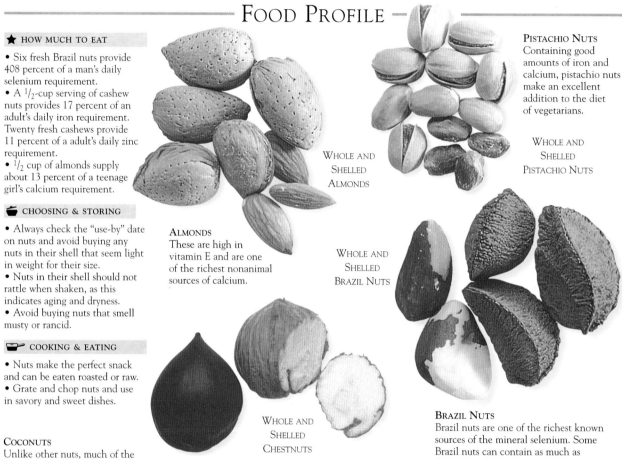

WHOLE AND SHELLED ALMONDS

ALMONDS
These are high in vitamin E and are one of the richest nonanimal sources of calcium.

PISTACHIO NUTS
Containing good amounts of iron and calcium, pistachio nuts make an excellent addition to the diet of vegetarians.

WHOLE AND SHELLED PISTACHIO NUTS

WHOLE AND SHELLED BRAZIL NUTS

WHOLE AND SHELLED CHESTNUTS

CHESTNUTS
A low-fat nut, more than 86 percent of a chestnut's calories come from carbohydrate. Chestnuts make an excellent low fat snack.

BRAZIL NUTS
Brazil nuts are one of the richest known sources of the mineral selenium. Some Brazil nuts can contain as much as 5,300mcg of selenium per 100g.

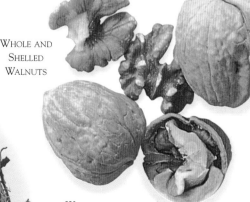

WHOLE AND SHELLED WALNUTS

WALNUTS
There are 15 different types of walnut. They contain a high level of linoleic acid, which is thought to give them cholesterol-lowering properties. (*See also page 102*)

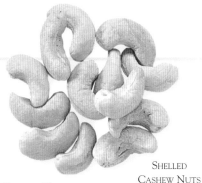

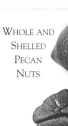

HAZELNUTS
The composition of the oil in hazelnuts is similar to olive oil. The very high levels of vitamin E help to protect hazelnuts from going rancid.

WHOLE AND
SHELLED
PECAN
NUTS

SHELLED
CASHEW NUTS

CASHEW NUTS
These nuts are particularly rich in potassium, phosphorus, and zinc, making them nutritious additions to main meals and snacks.

WHOLE AND
SHELLED
PEANUTS

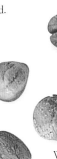

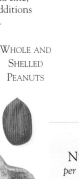

WHOLE AND
SHELLED
HAZELNUTS

PECANS
Bursting with zinc, pecan nuts are ideal for those needing to boost their immune systems and for men as part of preconceptual care.

PEANUTS
Also known as groundnuts, peanuts are part of the legume family. The unsaturated oleic and linoleic oils make up a high proportion of the fat in peanuts and supply good quantities of vitamin E.

KEY NUTRIENTS per 1 cup (100g)	CHESTNUTS	BRAZIL NUTS	ALMONDS	FRESH COCONUT	ROASTED PISTACHIO NUTS	PECANS	CASHEW NUTS	HAZELNUTS	PEANUTS	WALNUTS
Calories	170	682	612	351	601	689	573	650	564	688
Protein (g)	2	14	21	3	17	9	18	14	26	15
Fat (g)	3	68	56	36	55	70	48	64	46	69
Fiber (g)	4	4	7	7	6	5	3	7	6	4
Vitamin E (mg)	1	7	24	1	4	4	1	25	10	4
Calcium (mg)	46	170	240	1	110	61	32	140	60	94
Iron (mg)	1	3	3	2	3	2	6	3	3	3
Zinc (mg)	1	4	3	1	2	5	6	2	4	3
Selenium (mcg)	–	1,530	4	1	6	12	29	–	3	19
Folate (mcg)	–	21	48	26	58	39	67	72	110	66

HEALING PROPERTIES

OTHER FORM

✔ TRADITIONAL USES
In Chinese medicine, a drink made from ground almonds is given to alleviate coughs and asthma. In Indian Ayurvedic medicine, almonds are thought to build up a person's intellectual, spiritual, and reproductive abilities. Peanuts are used for lung conditions, and, raw and unsalted, are thought to help to stem bleeding. A drink made from the shells is given to those with high blood pressure. Walnuts are used in Chinese medicine to relieve inflammation and to help ease coughing and wheezing. They are thought to improve potency, enrich the sperm, and nourish the brain. The coconut is used to improve the nutrition of children and to calm a gaseous intestine.

✸ SPECIFIC BENEFITS
Impaired Immune System
Pecan nuts, peanuts, cashew nuts, and Brazil nuts are good sources of zinc. A lack of zinc is thought to impair immune system responses, especially those affecting the lymph system and the thymus gland.

High Cholesterol
Almonds have been shown to reduce total cholesterol. One study showed that after including almonds in the diet for three weeks, low-density lipoprotein (LDL) cholesterol (see page 25) had decreased by ten percent.

Heart Disease
Peanuts, walnuts, hazelnuts, and cashew nuts supply folate, which may reduce the risk of heart disease.

Infertility in Men
Male fertility has been found to be affected by a poor intake of the trace element selenium. Tests have revealed that low selenium levels can decrease the number of sperm that a man produces. Increasing selenium in the diet improves sperm counts and mobility. Brazil nuts are very rich in selenium and just three to four nuts a day could help to improve low selenium levels.

Low Bone Density
Almonds, hazelnuts, Brazil nuts, and pistachio nuts are useful sources of calcium, especially for people who do not eat dairy products. A low calcium intake during the teenage years can lead to osteoporosis in later life.

Peanut Butter
The Kellogg brothers marketed peanut butter in the US in the 1800, as a health food. Made from ground roasted peanuts, it is rich in oils and all the nutrients found in whole or ground nuts. A nutritious spread, peanut butter is a useful source of calcium and iron for vegetarians. Low-fat versions are available.

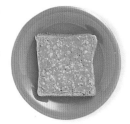

PEANUT BUTTER

SEE ALSO ANEMIA, PAGE 160; CANCER, PAGE 214; INFECTIONS, PAGE 212; INFERTILITY IN MEN, PAGE 227

WALNUTS

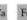 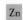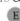
Grown in temperate climates, walnut trees belong to the *Juglandaceae* family of deciduous trees. There are 15 different species of edible walnut. Commercially, the common, or Persian, walnut, the black walnut, and the butternut walnut are the most important. First cultivated thousands of years ago in what is now Iran, most Persian walnuts are grown in California.

KEY BENEFITS

- HELP TO PREVENT HEART DISEASE
- MAY ALLEVIATE PREMENSTRUAL TENSION
- MAINTAIN A HEALTHY IMMUNE SYSTEM
- PREVENT THE SKIN FROM DEHYDRATING
- MAY HELP TO PREVENT ECZEMA

FOOD PROFILE

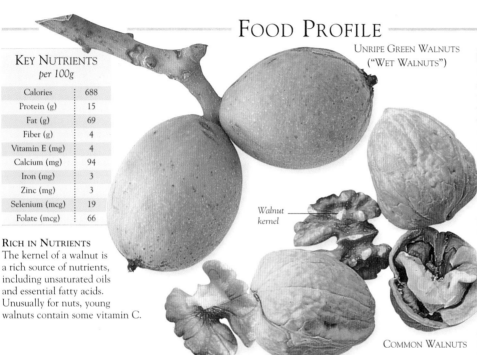

UNRIPE GREEN WALNUTS
("WET WALNUTS")

Walnut kernel

COMMON WALNUTS

KEY NUTRIENTS
per 100g

Calories	688
Protein (g)	15
Fat (g)	69
Fiber (g)	4
Vitamin E (mg)	4
Calcium (mg)	94
Iron (mg)	3
Zinc (mg)	3
Selenium (mcg)	19
Folate (mcg)	66

RICH IN NUTRIENTS
The kernel of a walnut is a rich source of nutrients, including unsaturated oils and essential fatty acids. Unusually for nuts, young walnuts contain some vitamin C.

★ **HOW MUCH TO EAT**

- Six whole walnuts, weighing about 2oz, provide almost 2mg of vitamin E. The estimated daily requirement of vitamin E is 30iu for adults.
- 1 cup of walnuts supply more than 1mg of copper, which is half an adult's daily requirement.

CHOOSING & STORING

- Buy walnuts in their shells, if possible, because they are usually fresher than shelled ones.
- Store in the refrigerator for up to six months.

COOKING & EATING

- Remove the shells with nutcrackers and eat the kernels raw.
- Add to meat dishes, salads, cakes, cookies, and stuffings.
- Use ground walnuts in pastries, cakes, and cookies.

HEALING PROPERTIES

✍ TRADITIONAL USES
Walnuts have been used extensively in Chinese medicine to treat impotency and to improve the quality of sperm. These nuts are also thought to be useful for reducing symptoms of inflammation in the back and knees. Herbalists in the West have traditionally used walnut leaf infusions to treat intestinal worms.

✴ SPECIFIC BENEFITS
High Cholesterol
It has been observed that in people who eat walnuts at least four times a week, deaths from heart attacks are half of those in people who do not eat walnuts regularly. Scientists have discovered that people who add walnuts to a cholesterol lowering diet can reduce their low-density lipoprotein (LDL) cholesterol (*see page 25*) by an extra 16.4 percent. This is probably due to the unsaturated fats in walnuts, especially linoleic acid. The latter is converted into gamma linoleic acid and then into hormonelike prostaglandins, which help to keep the blood thin, prevent clots and blockages, relax the blood vessels, and lower blood pressure.

Premenstrual Syndrome
A regular intake of the B vitamins is known to be crucial for maintaining a robust nervous system. Walnuts supply useful amounts of vitamin B_6, believed to be a useful substance for women who suffer regularly from premenstrual syndrome (PMS).

Infections
Walnuts, and nuts in general, are particularly good sources of copper, which is essential for keeping the immune system functioning correctly. Even small deficiencies of copper decrease the amount of the substance called interleukin, which is needed to help the immune system fight bacterial and viral infections. A reduction in dietary copper intake has been shown to adversely affect the immune system. A low intake of copper also affects the immune system's ability to clear away waste products in the blood.

Dehydration of the Skin
Eating walnuts regularly is a good way to help to improve the general smoothness and softness of the skin. Walnut oils contain linoleic acid, which helps to maintain the skin's structure, keeping it watertight and well hydrated. Vitamin E and zinc, also found in walnuts, are good for the skin, too.

Eczema
Allergic inflammatory diseases, such as the skin condition eczema, are common ailments, particularly in children. Two of the main types of cell that cause eczema are keratinocytes and peripheral blood lymphid cells. There is some evidence to suggest that the substances known as polyphenolic compounds, which are found in walnut kernels, help to prevent these cells being stimulated by allergic triggers in the environment.

SEE ALSO ECZEMA, PAGE 165; HIGH CHOLESTEROL, PAGE 154; MENSTRUAL PROBLEMS, PAGE 222

SESAME SEEDS

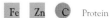
These small seeds were some of the first to be used as a source of oil in the human diet. The sesame plant was first cultivated in Africa, then introduced to India, and from there taken all over the world. The seeds are 20–25 percent protein and about 50 percent unsaturated oil. They have a perfect balance of potassium and sodium, and can help the body to maintain a good water balance.

KEY BENEFITS

- CAN HELP TO FIGHT FATIGUE AND ANEMIA
- PROVIDE VEGETARIANS WITH CALCIUM AND MAY HELP TO PREVENT OSTEOPOROSIS IN LATER LIFE
- MAY HELP TO BOOST MALE FERTILITY

FOOD PROFILE

KEY NUTRIENTS
per 8 tablespoons (100g)

Calories	598
Protein (g)	18
Fat (g)	58
Calcium (mg)	670
Iron (mg)	10
Zinc (mg)	5
Vitamin B$_3$ (mg)	5
Vitamin E (mg)	3
Folate (mg)	97

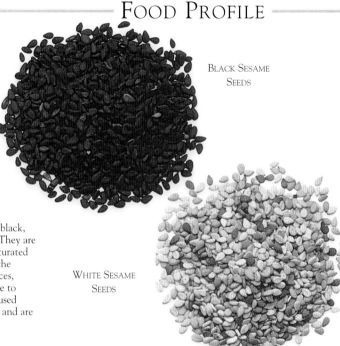

BLACK SESAME SEEDS

WHITE SESAME SEEDS

BLACK AND WHITE SEEDS
Sesame seeds can be white, black, brown, yellow, red, or gray. They are a rich source of highly unsaturated oils which, combined with the presence of oxidant substances, makes them extremely prone to rancidity. Sesame seeds are used whole or ground in cooking and are pressed to make sesame oil.

★ HOW MUCH TO EAT

- A tablespoon of sesame seeds supplies 9 percent of a woman's daily calcium needs.
- A 4 tbsp serving provides 12 percent of a woman's daily requirement of folate in the diet.

🗋 CHOOSING & STORING

- Always buy sesame seeds from a reputable shop that has a fast turnover of stock.
- Choose a recognized brand.
- Store in an airtight glass jar in a dry area out of direct sunlight, for up to a year.

🍲 COOKING & EATING

- Use ground seeds for cooking and baking and in tahini.
- Toast whole seeds under the grill or in a skillet, and use them to coat rissoles, meat, and fish.
- Sprinkle raw seeds over baked foods and cereals or add to salads.

HEALING PROPERTIES

🖉 TRADITIONAL USES
Black sesame seeds are used in Chinese medicine to lubricate the heart, liver, kidneys, pancreas, and lungs. They are given to treat constipation and joint stiffness. Paler sesame seeds are attributed with similar, but slightly weaker, healing properties.

▦ SPECIFIC BENEFITS
Fatigue
Iron is needed by the body to make the oxygen carrying pigment hemoglobin. A lack of hemoglobin causes tiredness, general lassitude, and eventually sub- or full-blown anemia. Consuming the daily requirement of iron can be difficult for those who do not eat animal products. Sesame seeds are a very good vegetable source of iron.

Osteoporosis
Sesame seeds contain a large amount of calcium, which gives bones their strength. It is not thought to be as readily absorbed as the calcium in dairy foods, but sesame seeds are still a useful source of calcium for vegetarians. Good intakes of this mineral are crucial during the teenage years, when it is being deposited in bones. If peak bone density is not achieved during this time, there is an increased risk of developing osteoporosis in later life.

Male Infertility
A regular daily intake of a mixture of seeds can help to keep zinc stores in the body topped up. Semen is very rich in zinc, and 8 tablespoons of sesame seeds will replenish

what is lost in ejaculation – about 5mg. Zinc plays an important role in maintaining sperm health. It helps to defend sperm against free radical attack, which can damage them, and protects their genetic material. A high concentration of zinc also helps to keep sperm activity low just before ejaculation. This lowers their oxygen consumption and conserves the energy that they need once in the female reproductive tract. Finally, zinc is needed for the correct timing of the "acrosome reaction." This occurs when a sperm attaches itself to an egg. Enzymes in the tip of the sperm are released, which enable it to penetrate the egg wall, allowing the sperm's genetic material to enter.

OTHER FORM

Tahini
Toasted, ground sesame seeds can be used to make tahini. This is added to chickpeas to make hummus. Tahini can be stirred into dips and sauces, spread on bread instead of peanut butter, and used in cakes and cookies. The nutty, slightly bitter flavor is an acquired taste.

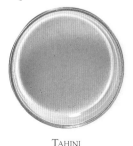

TAHINI

SEE ALSO FATIGUE, PAGE 235; INFERTILITY IN MEN, PAGE 227; OSTEOPOROSIS, PAGE 198

SEEDS

  Zn E Ca Protein, Omega fatty acids

Sources of protein, unsaturated fats, and a range of minerals and vitamins, seeds have a similar nutritional content to nuts. There are many different edible varieties of seeds that can be added to the diet, raw or cooked. They are particularly useful to people who do not eat animal products because they provide alternative supplies of iron and calcium.

KEY BENEFITS

- CAN HELP TO MAINTAIN PROSTATE HEALTH
- RELIEVE PROBLEMS OF THE BOWEL
- MAY REDUCE THE RISK OF HEART DISEASE
- MAY HELP TO PREVENT ANEMIA
- SOOTHE SYMPTOMS OF PSORIASIS AND ECZEMA

FOOD PROFILE

★ HOW MUCH TO EAT

- 1 tablespoon of pumpkin seeds supply 10 percent of a woman's daily iron requirement.
- 3 tablespoons of pumpkin seeds supply 25 percent of an adult's daily requirement of zinc.
- 1 tablespoon of sunflower seeds supplies 6mg of vitamin E.

🥣 CHOOSING & STORING

- Always buy in clear, sealed containers from a reputable outlet.
- Store, for no more than one year, in an airtight jar in a dry place, away from direct sunlight.

🍳 COOKING & EATING

- Eat sunflower and melon seeds as a healthy snack.
- Toasted sesame seeds can be added to salads and cereals.
- Use poppy and caraway seeds in homemade bread and cakes.
- Sprinkle dill seeds over fish dishes or bake on bread rolls.

CARAWAY SEEDS
Said to stimulate saliva production, caraway seeds are considered to aid digestion. Strongly aromatic, they are used to make liqueurs.

ANISE SEEDS
The ancient Romans used anise seeds to make cakes that were served as a digestive at the end of a meal. The seeds come from the anise plant.

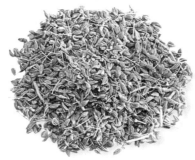

SUNFLOWER SEEDS
Native to Central America and Peru, sunflowers produce seeds that are rich in vitamin E. Regular intakes may help to boost the strength of the immune system.

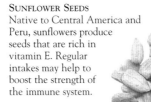

PUMPKIN SEEDS
These seeds are rich in the minerals zinc, iron, and selenium. They should be chewed thoroughly to make it easier for the body to absorb their valuable nutrients.

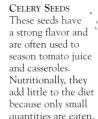

CELERY SEEDS
These seeds have a strong flavor and are often used to season tomato juice and casseroles. Nutritionally, they add little to the diet because only small quantities are eaten.

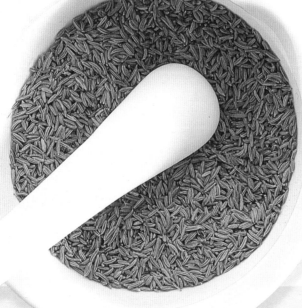

KEY NUTRIENTS

Many seeds are used in such small amounts that their nutritional contribution is not known. Other seeds can be used in larger quantities and may add significant amounts of vitamins, minerals, essential fats, and protein. Seeds provide unsaturated fatty acids from the omega-3 and omega-6 family, and are an important source of these nutrients for vegetarians.

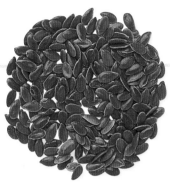

FLAX SEEDS
Unusually in the plant world, flax seeds contain omega-3 polyunsaturated fatty acids. These fats are more common in animal products, such as oily fish.

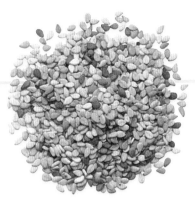

SESAME SEEDS
Rich in calcium, and nutty in flavor, these seeds can be roasted and then ground to make a cooking paste called tahini. (*See also page 103*)

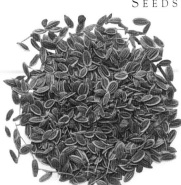

DILL SEEDS
Oil of dill seeds can be used to treat indigestion. The seeds are often cooked with cabbage, Brussels sprouts, and legumes to help prevent flatulence.

PSYLLIUM SEEDS
These seeds from the plantain plant are known for their laxative properties. They may be eaten whole or used to make an infusion. This should be drunk when cool, preferably at bedtime.

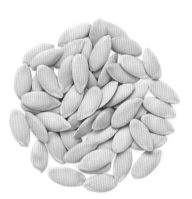

MELON SEEDS
Particularly rich in magnesium, and supplying good amounts of iron, melon seeds also provide zinc and folate, making them an all-around useful source of nutrients, especially for vegans.

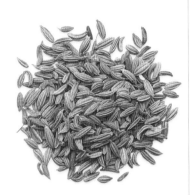

FENNEL SEEDS
Similar to anise seeds in flavor, fennel seeds have long been used as a treatment for weight problems. They are often ground, and may be sprinkled directly on to foods such as bread, or added to curry.

HEALING PROPERTIES

OTHER FORM

▣ TRADITIONAL USES
Fenugreek seeds are used in China to treat impotence and to help to relieve symptoms associated with menstruation and menopause. Flax seeds were used in the past to treat irregular menstruation and to brighten the vision. In the Middle East, sprouting fenugreek seeds are used to treat abdominal cramps and gastroenteritis, and to ease the pain of labor. Fennel seeds are used by herbalists in the West to soothe digestive disorders and to promote a new mother's breast milk. They are also used for treating colic in babies.

✜ SPECIFIC BENEFITS
Prostate Problems
Zinc is crucial for the health of the prostate gland, and men should take in at least 15mg a day. A handful of pumpkin, sesame, sunflower, or melon seeds, added to breakfast cereals or eaten as a snack, supplies about 1mg.

Constipation
Psyllium seeds are widely recommended for their laxative properties and for their ability to relieve the symptoms of irritable bowel syndrome. They bulk up the stools and, during digestion, speed the movement of stools through the colon.

Heart Disease
Flax, hemp, and pumpkin seeds supply omega-3 fatty acids. These thin the blood and reduce blood clotting, lessening the risk of heart disease and stroke. Sunflower, pumpkin, and sesame seeds contain omega-6 fatty acids. These are converted into substances called prostaglandins, which help to lower blood pressure. Sunflower seeds are rich in vitamin E, which reduces damage to artery walls.

Anemia
A major cause of chronic tiredness in many vegetarians is a low intake of iron. A lack of iron leads eventually to anemia. Sesame and pumpkin seeds are particularly good sources of iron, and melon and sunflower seeds also contain useful amounts.

Eczema and Psoriasis
A combination of hemp, flax, and pumpkin seeds may help to improve the skin. They can all decrease the inflammation associated with psoriasis. Combined with sesame and sunflower seeds, which supply omega-6 fats, these seeds may also help to improve eczema.

Hempseed Oil
The best source of omega-3 and omega-6 fatty acids are the seeds of the hemp, or marijuana plant. Hempseed oil contains 19 percent omega-3 fats, 57 percent omega-6 fats, and two percent gamma linoleic acid. This oil therefore supplies an adult's recommended daily intake of these essential fatty acids.

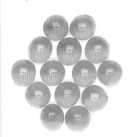

HEMPSEED OIL CAPSULES

SEE ALSO ANEMIA, PAGE 160; CONSTIPATION, PAGE 175; ECZEMA, PAGE 165; HEART DISEASE, PAGE 152

OILS

All oils, from both plant and fish sources, are a mixture of saturated, polyunsaturated, and monounsaturated fats. The most predominant group of fats present determines how the oil is described. For example, olive oil contains 14 percent saturated, 11 percent polyunsaturated, and 75 percent monounsaturated fat. It is therefore known as a monounsaturated oil.

KEY BENEFITS

- CAN REDUCE CHOLESTEROL AND MAY PROTECT AGAINST HEART DISEASE
- SLOW THE AGING PROCESS
- MAY HELP TO FIGHT INFECTIONS AND INFLAMMATORY SKIN DISEASES

FOOD PROFILE

★ HOW MUCH TO EAT

- All oils are dense sources of calories, and also supply vitamins A and E.
- Olive oil is particularly rich in monounsaturated fats. Using olive oil in place of other types of oil may help to lower blood cholesterol and reduce the risk of heart disease.

🥘 CHOOSING & STORING

- Buy oil from a reputable store, decanted or in a sealed bottle.
- Oils vary in color, aroma, and flavor, depending on the sources. Check the aroma and flavor of decanted oils. Do not buy them if they have unpleasant smells.
- Store oils at room temperature in order to keep them in a liquid form, and place bottles away from direct sunlight.

🍲 COOKING & EATING

- Different oils have different uses. Some, such as walnut oil, sesame seed oil, and extra virgin olive oil are ideal for seasoning. Others, such as sunflower oil, can be used in salad dressings.
- Some oils, including corn oil, are particularly good for cooking.

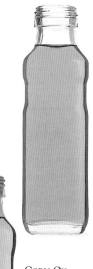
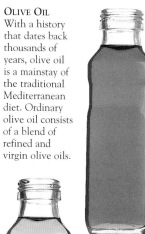
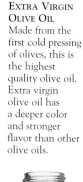
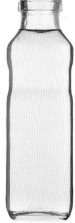

OLIVE OIL
With a history that dates back thousands of years, olive oil is a mainstay of the traditional Mediterranean diet. Ordinary olive oil consists of a blend of refined and virgin olive oils.

EXTRA VIRGIN OLIVE OIL
Made from the first cold pressing of olives, this is the highest quality olive oil. Extra virgin olive oil has a deeper color and stronger flavor than other olive oils.

CORN OIL
Pressed from the kernels of corn, this is mostly polyunsaturated and contains vitamin E. Corn oil is popular for salad dressings and is also used in margarine manufacturing.

SUNFLOWER OIL
Particularly high in essential polyunsaturated fat, sunflower oil also contains an especially large amount of vitamin E. This helps to prevent the oil from going rancid.

PEANUT, OIL
Used in South American and African cooking for thousands of years, this oil is mostly monounsaturated, and supplies useful amounts of vitamin E.

HEALING PROPERTIES

📖 TRADITIONAL USES

In Chinese medicine, oils are believed to increase "yin" in the body, and to be helpful for the nerves. Olive oil has been produced in Greece since at least 3000 BC. Its continued use through the ages is said to be partly responsible for the low rates of heart disease in Greece.

⊞ SPECIFIC BENEFITS

Heart Disease and Stroke
Reducing consumption of solid yellow fats by replacing them with olive oil may decrease cholesterol levels in

the blood by approximately ten percent. It is predicted that for every one percent reduction in cholesterol, the risk of coronary heart disease decreases by two percent. Rice bran oil contains an active ingredient called oryzanol, which helps to prevent the absorption of cholesterol into the body.

Blood Clotting
Hemp (see page 105), flax, and fish oils supply omega-3 fatty acids. These appear to help to keep the blood thin, reducing the risk of clots

forming. The blood is then less likely to coagulate and stick to any damaged areas on the artery walls.

Aging
Antioxidant properties in thyme oil appear to slow the aging process. Aging in all animals is linked to a progressive decline in the levels of long-chain polyunsaturated fatty acids in the body's tissues. This is caused by oxidation. These fatty acids normally help to keep cell membranes flexible and intact. They are also

involved in the production of certain hormonelike substances that are active in the eyes, brain, heart, joints, skin, and reproductive system. Thyme oil antioxidants restrict the oxidation of the fatty acids.

In studies in which animals were fed thyme oil, they retained better sight, firmer muscle tissue, and greater alertness in old age. An irritant if taken neat, thyme oil can be purchased as a supplement, commonly encapsulated with evening primrose oil (see page 25).

SEE ALSO ECZEMA, PAGE 165; HEART DISEASE, PAGE 152; HIGH CHOLESTEROL, PAGE 154; INFECTIONS, PAGE 212

KEY NUTRIENTS per ¹/₂ cup (100g)	OLIVE OIL	SUNFLOWER OIL	SOY OIL	SESAME SEED OIL	CORN OIL	COCONUT OIL	RAPESEED OIL	PALM OIL	PEANUT OIL	WALNUT OIL	COD-LIVER OIL
Calories	899	899	899	881	899	899	899	899	899	899	899
Fat (g)	99.9	99.9	99.9	99.7	99.9	99.9	99.9	99.9	99.9	99.9	99.9
Saturated fats (g)	14	11.9	14.5	14.2	12.7	85.2	6.6	45.3	18.8	9.1	20.2
Monounsaturated fats (g)	69.7	20.2	23.2	37.3	24.7	6.6	57.2	41.6	47.8	16.5	44.6
Polyunsaturated fats (g)	11.2	63	56.5	43.9	57.8	1.7	31.5	8.3	28.5	69.9	29.9
Vitamin E (mg)	5	49	16	–	17	1	22	–	15	–	20

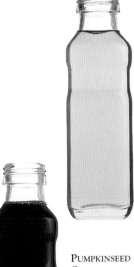

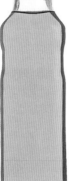

SOY OIL
Obtained from soybeans, this is pale yellow in color, with a bland taste. Used widely in the food industry, soy oil is found in dressings, margarines, and cooking fats.

SESAME OIL
Refined sesame oil is a mixture of mono- and polyunsaturated fats. It is golden amber in color and has a nutty flavor, which makes it ideal for stir-fries, salad dressings, and cooked dishes.

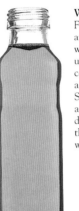

WALNUT OIL
First used in ancient Greece, walnut oil is used mainly in cooking and as a salad dressing. Several versions are available, depending on the type of walnut pressed.

PUMPKINSEED OIL
Pumpkin seeds contain 30 to 40 percent oil. If they are roasted before the oil is extracted, the end product is darker and has more flavor than other oils.

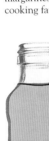

COD-LIVER OIL
This oil is extracted from the liver of the white fish, and is a rich source of vitamin A. It supplies a total of 18,000mcg per 100g, but should be avoided by pregnant women.

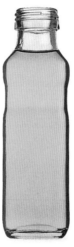

COCONUT OIL
This oil contains mostly saturated fat, but it is cholesterol-free. Found in cooking oils, margarines, and confectionery, it is semisolid if kept at room temperature.

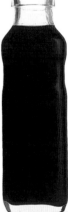

PALM OIL
Extracted from the palm nut, the color of this oil is due to the large amounts of alpha and beta carotene. Used in African cooking, it is a component of cooking fats and margarines.

Infections
Garlic oil can be used to help to prevent and treat bacterial, viral, and fungal infections, including those associated with the common cold and yeast infections. Garlic (see page 66) has antibiotic properties that seem to stimulate the immune system.

Inflammatory Disorders
Flax, hemp, evening primrose, and fish oils all contain essential fatty acids. These have an anti-inflammatory effect on the body and may relieve the symptoms of

rheumatoid arthritis, psoriasis, and eczema, the root causes of which are inflammatory. The body converts fatty acids into hormonelike prostaglandins which, in turn, combat inflammation in the cells.

CAUTION
Margarines contain saturated fats and "trans" fats (see page 24). Margarines that are rich in polyunsaturates contain five to seven percent trans fats, but hard margarines can contain as much as 40 percent trans fats.

OTHER FORMS

Margarines
Invented in 1869 by a French chemist, margarine was created as a cheap alternative to butter. It is now fortified with vitamins A and D and has the same fat and calorie contents as butter. A variety of oils can be used to make margarine, including soybean, sunflower, and palm oil. Unless the oil is specified on the pack, the blend usually depends on which oils are the cheapest on the world market. Margarines can be soft or hard. Soft versions are considered to be healthier than hard ones because they contain fewer trans fats, which are created as the margarine is made.

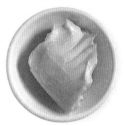

SOFT MARGARINE

SEE ALSO PSORIASIS, PAGE 166; RHEUMATOID ARTHRITIS, PAGE 197; STROKE, PAGE 156

HERBS

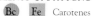

There are more than 200 different plants known as herbs that can be put to culinary or medicinal use. These plants have played an important role in nutritional healing for thousands of years. Many of their ancient uses are still valid today. The medicinal use of herbs has grown in popularity as people turn away from orthodox drugs to gentler herbal remedies.

KEY BENEFITS

- MAY FIGHT FOOD-POISONING BACTERIA
- LESSEN THE AGING EFFECTS OF POLLUTION
- MAY HELP IN THE TREATMENT OF DIABETES
- CAN REDUCE CHOLESTEROL AND BLOOD PRESSURE AND MAY PROTECT AGAINST CANCER

FOOD PROFILE

★ HOW MUCH TO EAT

- A 1oz bunch of fresh parsley provides 25 percent of an adult's recommended daily requirement of vitamin C. Regular consumption may play a role the prevention of cancer.
- A 1oz bunch of chopped chives added to savory dishes supplies good amounts of the plant nutrient allicin.

CHOOSING & STORING

- Buy fresh, dried, and ground herbs from a reliable source. Avoid buying dried parsley.
- Storage depends on the herb. Keep fresh mint for up to two weeks in cold water. Change the water every three days. Rosemary and thyme will survive for only five days in similar conditions.

COOKING & EATING

- Herbs can be used in salads and a variety of cooked dishes.
- Make herbal teas by infusing fresh leaves and flowers in water.
- Simmer the roots, bark, seeds, or stems for about 30 minutes to make an herbal decoction.

FENNEL
This is a classic herb to serve with oily fish such as mackerel and trout. Fennel is known for its diuretic effect.

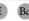

CHAMOMILE
This herb has a slightly bitter taste and the flowers have a rich, pungent smell. Chamomile has a wide variety of uses, from relieving pain and fever to treating skin problems, such as rashes and chilblains. It can be drunk in the form of tea to aid sleep.

CHIVES
Members of the onion family, chives are good added to omelettes, potato salad, cream cheese, and yogurt. If eaten regularly, they are believed to stimulate the appetite.

MINT
Deemed "profitable to the stomach" by the British herbalist Nicholas Culpeper (1616–54), mint is a popular medicinal herb. Use in drinks, sauces, and relishes, and in the water when boiling new potatoes.

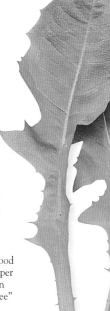

ROSEMARY
This evergreen shrub grows up to 4.5ft high. The needle-like leaves are covered with a layer of volatile oils that help to keep in the moisture. Rosemary's strong and pungent flavor goes well with lamb and chicken.

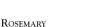

ANGELICA
The angelica plant is native to Lapland. The stalks and roots are often candied, and are believed to fight infections. The herb can be added to drinks such as vermouth.

DANDELION
The name "dandelion" comes from the French *dents de lion*, meaning "teeth of the lion" and describing the leaves. Dandelion leaves are good sources of iron and copper and can be used fresh in salads. Dandelion "coffee" can be made from the chopped and roasted roots.

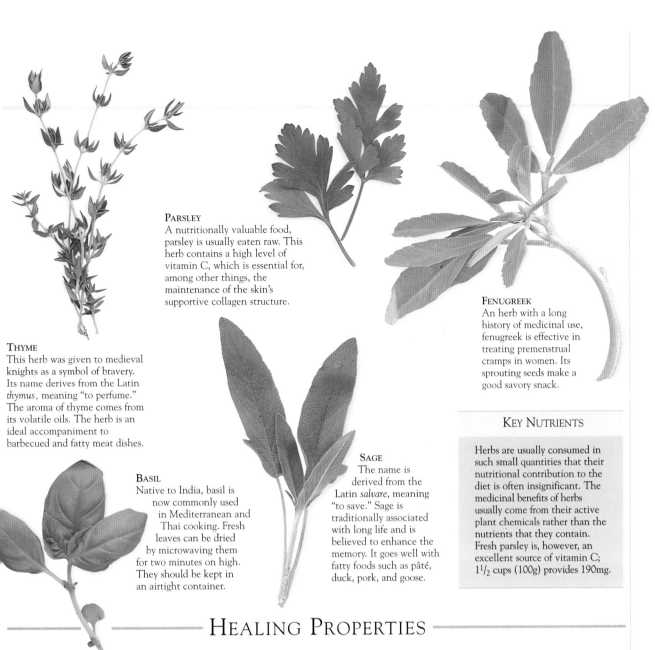

PARSLEY
A nutritionally valuable food, parsley is usually eaten raw. This herb contains a high level of vitamin C, which is essential for, among other things, the maintenance of the skin's supportive collagen structure.

FENUGREEK
An herb with a long history of medicinal use, fenugreek is effective in treating premenstrual cramps in women. Its sprouting seeds make a good savory snack.

THYME
This herb was given to medieval knights as a symbol of bravery. Its name derives from the Latin *thymus*, meaning "to perfume." The aroma of thyme comes from its volatile oils. The herb is an ideal accompaniment to barbecued and fatty meat dishes.

BASIL
Native to India, basil is now commonly used in Mediterranean and Thai cooking. Fresh leaves can be dried by microwaving them for two minutes on high. They should be kept in an airtight container.

SAGE
The name is derived from the Latin *salvare*, meaning "to save." Sage is traditionally associated with long life and is believed to enhance memory. It goes well with fatty foods such as pâté, duck, pork, and goose.

KEY NUTRIENTS

Herbs are usually consumed in such small quantities that their nutritional contribution to the diet is often insignificant. The medicinal benefits of herbs usually come from their active plant chemicals rather than the nutrients that they contain. Fresh parsley is, however, an excellent source of vitamin C; $1^1/_2$ cups (100g) provides 190mg.

HEALING PROPERTIES

✅ TRADITIONAL USES

An infusion of dried or fresh basil leaves is believed by herbalists to be a good remedy for vomiting, cramps, indigestion, and flatulence. After childbirth it can also help to prevent the placenta from being retained. Sage is beneficial to digestion and is believed to assist the body to break down the fats in rich foods. Mint is a stomach-calming herb that can relieve motion sickness. Chewing fennel seeds is recommended for soothing digestion, and an infusion of the leaves can alleviate colic. Mothers can relieve colic symptoms in babies by drinking fennel tea and passing on its soothing properties through their breast milk. Rosemary tea is recommended by herbalists for treating colds, influenza, and rheumatic pains. Believed to be a stimulating tonic, rosemary has uplifting and energizing properties. Chamomile tea is believed to have a calming and sedative effect and is useful in treating insomnia. It is also thought to help with premenstrual problems, anxiety, and stress.

✳️ SPECIFIC BENEFITS

Food Poisoning
Under laboratory conditions, rosemary has been shown to fight food poisoning bacteria, including *Staphylococcus*, and the dangerous *Escherichia coli*.

Aging
Scientific research suggests that thyme has particularly powerful antioxidant properties. In experiments, aging mice fed oil of thyme became more lively than those deprived of the oil. It is thought that thyme helps to stop the breakdown of long-chain fatty acids present in the walls of cells. By helping these fats to resist oxidation, thyme may protect against the aging effects of pollution and sun damage.

Diabetes
Active constituents in fenugreek have properties that appear to reduce blood sugar levels in some people with diabetes. Trials have revealed that a daily intake of 1oz of fenugreek seed powder can reduce sugar levels in the blood and urine, making it possible for those with diabetes to decrease their regular dosage of insulin.

Fluid Retention
Fresh dandelion leaves contain 297mg of potassium per 100g. They are known to increase urination and can be used to treat fluid retention and high blood pressure.

Heart Disease and Cancer
Related to onions and garlic, chives contain chemicals called sulfurous compounds, which seem to be capable of lowering blood cholesterol and triglyceride levels and possibly of leading to a reduction in blood-clotting. Studies have also indicated that these substances are able to prevent cells becoming cancerous. Increasing dietary intake of chives, garlic, and onions may help to reduce the risk of developing heart disease and cancer.

SEE ALSO CANCER, PAGE 214; DIABETES, PAGE 218; FLUID RETENTION, PAGE 153; HEART DISEASE, PAGE 152

TEA

STAR NUTRIENTS & PHYTONUTRIENTS

Polyphenols, Caffeine

Tea is one of the most widely consumed beverages in the world. A small, evergreen, shrublike tree, the tea plant is native to Southeast Asia. Tea has traditionally been used to treat ailments such as flatulence and fluid retention. Herbal or fruit "teas," made from ingredients such as mint and black currant, are known for their calming properties.

KEY BENEFITS

- APPEARS TO HELP PREVENT HEART DISEASE
- MAY LOWER STROKE RISK IN ELDERLY MEN
- MAY HELP TO PREVENT KIDNEY FAILURE
- POSSIBLY HELPS TO STOP CANCERS FROM GROWING

FOOD PROFILE

KEY NUTRIENTS

An infusion of tea contains only traces of most nutrients. Adding milk, cream, or sugar to a cup of tea will boost the nutrients present.

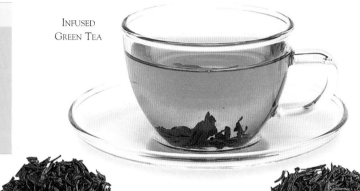

INFUSED GREEN TEA

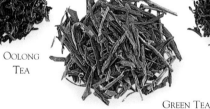

TEA TYPES
The three main types of tea are green, black, and oolong. Green tea is made from the fresh tips, or shoots, of the plant. Black tea is made by withering, rolling, then drying the leaves. Oolong tea is made by semifermenting the shoots.

OOLONG TEA

BLACK TEA

GREEN TEA

★ HOW MUCH TO DRINK
- Two or more cups of tea daily may help to reduce the risk of heart disease because tea contains a range of important antioxidant phytonutrients such as quercetin.
- A 7fl oz-serving of tea contains on average 44mg of caffeine. The exact amount depends on the brewing time.

🍵 CHOOSING & STORING
- Choose the type of tea according to your personal preference. Decaffeinated tea is also available.
- Store in an airtight container in a cool place for up to a few months.

🥘 MAKING TEA
- Always make tea with boiling water. Allow one teaspoon of fresh tea per person plus one more "for the pot."

HEALING PROPERTIES

📖 TRADITIONAL USES
Chinese herbalists have traditionally recommended green tea for a wide variety of ailments, including flatulence, indigestion, and water retention. Tea is also thought to be good for diarrhea, gastritis, and dysentery. Tea can also be used as a mild stimulant, although its effects are less strong than those of coffee.

⚙ SPECIFIC BENEFITS
Heart Disease
The intake of tea has been shown to be related to the amount of coronary heart disease in humans. There are antioxidant substances in tea called flavonoids, such as catechin, epicatechin, and epigallocatechin. These are thought to help to stop low-density lipoprotein (LDL) cholesterol (*see page 25*) from being damaged, thereby reducing the risk of blocked arteries. Studies on humans have shown that drinking either green or black tea produces a significant increase in the blood's antioxidant capacity, which peaks within 30 to 50 minutes of drinking the tea. Adding milk to tea does not neutralize this beneficial effect. Other plant chemicals in tea, such as lignans, may also help to protect against heart disease.

Stroke
It has been shown in various studies that the risk of stroke in elderly men decreases as the intake of flavonoids increases. One study carried out over ten years revealed that black tea with milk accounted for 70 percent of the flavonoid intake. In those who drank more than 4.7 cups of black tea a day, the risk of stroke was reduced by 69 percent compared with that in those who drank less than 2.6 cups. These results, as in the case of heart disease, can probably be explained by the ability of the flavonoids in tea to act as antioxidants and prevent damage to beneficial LDL cholesterol.

Kidney Disease
Studies have shown that green tea extracts, including tannin, can help to protect cells in the kidneys from damage by free radicals, and decrease the amount of toxins produced by the kidneys. The researchers concluded that certain green tea extracts prevent the progression of kidney failure, but this has not yet been proved outside the laboratory.

Cancer
No clear cut conclusions can be drawn about tea's role in the prevention of cancer. The most convincing evidence suggests that green tea decreases the risk of stomach cancer. Many laboratory studies have shown that tea polyphenol extracts inhibit tumor formation and growth. This is believed to be due to the antioxidant effects of the polyphenols. Tea polyphenol extracts may also suppress carcinogens and block the formation of cancer causing substances called N-nitroso compounds.

SEE ALSO CANCER, PAGE 214; HEART DISEASE, PAGE 152; KIDNEY DISORDERS, PAGE 192; STROKE, PAGE 156

COFFEE

STAR NUTRIENTS & PHYTONUTRIENTS

Caffeine

The first cultivated coffee tree was *Coffea arabica*. It originated in Ethiopia and began to be grown for consumption around 570 AD. *Coffea* seeds, called coffee beans, are one of the world's most important crops. *Coffea arabica* accounts for 90 percent of the coffee produced today with *Coffea robusta* supplying a further nine percent, and the remainder coming from *Coffea liberica*.

KEY BENEFITS

- PROVIDES A REFRESHING, STIMULATING DRINK AND CAN IMPROVE ALERTNESS
- INCREASES THE METABOLIC RATE
- MAY REDUCE ASTHMA ATTACKS
- HELPS THE BODY TO PRODUCE ENERGY

FOOD PROFILE

KEY NUTRIENTS

Unsweetened black coffee contains a small amount of niacin (vitamin B₃). Adding sugar, milk, or cream will increase its nutritional value.

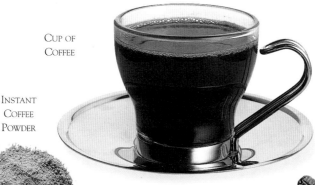

CUP OF COFFEE

INSTANT COFFEE POWDER

"REAL" AND INSTANT COFFEE
Coffee beans are roasted and ground to make "real" coffee. Instant coffee is made from ground, freeze-dried beans. A cup of "real" coffee contains nearly double the caffeine of a cup of instant coffee.

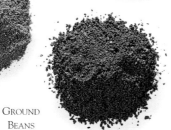

GROUND BEANS

ROASTED BEANS

★ HOW MUCH TO DRINK

- A maximum of six cups of coffee drunk throughout the day can help to stimulate the immune system and aid concentration.
- One cup of coffee made from ground coffee supplies 115mg of caffeine. One cup of instant coffee supplies 65mg. One cup of decaffeinated coffee supplies 3mg.

CHOOSING & STORING

- Buy decaffeinated coffee that has had the caffeine removed by the Swiss Water Process, rather than with solvents, because some residues from the solvents may remain.
- Store whole and ground coffee beans in an airtight container in the refrigerator.

MAKING COFFEE

- Make sure coffee grounds are the right size for the method used to make the drink.

HEALING PROPERTIES

TRADITIONAL USES
Coffee has traditionally been used for its stimulating effects and is often given to people when they wake up from an alcohol-induced sleep. It has been used in Chinese medicine for treating asthma, jaundice, and headaches. It has a laxative effect, and is often given to people to relieve constipation.

SPECIFIC BENEFITS
Fatigue and Depression
Caffeine has been shown to increase the speed of rapid information processing by the brain by ten percent. A regular cup of coffee after lunch helps to counteract the normal "post-lunch dip" in concentration that many people experience. Caffeine has also been shown in tests

to improve reaction times, resulting in increases in vigor, alertness, and efficiency, and a noticeable decline in depression and anxiety levels.

Low Metabolic Rate
The consumption of caffeine has been shown to lead to a temporary increase in the metabolic rate and in the rate at which fat is broken down in the body. Some studies show that the larger the amount of coffee drunk, the greater these effects will be. Although caffeine increases the burning of calories by only a small amount, a sensible intake may still be useful to those trying to lose weight. It should, however, be remembered that two cups a day is the recommended maximum intake.

Asthma
Caffeine has long been known to relieve asthma, and many people have found that the regular consumption of coffee helps to moderate their attacks. This theory has been supported by two large scientific studies in the US and in Italy, in which three or more cups of coffee per day were found to reduce the number of attacks in asthma sufferers. Studies of people whose bronchial asthma is brought on by exercise, show that coffee improves the function of the lungs, but about six cups of coffee were needed to have any effect. Coffee appears to help reduce the onset of bronchial asthma, although this is not widely accepted by the medical profession.

Low Energy Levels
In addition to providing caffeine, coffee supplies the B vitamin niacin, which is needed by the body for the efficient production and boosting of energy in cells. The more energy that the body burns, the more niacin it requires. A typical cup of coffee made from ground beans provides 1mg of niacin. The recommended daily intake of niacin is 13mg for women and 17mg for men.

CAUTION
Moderation is the key. Too much caffeine can lead to tremors, sweating, insomnia, and palpitations. Drinking too much percolated or boiled coffee can increase levels of cholesterol.

SEE ALSO ASTHMA, PAGE 187; DEPRESSION, PAGE 233; FATIGUE, PAGE 235

SPICES

The word "spices" is derived from the Latin *species*, meaning "fruits of the earth." Spices come from plants that flourish in semitropical and tropical climates. They derive from the bark, buds, flowers, fruits, or roots, and are highly aromatic due to their essential oils. Spices have played a role in the world's history. At one time, they were so valuable that they were used as currency.

KEY BENEFITS

- CAN REDUCE INFLAMMATION
- MAY HELP TO REDUCE AND FIGHT CANCER
- MAY HELP TO RELIEVE SYMPTOMS OF MENOPAUSE
- HELP TO RELIEVE COLDS AND CHILLS

FOOD PROFILE

★ HOW MUCH TO EAT

- These strongly flavored aromatic substances are used in food preparation according to individual taste. They may be used whole or ground.

CHOOSING & STORING

- Buy whole or ground spices from sources with a regular turnover so that they are fresh. The flavor of spices gradually diminishes.
- Store spices in airtight containers in cool conditions and away from direct sunlight.
- Buy cardamom in the pod and remove it before using.

COOKING & EATING

- Use whole spices to provide flavor, aroma, and visual and textural effects to food.
- Crush or grind spices and add to food during cooking.
- Use cardamom in anything from curries to ice cream.
- Color soups, condiments, and pickled foods with turmeric.
- Use allspice whole in pickling and chicken dishes, and ground in cakes and soups.
- Grate nutmeg and add a little to ice cream and baked foods.
- Spice cooked apples and mulled wine with cinnamon and cloves.

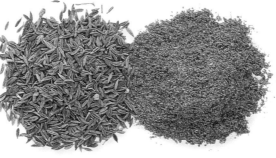

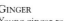 WHOLE CUMIN   GROUND CUMIN

CUMIN
This aromatic spice is made from the dried, ripe fruits of an herb belonging to the parsley family. Cumin is a key constituent of curry powder. The flavor can be described as warm, heavy, spicy, and bitter.

CLOVES
The dried, unopened flower buds of an evergreen tree of the myrtle family, cloves have a warm, spicy, fruity flavor. They also have a slightly numbing effect, which explains the traditional use of tincture of cloves to treat toothaches.

GINGER
Young ginger roots are used fresh, either sliced or grated, while older roots are dried and powdered. Ginger contains oleoresins, extracts used to flavor foods and drinks.
(*See also page 114*)

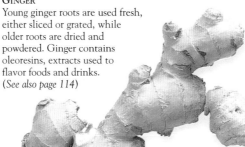

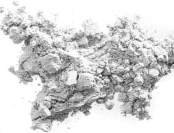

GROUND GINGER

GINGER ROOT

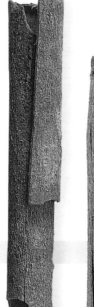
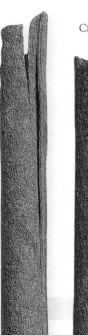

CINNAMON STICKS

CINNAMON
One of the oldest spices, cinnamon comes from the inner bark of a tree of the laurel family. A constituent of curry powder, it is often used to spice cooked apples and mulled wine.

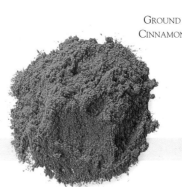

GROUND CINNAMON

CARDAMOM
The seeds come from the fruits of a perennial herb of the ginger family. Cardamom has a sweet, pungent, spicy flavor. Some people chew the seeds to sweeten the breath.

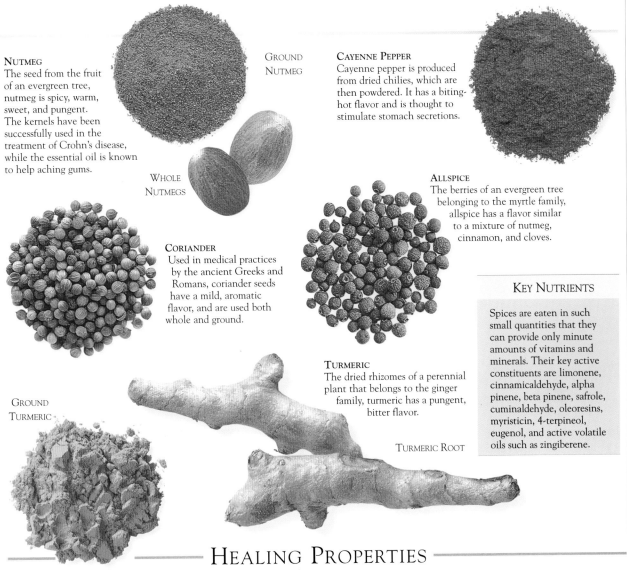

NUTMEG
The seed from the fruit of an evergreen tree, nutmeg is spicy, warm, sweet, and pungent. The kernels have been successfully used in the treatment of Crohn's disease, while the essential oil is known to help aching gums.

GROUND NUTMEG

WHOLE NUTMEGS

CAYENNE PEPPER
Cayenne pepper is produced from dried chilies, which are then powdered. It has a biting-hot flavor and is thought to stimulate stomach secretions.

ALLSPICE
The berries of an evergreen tree belonging to the myrtle family, allspice has a flavor similar to a mixture of nutmeg, cinnamon, and cloves.

CORIANDER
Used in medical practices by the ancient Greeks and Romans, coriander seeds have a mild, aromatic flavor, and are used both whole and ground.

TURMERIC
The dried rhizomes of a perennial plant that belongs to the ginger family, turmeric has a pungent, bitter flavor.

GROUND TURMERIC

TURMERIC ROOT

KEY NUTRIENTS

Spices are eaten in such small quantities that they can provide only minute amounts of vitamins and minerals. Their key active constituents are limonene, cinnamicaldehyde, alpha pinene, beta pinene, safrole, cuminaldehyde, oleoresins, myristicin, 4-terpineol, eugenol, and active volatile oils such as zingiberene.

HEALING PROPERTIES

✍ TRADITIONAL USES

In ancient Egypt, cumin was used in the mummification of bodies. In ancient Rome, Pliny referred to cumin as a good appetizer. Today, cumin is thought to aid digestion. Cinnamon has long been used to treat colds, stomach chills, arthritis, and poor circulation. It is used in Chinese medicine to relieve symptoms of menopause and asthma. Herbalists in the West recommend it for indigestion and diarrhea. Spices are often used in Indian medicine: Turmeric is given to improve blood conditions and to induce the flow of bile, which in turn helps to break down fats. It is also applied to infected wounds because of its antiseptic qualities. Ginger is known for its warming action

and in Chinese medicine it is used to treat respiratory conditions such as coughs and colds. Nutmeg is used in Chinese medicine as a digestive remedy and to improve general weakness. In the West, a decoction of the kernel is thought to help in the treatment of diarrhea. Clove oil has long been used by herbalists in the West for its local anesthetic actions, which come from its volatile oil known as eugenol. Oil of cloves is also used for treating colic and toothaches.

✦ SPECIFIC BENEFITS
Inflammatory Conditions
The spice that has been most widely researched by scientists in the West is turmeric. Its active constituent, known as curcumin, has been shown to

have anti-inflammatory effects. Curcumin works by directly "dampening down" the mechanisms involved in the inflammatory process. This helps to explain the use of turmeric to treat sprains and arthritis in Ayurveda, the Indian system of medicine.

Cancer
Recent research indicates that curcumin in turmeric may reduce the risk of cancer. Some scientists also believe that curcumin may encourage the regression of cancer. The cancer fighting effects seem to come from a combination of factors, including the antioxidant effects of a bioactive peptide called turmerin, which helps to protect the genetic material DNA from injury. A study in

Israel has observed that people who eat cumin have fewer bladder cancers than those who do not eat it. Evidence of cumin's ability to fight cancer is not conclusive.

Menopause
It is possible that the plant estrogens present in turmeric may reduce the severity of some of the symptoms that are associated with a decline in estrogen levels in women at the time of menopause.

CAUTION

Nutmeg contains myristicin and elemicin, which both have mild anaesthetic and sedative properties. Amounts greater than 1 tablespoon are not recommended.

SEE ALSO CANCER, PAGE 214; MENOPAUSAL PROBLEMS, PAGE 223

GINGER

A brown tropical root native to Southeast Asia, ginger has been used as a spice and as a medicine for centuries. Known to the ancient Greeks and Romans, it was available throughout Europe by the 10th century. Ginger was traditionally used by doctors in the East to warm the system and deal with digestive disorders. It is still recognized for its warming, stimulant properties today.

KEY BENEFITS

- APPEARS TO HELP OVERCOME MOTION SICKNESS
- MAY IMPROVE SYMPTOMS OF MORNING SICKNESS
- MAY ALLEVIATE SYMPTOMS OF RHEUMATOID ARTHRITIS
- CAN BE USED TO TREAT FLATULENCE

FOOD PROFILE

KEY NUTRIENTS

Ginger is eaten in such small quantities that it can provide only minute amounts of vitamins and minerals. Its key active constituents are oleoresins and active, volatile oils such as zingiberene.

COLD COMFORT

For a warming drink to fight colds and chills and to improve the circulation, simmer two slices of fresh ginger root for ten minutes in a small pan of water. Add honey for sweetness.

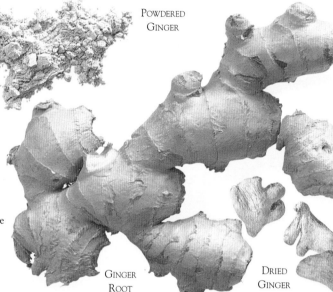

POWDERED GINGER

GINGER ROOT

DRIED GINGER

★ HOW MUCH TO EAT

- Adding fresh ginger to foods and drinks on a regular basis may help to overcome nausea and motion sickness.

CHOOSING & STORING

- Choose young, creamy yellow roots. Avoid old, fibrous ones.
- Wrap ginger in foil and keep in the refrigerator for several days. Do not peel before storing.
- Powdered ginger should not be stored for more than a week or so once it is opened.

COOKING & EATING

- Peel fresh ginger, then grate or slice thinly and use in stir-fries and curries. Use dried ginger in baking or as a tenderizer for meat.
- Sliced ginger can be used in cakes and cookies and added to tea for a spicy, warming drink.

HEALING PROPERTIES

✒ TRADITIONAL USES

Ginger has a warming, stimulating effect on the body. It is highly regarded by practitioners of Ayurvedic medicine in India, who have traditionally used it to help all the body tissues, especially those of the respiratory and digestive tracts, to dislodge congestion. Similar uses for ginger were recognized thousands of years ago in China. Ginger oil has been used in many parts of the world for hundreds of years to deal with flatulence, and it is rubbed directly on to areas of aches and pains. Roasted ginger was recommended in traditional Chinese medicine to treat diarrhea. The peeled root was also given for water retention and bloating in the stomach area.

❊ SPECIFIC BENEFITS

Motion Sickness

Studies have shown that ginger can help to improve the symptoms of motion sickness. In one trial in Utah in 1982, 36 people who were susceptible to motion sickness were seated in a tilting, rotating chair, and blindfolded. Their degree of stomach upset was monitored every 15 seconds for six minutes. Those who took powdered root ginger experienced less sickness than those who were taking an antihistamine. This works by blocking the signals of motion sickness to the brain. Scientists suspect that powdered ginger is more likely to work by affecting the stomach itself, possibly by increasing stomach activity and by absorbing toxins and acids that would otherwise trigger signals of nausea to the brain. Not all the studies on motion sickness show an improvement after taking ginger, but it appears to work for some people.

Vertigo and Nausea

Ginger has been shown to improve the symptoms of vertigo and nausea, as well as morning sickness during pregnancy. Ginger is also believed to be effective in treating the nausea that is associated with excessive consumption of alcohol.

Rheumatoid Arthritis

In studying patients with osteoarthritis, rheumatoid arthritis, and muscular discomfort, it was observed that more than 75 percent of those with rheumatoid arthritis experienced relief in pain and swelling when given powdered ginger. Those with muscular discomfort also experienced pain relief. The ginger did not seem to affect those with osteoarthritis. Even though this trial was based on a questionnaire, the results are nonetheless interesting. Scientists believe that ginger may bring about pain relief by inhibiting the production of inflammatory substances known as prostaglandins (particularly PGE2) and leukotrienes (particularly LTB4), which cause many arthritic symptoms. Other work on rheumatoid arthritis has shown that eating raw ginger can bring about improvements in symptoms.

SEE ALSO NAUSEA, PAGE 180; RHEUMATOID ARTHRITIS, PAGE 197

HONEY

STAR NUTRIENTS & PHYTONUTRIENTS

K   Carbohydrate, Sugar

This sweet, syrupy liquid is made by bees from the nectar of flowers. Known as the "nectar of the gods," honey has been highly regarded for its healing properties for thousands of years. The flavor and color of honey depends on the flowers and trees from which the nectar is obtained. Honey is digested and absorbed into the blood almost as rapidly as refined sugar.

KEY BENEFITS

- MAY REDUCE STOMACH ULCERS
- COULD HELP TO TREAT GASTROENTERITIS
- A SOOTHING REMEDY FOR MINOR WOUNDS AND BURNS

FOOD PROFILE

KEY NUTRIENTS
per 5 tablespoons (100g)

Calories	288
Carbohydrate (g)	76
Sugars (g)	76
Iron (mg)	0.4
Copper (mg)	0.1
Protein (g)	0.4
Sodium (mg)	11
Potassium (mg)	51
Phosphorus (mg)	17

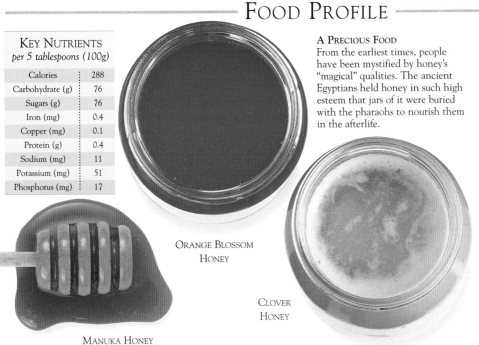

ORANGE BLOSSOM HONEY

CLOVER HONEY

MANUKA HONEY

A PRECIOUS FOOD
From the earliest times, people have been mystified by honey's "magical" qualities. The ancient Egyptians held honey in such high esteem that jars of it were buried with the pharaohs to nourish them in the afterlife.

★ HOW MUCH TO EAT

- An average 1oz spreading of honey on bread supplies 15g of quickly absorbed sugar. For those needing instant energy, such as athletes after training, eating honey on a regular basis may help them to maintain energy levels and improve performance.

CHOOSING & STORING

- Clover honey is creamy, with a smooth, buttery texture, Manuka is robust and aromatic, and Orange Blossom is golden orange in color, with a citrus fragrance.
- Store honey in a warm place or put the jar in hot water for an hour before using, to soften it. Honey can be made firmer by storing it in the refrigerator.

COOKING & EATING

- Use in baking, in desserts, as a spread, or as a sweetener for hot drinks and cereals.

HEALING PROPERTIES

⬛ TRADITIONAL USES
The use of honey in the treatment of ailments is legendary. It has been known to relieve disorders ranging from coughs and hayfever to influenza and hangovers. In Chinese medicine, honey is used to harmonize the liver, neutralize toxins, and relieve pain. Said to have a "neutral energy," honey is added to hot drinks, for treating dry coughs or hoarse throats. Interestingly, however, it is claimed in Indian Ayurvedic medicine that honey's beneficial effects are lost once it is heated. Honey has traditionally been used in Chinese medicine to treat stomach ulcers, high blood pressure, and constipation. It can be applied directly to minor burns and wounds.

⬛ SPECIFIC BENEFITS
Stomach Ulcers
Scientists investigating the traditional Chinese treatment of stomach ulcers with honey have discovered that the benefit appears to come from its antibacterial effect on the bacterium *Helicobacter pylori*. This bacterium is probably responsible for many cases of stomach ulcers. In the laboratory, it has been discovered that the action of *H. pylori* can be inhibited by concentrations of Manuka honey. The effectiveness of Manuka honey needs to be fully tested in people with gastric ulcers caused by *H. pylori* before scientists can prove what traditional medicine believes is an effective treatment for this distressing condition.

Gastritis and Duodenitis
People have reported an improvement in both of these conditions through the consumption of honey. While nothing has been clinically proven so far, it is possible that the antibacterial effect of the hydrogen peroxide and the phytonutrients in honey could be responsible for this beneficial effect.

Hangovers
While no scientific proof exists as yet, it is widely held that honey can help to sober up drunken or hungover people through the effect of fructose on the liver. It is thought that the fructose in honey stimulates the oxidation of alcohol by the liver, thereby speeding up the cleansing of the system.

Minor Wounds and Burns
Applying raw honey to minor wounds and superficial burns on the skin appears to improve the healing process. The honey helps to absorb moisture and prevents the growth of bacteria.

WARNING
Do not give honey to babies who are less than one year old.
Cases of botulism affecting babies in this age group have been traced to bacterial spores in honey.

SEE ALSO ALCOHOL, PAGE 19; BURNS, PAGE 167; DIARRHEA, PAGE 176; PEPTIC ULCERS, PAGE 171; WOUND HEALING, PAGE 167

MEATS, FISH & DAIRY

HEALTHY EATING GUIDELINES suggest that between two and four servings of meats, fish, or other protein sources be consumed on a daily basis. In practice, a mix of protein sources is advisable, with some days that include fish, others that include meats and poultry, and yet others when vegetable sources of protein are consumed. Meats should be lean, and poultry should be eaten without the skin. All meats and fish should be prepared with as little fat or oil as possible. Meat products tend to be fatty and should only be eaten occasionally. Reduced-fat versions of most dairy foods are available and are advisable whenever possible. Check with your child's doctor about lowfat milk for children under two years old.

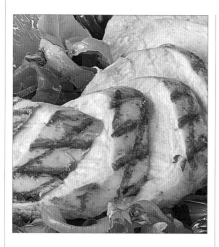

LEAN MEATS

During the last 20 years, the fat content of lean red meat has fallen on average, by 30 percent. While this reduces the total number of calories provided by meats, all of the essential nutrients are found in the lean part and, therefore, remain intact. Fatty cuts of meat and meat products, such as sausages and burgers, tend to be high in saturated fats. About half the fat in lean red meats is, however, unsaturated, which makes them one of the main sources of monounsaturated fat in the diet.

WAYS OF PRESERVING MEAT

Historically, fresh meats were preserved by salting, smoking, curing, or processing into sausages and pâtés. Although modern cold storage means that meats can be kept for months or years, the unique flavors and textures of old-fashioned methods make preserved meat products popular today. These can be high in fat and should be eaten in moderation. In Japan, large amounts of salted meat are eaten, and high rates of stomach cancer have been observed.

OTHER MEATS

Cultural preferences for meat vary greatly around the globe. While kangaroo meat and emu may be acceptable to some Australians, and the French enjoy horse meat and frog's legs, people living in other countries may feel uneasy about eating these less common types of meat.

MEATS

Humans have eaten meat since the earliest times. Once the art of hunting wild animals was mastered and various species were gradually domesticated, meat began to play an important role in the diet. Today cattle, sheep, and pigs are the main animals reared and consumed in Europe and the US, while goats, camels, and water buffalo are important food sources in the Middle East, India, and Africa. Poultry has risen in popularity since intensive farming has made chicken a readily available and inexpensive source of animal protein. Liver, kidneys, oxtail, and other organ meats are less popular, but are still consumed. Fatty cuts and meat products tend to be high in fat, particularly saturated fats that raise cholesterol. With the increasing demand for leaner meats has come the introduction of "new" meats, such as emu, ostrich, and buffalo. These red meats are exceptionally low in fat and high in protein and iron.

HEALTH BENEFITS OF MEAT

In population studies around the world, eating meat has been found to be associated with a lower prevalence of iron deficiency. Iron is a vital constituent of two proteins, hemoglobin and myoglobin. Hemoglobin carries oxygen in the blood, while myoglobin stores oxygen in muscle tissue. Meats contain a type of iron, known as haem iron, that the body finds easy to absorb. Haem iron increases the absorption of nonhaem iron, which is found in some grains and vegetables. Oily fish contain smaller amounts of haem iron than meats. Zinc and selenium, two minerals that are crucial for the correct development of sperm, are both provided by meat. Male fertility may be protected by the regular consumption of meat.

FISH

People eat many types of fish, including white, bony varieties, such as cod and haddock; oily, bony fish, such as herring, mackerel, and salmon; cartilaginous fish, such as skate; mollusks, such as mussels, oysters, and squid; and crustaceans, including crab, shrimp, and lobster. The amount of oils, essential fats, and minerals they supply vary, but all are good sources of protein. With the exception of farmed trout, salmon, and some shellfish, fish are the only animal foods consumed in the West that are still hunted.

HEALTH BENEFITS OF FISH

The consumption of large quantities of oily fish is linked with low rates of heart disease. It is thought that the essential oils in these fish help to lower the risk of blood clotting and decrease inflammation. This reduces the buildup of atherosclerotic fatty plaques on the artery walls. Oily fish supply some of the best sources of vitamin D, which is needed for the absorption of calcium from foods. Canned oily fish, which have soft bones, are excellent suppliers of calcium. Regular intakes of these fish throughout life can help to build and maintain strong bones, and reduce the risk of the bone condition osteoporosis.

DAIRY PRODUCTS

Milk and its byproducts began to feature in the human diet when people domesticated animals and exploited them for more than their meat and skins. While dairy foods are popular in Europe and the Americas, they are rarely consumed in some countries in the Far East, where people lose the ability to digest milk after being weaned. Cow's milk, cheese, and yogurt are the most commonly consumed dairy products. Milk provides calcium and phosphorus in the diet, along with protein. With the increasing trend for drinking skim and lowfat varieties, milk is a less important source of fat.

HEALTH BENEFITS OF DAIRY PRODUCTS

Dairy products are rich in calcium, which is needed for the development and maintenance of strong bones. A diet low in calcium during childhood and adolescence can contribute to weak bones in adulthood. The live, "friendly" bacteria in some yogurts can reproduce in the large intestine and replace "unfriendly" bacteria, the cause of flatulence and bloating.

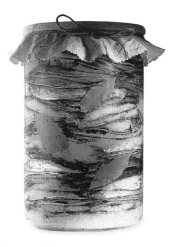

WAYS OF PRESERVING FISH

In the past, fish had to be pickled, dried, salted, or smoked in order to preserve it. Today, freezing and canning are the main methods of preservation. Many fish are available canned, including sardines, salmon, and tuna, which provide calcium when canned with their bones. Eel, salmon, cod, and haddock can be smoked, and cod is also dried and salted. Salted and dried fish are popular in the East. They are, however, high in sodium, so are best eaten in moderation.

FISH FARMING

Most fish produced globally is caught in the world's oceans, but farming fish can be more efficient than hunting. Fish are bred on farms to produce good-quality stock and to provide protection from predators. Carp and trout are the main freshwater farmed fish.

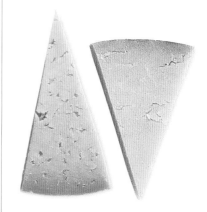

CHEESE

The earliest cheese is thought to have been made accidentally by travelers whose milk turned sour, forming a type of cottage or curd cheese. It was soon realized that cheese kept better once the whey was removed and sodium added. There are now five main types of cheese: curd, cream, soft, semi-hard, and hard.

OILY FISH

Found in seas, lakes, and rivers, oily fish are so named because their body fat is distributed throughout their flesh; in white fish, such as cod, fat is stored in the liver. Fish oils are rich sources of the fatty acids eicosapentanoeic acid (EPA) and docosahexaenoic acid (DHA). These appear to be the main reasons why eating oily fish provides many health benefits.

> ### KEY BENEFITS
>
> • HELP TO RELIEVE SYMPTOMS OF PSORIASIS
> • MAY REDUCE THE RISK OF HEART DISEASE
> • HELP TO MAINTAIN PEAK BONE DENSITY
> • CAN HELP TO PREVENT ANEMIA

FOOD PROFILE

★ HOW MUCH TO EAT

• Between 4 and 6oz of oily fish, three times a week, may help to reduce the risk of blood clots and heart disease.
• 4oz of oily fish supply more than 9 percent of the daily recommended intake of the mineral iron.
• 4oz of canned sardines hold more than 38 percent of the daily recommended intake of calcium.

🍲 CHOOSING & STORING

• Fresh fish should have bright, bulging eyes and firm flesh.
• Remove the scales, gills, and guts from fresh fish before storing for up to three days in the refrigerator.
• Oily fish can be frozen safely, but must be defrosted and eaten within six months.

🥘 COOKING & EATING

• Bake, grill, poach, pan fry, or cook on a barbecue.

KIPPERS
These are herrings that have been smoked. In the UK, they are traditionally served grilled at breakfast. They contain quite high levels of sodium so need no added salt.

MACKEREL
The fat content of mackerel varies between 6g and 23g per 4oz. Smoked mackerel has a strong flavor and makes delicious pâté.

BROWN TROUT
This fish has one of the lowest levels of fat among oily fish and one of the highest levels of the mineral potassium.

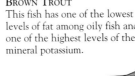

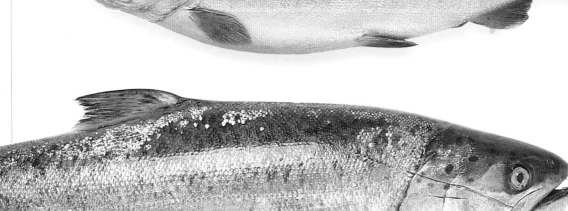

SALMON
Pacific salmon contain more vitamin D than Atlantic salmon, with up to 20mg per 4oz. Smoked and canned salmon are higher in salt than fresh salmon.

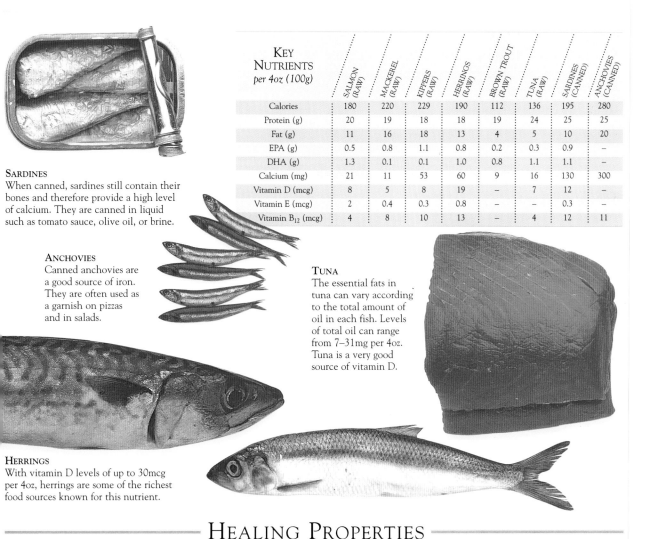

KEY NUTRIENTS per 4oz (100g)	SALMON (RAW)	MACKEREL (RAW)	KIPPERS (RAW)	HERRINGS (RAW)	BROWN TROUT (RAW)	TUNA (RAW)	SARDINES (CANNED)	ANCHOVIES (CANNED)
Calories	180	220	229	190	112	136	195	280
Protein (g)	20	19	18	18	19	24	25	25
Fat (g)	11	16	18	13	4	5	10	20
EPA (g)	0.5	0.8	1.1	0.8	0.2	0.3	0.9	–
DHA (g)	1.3	0.1	0.1	1.0	0.8	1.1	1.1	–
Calcium (mg)	21	11	53	60	9	16	130	300
Vitamin D (mcg)	8	5	8	19	–	7	12	–
Vitamin E (mcg)	2	0.4	0.3	0.8	–	–	0.3	–
Vitamin B$_{12}$ (mcg)	4	8	10	13	–	4	12	11

SARDINES
When canned, sardines still contain their bones and therefore provide a high level of calcium. They are canned in liquid such as tomato sauce, olive oil, or brine.

ANCHOVIES
Canned anchovies are a good source of iron. They are often used as a garnish on pizzas and in salads.

TUNA
The essential fats in tuna can vary according to the total amount of oil in each fish. Levels of total oil can range from 7–31mg per 4oz. Tuna is a very good source of vitamin D.

HERRINGS
With vitamin D levels of up to 30mcg per 4oz, herrings are some of the richest food sources known for this nutrient.

HEALING PROPERTIES

🗹 TRADITIONAL USES
In Chinese medicine, herrings are often recommended for detoxifying the body, while sardines are believed to fortify the sinews and bones, act as a mild diuretic, and improve blood circulation. Mackerel are prescribed for conditions that are connected with damp, such as rheumatism.

❇ SPECIFIC BENEFITS
Psoriasis
Research has revealed that 6oz of oily fish eaten on a daily basis can help to relieve the symptoms in some people of the chronic skin disease psoriasis. Whole oily fish and fish oil supplements contain the fatty acids EPA and DHA which, it is believed, are converted into prostaglandins. These substances then "dampen down" the underlying inflammatory process of psoriatic outbreaks.

Heart Disease
Death from heart disease is less common among those who eat large amounts of oily fish, such as the Inuit people of Greenland, than among other people. This has been attributed to EPA and DHA in the fish. These lower the risk of clots forming and help to prevent fatty buildups in blood vessels. It has been shown that, when eaten regularly, oily fish can help to prevent second heart attacks.

Calcium Deficiency
Teenagers, pregnant and breast-feeding women, the elderly, and those who get little exposure to the sun may particularly benefit from regularly including oily fish in the diet. Oily fish are sources of vitamin D, calcium, and phosphorus, all of which are important for building and maintaining strong bones. Vitamin D is essential for calcium to be absorbed into the blood. A shortage of calcium in teenage years may stunt growth, and bones will not reach peak bone density. This increases the risk of osteoporosis in later life. Canned fish that retain their softened bones, such as sardines and pilchards, are the best sources of all three bone building nutrients.

Anemia
Regular consumption of oily fish can significantly improve intakes of the mineral iron. If the body has inadequate iron stores on which to draw, anemia can develop. Like meat, fish contains "hem" iron (see page 160), which is up to 30 times more readily absorbed than iron from plant sources.

Rheumatoid Arthritis
Studies have shown that fish oil supplements help to relieve the pain and swelling associated with rheumatoid arthritis. The fish oil appears to "dampen down" the inflammatory process through the production of substances called prostaglandins. There is no hard evidence that intakes of oily fish have the same effect, but people with rheumatoid arthritis may find that adding this type of fish regularly to the diet will help to relieve symptoms.

SEE ALSO ANEMIA, PAGE 160; HEART DISEASE, PAGE 152; PSORIASIS, PAGE 166; RHEUMATOID ARTHRITIS, PAGE 197

SHELLFISH

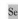

Common inhabitants of the shoreline, shellfish fall into two groups: crustaceans and mollusks. Crustaceans include shrimp, crabs, lobsters, and crayfish, and all have jointed external skeletons. Mollusks such as oysters, scallops, cockles, and mussels live inside a shell, while cuttlefish, squid, and octopuses do not. All shellfish are rich in minerals and good sources of protein.

KEY BENEFITS

- USEFUL FOR THOSE ON WEIGHT-LOSS DIETS
- IMPORTANT FOR MALE FERTILITY
- PROVIDE NUTRIENTS FOR BLOOD, BONE, AND MUSCLE FUNCTION
- MAY HELP TO PREVENT CANCER

FOOD PROFILE

★ HOW MUCH TO EAT

- All shellfish are low in calories and fat, yet rich in minerals. An average 4oz serving of oysters can provide up to 90mg of an adult's daily requirement of zinc.

CHOOSING & STORING

- Avoid buying crabs and lobsters that are discolored or damaged.
- Avoid cooked shrimp that are black. Uncooked shrimp should be firm.
- Buy live oysters in their shells. Shelled oysters should be plump and creamy gray in color.
- When buying scallops, make sure that the shells are tightly closed. Avoid those with brown markings.
- Live lobsters should be kept in damp cloth bags, as they drown if kept in water for too long.

COOKING & EATING

- Drown or freeze live crabs and lobsters, then put them in a pan of water and bring to the boil. Simmer for five to 20 minutes.
- Rinse oysters, remove the top shell, and eat with lemon.
- Wash scallops and remove the brown veins. Pan fry or poach.
- Grill, barbecue, or stir-fry shrimp.

MUSSELS
These shellfish are a good source of iron. Green-lipped mussels, found off the coast of New Zealand, may help to relieve symptoms of rheumatoid arthritis.

OYSTERS
One of the richest food sources of zinc, oysters are also an excellent source of iron in a form that can be easily absorbed by the body.

LOBSTER
The color of lobsters varies, according to the species. They are all an excellent source of selenium.

COCKLES
Particularly low in calories and high in iron, cockles are sometimes nicknamed "the poor man's oyster."

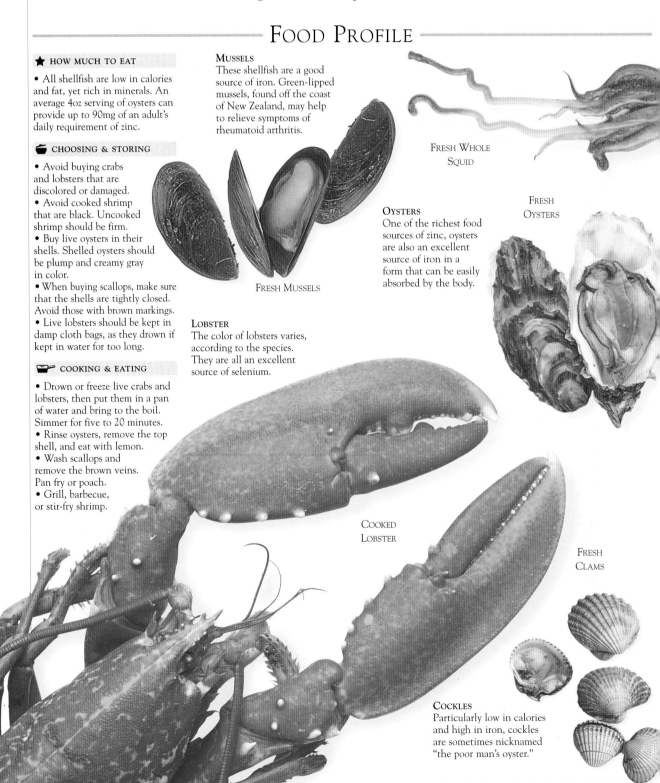

FRESH WHOLE SQUID

FRESH OYSTERS

FRESH MUSSELS

COOKED LOBSTER

FRESH CLAMS

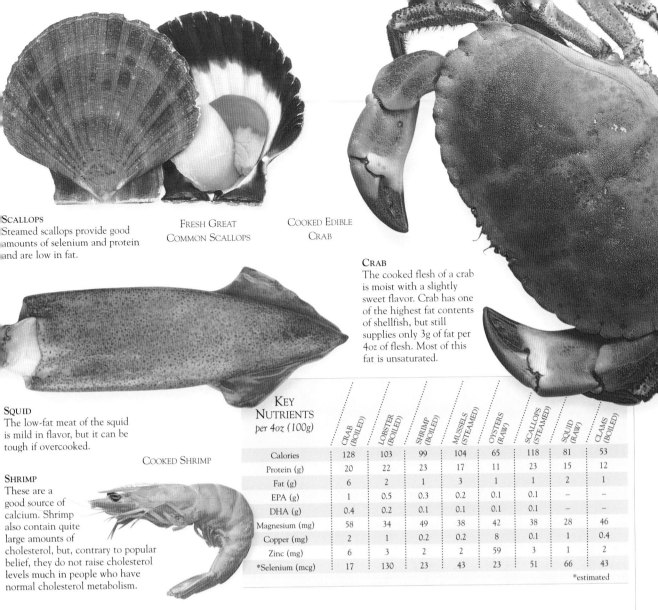

SCALLOPS
Steamed scallops provide good amounts of selenium and protein and are low in fat.

FRESH GREAT COMMON SCALLOPS

COOKED EDIBLE CRAB

CRAB
The cooked flesh of a crab is moist with a slightly sweet flavor. Crab has one of the highest fat contents of shellfish, but still supplies only 3g of fat per 4oz of flesh. Most of this fat is unsaturated.

SQUID
The low-fat meat of the squid is mild in flavor, but it can be tough if overcooked.

COOKED SHRIMP

SHRIMP
These are a good source of calcium. Shrimp also contain quite large amounts of cholesterol, but, contrary to popular belief, they do not raise cholesterol levels much in people who have normal cholesterol metabolism.

KEY NUTRIENTS per 4oz (100g)	CRAB (BOILED)	LOBSTER (BOILED)	SHRIMP (BOILED)	MUSSELS (STEAMED)	OYSTERS (RAW)	SCALLOPS (STEAMED)	SQUID (RAW)	CLAMS (BOILED)
Calories	128	103	99	104	65	118	81	53
Protein (g)	20	22	23	17	11	23	15	12
Fat (g)	6	2	1	3	1	1	2	1
EPA (g)	1	0.5	0.3	0.2	0.1	0.1	–	–
DHA (g)	0.4	0.2	0.1	0.1	0.1	0.1	–	–
Magnesium (mg)	58	34	49	38	42	38	28	46
Copper (mg)	2	1	0.2	0.2	8	0.1	1	0.4
Zinc (mg)	6	3	2	2	59	3	1	2
*Selenium (mcg)	17	130	23	43	23	51	66	43

*estimated

HEALING PROPERTIES

☑ TRADITIONAL USES

Oysters have long been associated with heightened virility. It is possible that they acquired this reputation because of their high zinc content. A lack of zinc causes impotence in men, and some men may have regained their sexual appetites after eating oysters. The ancient Romans noted that an open oyster has a visually stimulating aphrodisiac effect, and this may also have contributed to the oyster's reputation. In Chinese medicine, oysters are used to treat nervousness and insomnia. Mussels are believed to strengthen the liver. They are also used for kidney problems, abdominal swelling, and vertigo. Crab is believed to help those with broken bones.

✳ SPECIFIC BENEFITS

Weight Problems
All shellfish are relatively low in calories and fat and high in protein. This combination makes them ideal for inclusion in the diet of those who are trying to lose weight.

Male Infertility
A lack of zinc in the diet can cause infertility in men. Most shellfish, especially oysters, provide useful amounts of zinc. The high presence of this mineral in semen implies an important role in sperm health. Zinc maintains the genetic material of sperm, and keeps them in a quiet state, thereby preserving their energy prior to ejaculation. Zinc also stops sperm from releasing important enzymes before fusing with an ovum.

Shellfish additionally contain useful amounts of selenium, which improves the mobility of sperm in subfertile men.

Brittle Bones
Oysters and crabs are good sources of the mineral copper, which is crucial for the formation of many enzymes. A lack of copper is not common in well balanced diets, but inadequate intakes can retard growth in children and lead to bone fractures.

Weak Muscles
All shellfish supply good amounts of magnesium, which keeps the muscles toned and strong. A lack of magnesium can be caused by anorexia, problems with absorption, long periods of diarrhea or vomiting, and alcoholism.

Cancer
Research has shown that selenium may protect against lung cancer. This protection may come from selenium's antioxidant properties and its apparent ability to suppress abnormal cell growth. This mineral is also thought to enhance the immune system and to alter the action of carcinogens, making them less toxic. Lobster, squid, and scallops are particularly good sources of selenium.

CAUTION
Oysters, mussels, and cockles can contain toxins that are not destroyed by cooking. Commercially farmed mollusks are the safest to eat because they are tested for contaminants.

SEE ALSO ANOREXIA, PAGE 181; CANCER, PAGE 214; INFERTILITY IN MEN, PAGE 227; OBESITY, PAGE 178

MEATS

   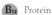

S ince prehistoric times, meats have been part of the human diet. They are an important source of protein, vitamins, and minerals, and, when eaten with vegetables, help the body to absorb plant sources of minerals, such as chromium, copper, selenium, zinc, and iron. More than half the fat in most meats is unsaturated, and very lean, low fat cuts of meat are now readily available.

KEY BENEFITS

- MAY HELP TO PREVENT ANEMIA
- HELP TO BUILD AND MAINTAIN BODY TISSUES
- MAY HELP IMPROVE MALE FERTILITY
- HELP TO MAINTAIN THE NERVOUS SYSTEM

FOOD PROFILE

★ HOW MUCH TO EAT

- Eating lean red meats about three times a week provides iron, protein, zinc, and B vitamins.
- 4oz of roast beef supplies 16 percent of the recommended daily intake of iron for adults.

🥄 CHOOSING & STORING

- Choose lean cuts of meat.
- Take meats home as quickly as possible and store, covered, in the lower section of the refrigerator.
- Store all types of raw meats away from any cooked foods.

🍲 COOKING & EATING

- Keep a separate chopping board for chopping raw meats.
- Trim off any excess fat.
- Dry-fry, broil, open roast, or casserole meats in order to avoid using extra fat when cooking.
- Try grilling or cooking meat steaks on a hot griddle.
- Serve with vegetables for a nutritionally balanced meal.

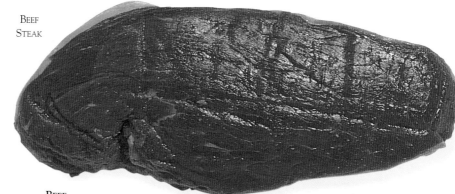

BEEF
STEAK

BEEF
Rump steak can contain as little as 4g of fat per 4oz and is rich in zinc.

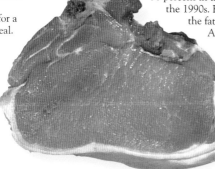

PORK
The fat content of pork has fallen from 30 percent in the 1950s to 20 percent in the 1990s. Further trimming brings the fat down to four percent. A lean pork steak can contain as little as 3g of fat per 4oz.

LOIN PORK
CHOP

VENISON
Deer meat, or venison, is an excellent source of iron and zinc. The buck, or male, tends to be tastier than the doe, or female.

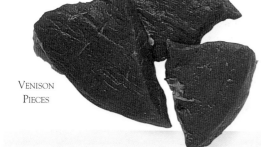

VENISON
PIECES

LAMB
Even though lamb is considered to be a fatty meat, a lean leg joint can contain as little as 2.2g of fat if it is trimmed. An average cut of lamb contains fractionally more saturated fat than unsaturated fat.

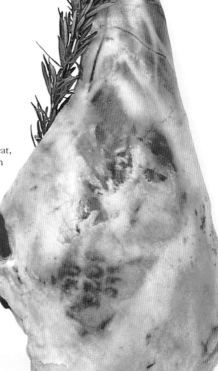

LEG OF LAMB

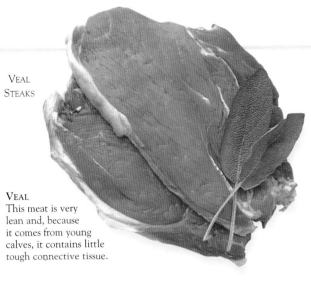

VEAL
STEAKS

VEAL
This meat is very
lean and, because
it comes from young
calves, it contains little
tough connective tissue.

CALF'S
LIVER

LIVER
Calf's liver is a rich source of
easily absorbable iron, zinc, and
selenium, and is also rich in
vitamin A. The strong flavor
of ox and pig's liver can be
reduced by soaking it in
milk. Pregnant women
should not eat liver
since its high levels
of vitamin A can
cause birth defects.

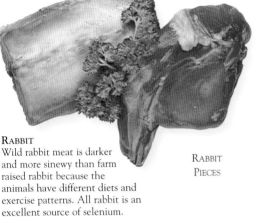

RABBIT
Wild rabbit meat is darker
and more sinewy than farm
raised rabbit because the
animals have different diets and
exercise patterns. All rabbit is an
excellent source of selenium.

RABBIT
PIECES

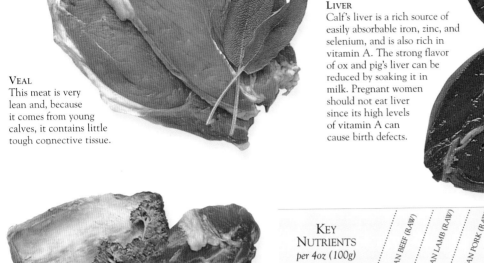

KEY NUTRIENTS per 4oz (100g)	LEAN BEEF (RAW)	LEAN LAMB (RAW)	LEAN PORK (RAW)	VENISON (RAW)	RABBIT (RAW)	VEAL (RAW)	LIVER (RAW)
Calories	123	162	123	103	137	106	153
Protein (g)	20	21	22	22	22	23	20
Fat (g)	5	9	4	2	6	2	7
Saturated fats (g)	1.9	4.2	1.4	0.8	2	0.6	2.2
Polyunsaturated fats (g)	0.2	0.4	0.7	0.4	1.8	0.3	1.9
Monounsaturated fats (g)	2.1	3.3	1.5	0.4	1.3	0.7	1.3
Iron (mg)	2	2	1	3	1	1	8
Zinc (mg)	4	4	2	42	1	2	8
Selenium (mcg)	3	1	13	9	17	9	22
Vitamin B_{12} (mg)	2	2	1	1	10	2	100

HEALING PROPERTIES

☑ TRADITIONAL USES
Ayurvedic teaching does not
recommend meats as a regular
part of the diet because they
are hard to digest. Meats are,
however, recommended for
those who are run down, in
order to strengthen the body,
as long as they are prepared
in an easily digestable way, for
example in soups. Chinese
doctors believe that beef is
good for the blood, the bones,
and lower back pain. Lamb is
prescribed for impotence and
kidney problems. Pork is
believed to be good for dry
coughs, and for those with a
weak or nervous constitution.

❖ SPECIFIC BENEFITS
Anemia
Iron deficiency, or anemia,
can be prevented and treated
through the regular inclusion
of red meats in the diet. These
are a good source of "hem"
iron (see page 160), of which
between 15 and 20 percent
is absorbed by the body.

Weight Problems
In recent years, meat has
become dramatically leaner
due to new breeding and
butchering techniques. As a
result, some red meats contain
less fat than skinless chicken.
Extra-lean cuts of meat are
rich, low fat sources of
protein that can be part
of a weight-loss diet.

Loss of Appetite
Meats supply all of the nine
essential amino acids and are
known as a high biological
value protein food. They are
a particularly useful source
of protein for young children,

convalescents, and the elderly,
who may have small appetites,
but who need to take in high
levels of protein to build up
or maintain their bodies.

Infertility in Men
Lean red meats are good
sources of easily absorbable
zinc and selenium, nutrients
that are essential for male
fertility. Up to 40 percent
of the zinc in red meats is
absorbed. Zinc has strong
antioxidant properties. It
helps to protect sperm from
free radical damage and is
involved in the structure of
sperm DNA. It reduces sperm
activity, conserving energy
until it is needed. Selenium
can decrease the number
of damaged sperm and can
increase the number and
mobility of viable sperm.

Nerve Damage
Meat is a very good source
of vitamin B_{12}. This vitamin
is needed for the formation
of myelin, the protective
sheath surrounding nerves.
A prolonged deficiency
of vitamin B_{12} leads to
irreversible nerve damage.

Osteoporosis
It is important that children
take in sufficient vitamin D
in order to help prevent bone
disorders such as osteoporosis
developing in later life. Recent
analysis of meat has shown
that it supplies a significant
amount of vitamin D. This
vitamin is needed for the
absorption of calcium and
for the development of strong
bones. Meats can contribute
up to 21 percent of a child's
daily requirement.

SEE ALSO ANEMIA, PAGE 160; INFERTILITY IN MEN, PAGE 227; OBESITY, PAGE 178

POULTRY & GAMEBIRDS

STAR NUTRIENTS & PHYTONUTRIENTS
   Fe Zn B₁₂ Protein, Monounsaturated fats

The focal point of many a celebratory meal, chickens, turkeys, ducks, geese, partridges, and pheasants have graced the grandest to the most humble tables throughout the ages. The nutritional value of poultry and gamebirds varies from bird to bird and depends on the cooking technique employed. All are excellent sources of protein, which is easily digested.

KEY BENEFITS

- CAN BE USED IN A WEIGHT-LOSS DIET
- MAY IMPROVE MOOD AND CONCENTRATION
- MAKE USEFUL ADDITIONS TO SPECIAL DIETS
- CAN HELP TO PREVENT ANEMIA

FOOD PROFILE

★ KEY PROPERTIES

- An average 5oz serving of chicken provides 35mg of protein, which is more than half an adult's daily requirement.
- A 4oz serving of pheasant supplies about 53 percent of an adult's daily iron requirement.

🥣 CHOOSING & STORING

- Buy from a reputable supplier.
- Store birds in the refrigerator or freezer immediately after buying.
- Store raw birds away from cooked foods in the refrigerator.

🍲 COOKING & EATING

- Cook until the juices run clear.
- Roast or microwave whole birds. Pieces, such as a leg or breast, can be broiled.
- Do not reheat cooked poultry more than once.

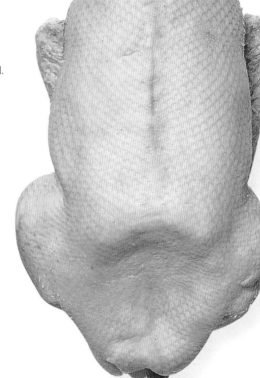

GOOSE
Goose is a naturally fatty bird. When it is cooked, remove the skin before serving to keep the consumption of fat to a minimum.

TURKEY
Dark turkey meat contains almost three times as much iron as the light meat.

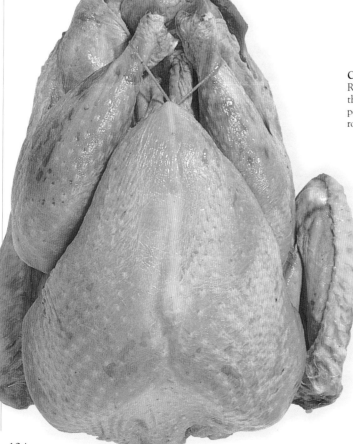

CHICKEN
Roast chicken eaten with the skin has 9g more fat per 4oz than skinless roast chicken.

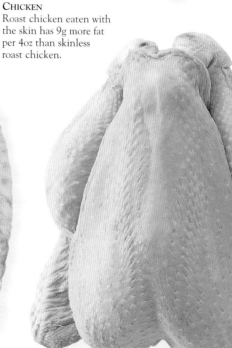

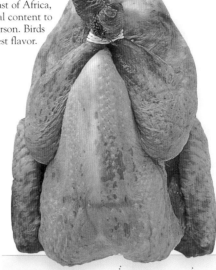

GUINEA FOWL
Originally from the Guinea coast of Africa, these birds are similar in nutritional content to pheasant. One bird is served per person. Birds that have been "hung" have the best flavor.

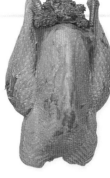

PHEASANT
A good source of iron, pheasant also contains a wide range of B vitamins, including B_6, B_{12}, and B_2. All of these are needed to maintain a healthy nervous system and to promote the release of energy.

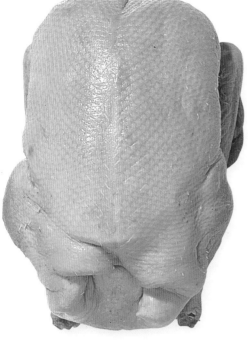

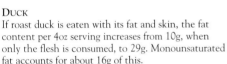

DUCK
If roast duck is eaten with its fat and skin, the fat content per 4oz serving increases from 10g, when only the flesh is consumed, to 29g. Monounsaturated fat accounts for about 16g of this.

KEY NUTRIENTS per 4oz (100g)	CHICKEN (RAW)	TURKEY (RAW)	DUCK (RAW)	GOOSE (ROAST)	PARTRIDGE (ROAST)	PHEASANT (ROAST)
Calories	106	105	137	319	212	220
Protein (g)	24	24	20	29	37	28
Fat (g)	1	1	7	22	7	12
Saturated fat (g)	0.3	0.3	2	unknown	1.9	41
Monounsaturated fat (g)	0.5	0.3	3	unknown	3.4	5.6
Polyunsaturated fat (g)	0.2	0.2	1	unknown	1.7	1.6
Iron (mg)	1	0.3	2	5	2	2
Zinc (mg)	1	1	2	3	1	1
Magnesium (mg)	29	27	19	31	26	26
Vitamin B_6 (mg)	0.5	0.8	0.3	0.4	–	1

HEALING PROPERTIES

◪ TRADITIONAL USES
Some Chinese therapists believe that chicken can relieve the symptoms of diarrhea, water retention, and poor appetite associated with spleen and pancreas imbalances. Today, therapists may advise against eating chickens that have been given antibiotics to prevent infections from spreading among birds kept together.

❖ SPECIFIC BENEFITS
Weight Problems
White turkey meat is a rich source of protein and has a low fat content. It is therefore an ideal food for those on a weight-loss diet. Lean chicken and duck cooked using a low-fat method and then served without the fat and skin are good alternatives. These protein-rich foods may also influence the appetite centers in the brain, helping to create a feeling of fullness.

Depression
Turkey is rich in the amino acid tryptophan, which is needed for the production of the neurotransmitter serotonin. This helps the body to maintain a feeling of well-being and it also controls appetite. A drop in levels of serotonin in the brain can lead to depression and hunger. Serotonin levels naturally dip in the winter, due to a reduction in sunlight. Eating turkey regularly during the winter may help those who are susceptible to this effect to maintain a high level of serotonin and thereby dispel depression and hunger.

Poor Concentration
All poultry and gamebirds contain good amounts of the amino acid tyrosine, which the brain uses to produce norepinephrine and dopamine. These substances trigger the brain cells that enhance concentration and mental alertness. For those whose concentration falters at certain times of the day, a snack containing poultry or game may provide a boost to mental abilities. Prepared turkey or chicken slices are useful "power sources" for quick snacks.

Food Allergies
Chicken and turkey do not have a strong flavor, so they are ideal for those who temporarily have no appetite. Both birds are known for rarely causing allergic reactions, so they can be used in exclusion diets (*see page 245*) by those trying to identify allergies. Poultry and gamebirds are ideal foods at all stages of life. They supply the nine essential amino acids that are needed for the growth and repair of tissues, and they are easy to digest.

Anemia
Duck, goose, partridge, and pheasant all provide some "hem" iron (*see page 160*), which is easily absorbed. These birds are especially useful to those who do not like red meats, the other good supplier of hem iron. It is important to maintain a good store of iron in the body to prevent the development of subclinical or full blown anemia.

SEE ALSO ANEMIA, PAGE 160; DEPRESSION, PAGE 233; FOOD ALLERGIES, PAGE 210; OBESITY, PAGE 178

DAIRY PRODUCTS

Ever since people first domesticated animals such as cattle, goats, and sheep, they have drunk their milk. A wide variety of foods are produced from animal milk, including cheeses, yogurts, milk shakes, cream, and ice cream. Products such as hard cheeses are rich in calcium and zinc, and high in saturated fat. Soft cheeses are often low or medium fat and contain less zinc and calcium.

> ### KEY BENEFITS
> - CAN REDUCE THE RISK OF BONE FRACTURES DUE TO OSTEOPOROSIS
> - MAY PREVENT CERTAIN CANCERS
> - HELP TO PREVENT TOOTH DECAY
> - MAY HELP TO MAINTAIN GENERAL GOOD HEALTH

FOOD PROFILE

★ HOW MUCH TO EAT
- 2 cups of skimmed milk supply more than 60 percent of an adult's daily needs of calcium.

🍲 CHOOSING & STORING
- Buy all dairy products from reputable outlets that have a regular turnover of stock.
- Store products in a refrigerator, only until their "use-by" date.

🍳 COOKING & EATING
- Drink fresh milk plain or as a milk shake. Pour it over cereals or use in sweet and savory sauces.
- Eat cheese in chunks, grated in salads and sandwiches, on toast, in sauces, or on top of pizzas.

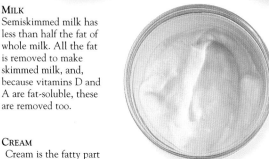

MILK
Semiskimmed milk has less than half the fat of whole milk. All the fat is removed to make skimmed milk, and, because vitamins D and A are fat-soluble, these are removed too.

CREAM
Cream is the fatty part of milk that separates out from the watery part when milk is left to stand. To make cream commercially, these two parts are separated out even more.

CREME FRAICHE
Meaning "fresh cream" in French, crème fraîche is cream mixed with sour cream. The fat content of both the whole and reduced fat versions is high.

LIVE NATURAL YOGURT
All yogurt is made by growing "live" bacterial culture in milk. Live yogurt is not heat-treated, as nonlive yogurt is, as this kills off the bacteria that are beneficial to the digestive system.
(See also page 128)

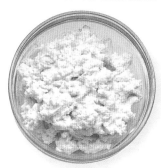

RICOTTA CHEESE
This soft cheese retains more of the watery part of the milk than hard cheese, and has a slightly sweet taste. It can be used in cooking as a low-fat alternative to cream cheese.

HEALING PROPERTIES

📖 TRADITIONAL USES
Cow's milk is often prescribed in Chinese medicine for a weak constitution and for those who need "building up." Goat's milk is recommended for stomach disorders. In the West, milk is recommended for those with a stomach ulcer or an upset stomach. It is also considered to be good for convalescents and for the elderly.

✤ SPECIFIC BENEFITS
Osteoporosis
There is increasing evidence that an adequate intake of calcium during early life is necessary for the development of maximum bone mass at maturity (between the ages of 30 and 40). The better the bone mass that people have at maturity, the less likely they are to have bone fractures in old age. Milk supplies an easily absorbable form of calcium and, if drunk daily in early life, may reduce the risk of osteoporosis in old age.

Rickets
If insufficient calcium is deposited on growing bones in childhood the bones may become weak, leading to rickets. The bowing of leg bones beneath the weight of a child is a symptom. Rickets is caused by a lack of vitamin D, which is needed by the body to absorb calcium from the intestines. Whole milk supplies this vitamin, especially for children who do not have enough exposure to the sun. Without sunlight to make vitamin D, they have to rely on dietary sources.

Cancer of the Colon
Researchers have noticed that there is a lower risk of colonic cancer in populations in which people consume large amounts of calcium. It is thought that the calcium may combine with bile acids and prevent them from promoting cancerous cells in the colon. It is possible that a regular intake of milk could help to prevent other cancers too. Milk contains a fatty acid called conjugated linoleic acid, or CLA. Studies in the laboratory have shown that CLA reduces the incidence of some cancers by up to 50 percent. CLA may also boost the immune system and slow the development of diseases such as atherosclerosis, which affect the arteries, particularly in later life.

SEE ALSO CANCER, PAGE 214; CHILDREN & NUTRITION, PAGE 136; HIGH BLOOD PRESSURE, PAGE 155

KEY NUTRIENTS per 4oz (100g)	WHOLE MILK	SKIMMED MILK	GOAT'S CHEESE	COTTAGE CHEESE	FROMAGE FRAIS	WHIPPING CREAM	RICOTTA CHEESE	CHEDDAR CHEESE	BRIE	LOW-FAT NATURAL YOGURT	BUTTER
Calories	66	33	60	98	113	373	144	412	319	56	737
Protein (g)	3	3	3	14	7	2	9	26	19	5	0.5
Fat (g)	4	0.1	4	4	7	39	11	34	27	1	82
Saturated fat (g)	2.4	0.1	2.3	2.4	4.4	24.6	6.9	21.7	16.8	0.5	54
Monounsaturated fat (g)	1.1	–	0.8	1.1	2.1	11.4	2.7	9.4	7.8	0.2	19.8
Polyunsaturated fat (g)	0.1	–	0.1	0.1	0.2	1.1	0.5	1.4	0.8	–	2.6
Calcium (mg)	115	120	100	73	89	62	240	720	540	190	15
Phosphorus (mg)	92	94	90	160	110	58	170	490	390	160	24
Vitamin A (mcg)	52	1	44	44	100	565	185	325	285	8	815
Vitamin D (mcg)	0.03	–	0.1	0.03	0.1	0.2	–	0.3	0.2	0.01	1.0

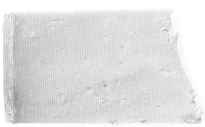

HARD CHEESE
After milk has separated into curds and whey, caused by the action of rennet, the solid curds are pressed to create hard cheeses, such as cheddar. All hard cheeses keep well.

BRIE

SOFT CHEESE
Soft cheeses are made in the same way as hard cheeses, except that the curds are not pressed. Examples of soft cheeses are brie and camembert.

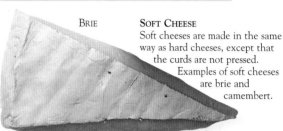

CHEDDAR CHEESE

BUTTER

COTTAGE CHEESE
This is white, unripened curd cheese. Very low-fat cottage cheese can be made using skimmed milk, but this can be bland in flavor.

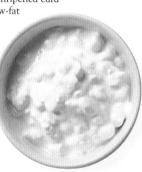

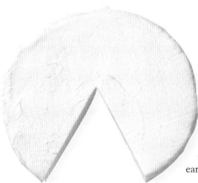

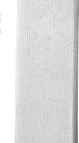

BUTTER
The minimum amount of milk fat that butter should contain is 80 percent. The color of butter depends on the amount of carotene present in the cows' feed.

GOAT'S CHEESE
There are about 400 varieties of goat's cheese throughout the world. Goat's milk has been used to produce cheeses since early Roman times.

Tooth Decay
The ability of foods and drinks to cause tooth decay depends on their composition and texture, how easily they dissolve in the mouth, how long they are retained in the mouth, and how well they stimulate saliva production. Cheese may help to stop tooth decay by preventing the tooth enamel from being attacked by acids which are formed when bacteria in the mouth begin to break down food. Cheese does this by stimulating the flow of alkaline saliva, which returns the acidity levels of the mouth to normal. In addition the calcium in cheese can stop the tooth enamel from dissolving. It is thought that cheese proteins may coat the surface of the enamel and protect it, and that fatty acids in cheese may be antibacterial. As little as 5–10g of hard cheese eaten after a meal is believed to be enough to help protect the teeth from decay.

Energy Deficiency
Milk supplies the body with vitamins B_1 and B_2, pantothenic acid, and niacin. It also contains the minerals phosphorus and magnesium. These nutrients all play a role in releasing energy from food and producing enzymes that utilize the energy in food.

Weight Problems
Full-fat dairy products are good sources of calories. They are particularly valuable to the young and elderly, who do not eat large volumes of food.

High Blood Pressure
Low intakes of calcium may contribute to high blood pressure. Studies show that when people took calcium supplements their blood pressure dropped.

Protein Deficiency
Protein is necessary for the general growth, maintenance and repair of body tissue. Dairy products such as milk and cheese contain all eight essential amino acids, so they are good sources of "high biological value" protein.

CAUTION
Some people cannot digest lactose, the sugar in milk. A rarer complaint is an allergy to the protein in milk. People with either condition should exclude milk and milk products from the diet.

SEE ALSO MINERALS, PAGE 30; OSTEOPOROSIS, PAGE 199; PROTEINS, PAGE 20; TOOTH DECAY, PAGE 207

YOGURT

STAR NUTRIENTS & PHYTONUTRIENTS

 Ca P B₁₂ Protein, Monounsaturated fats

To make yogurt, a bacterial culture is added to warm milk. The bacteria feed on the milk sugar, called lactose, and release lactic acid, which thickens the milk into the familiar creamy texture of yogurt. Originally developed as a means of preserving milk, the nutritional value of yogurt depends on the type of milk used, and whether or not sugar and fruit are added.

KEY BENEFITS

- MAY HELP TO REDUCE HEART DISEASE
- CAN BE USED TO TREAT DIARRHEA
- HELPS THE PASSAGE OF STOOLS THROUGH THE INTESTINE
- HELPS TO RELIEVE IRRITABLE BOWEL SYNDROME

FOOD PROFILE

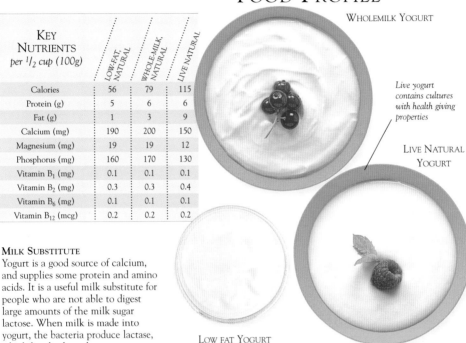

WHOLEMILK YOGURT

Live yogurt contains cultures with health giving properties

LIVE NATURAL YOGURT

LOW FAT YOGURT

KEY NUTRIENTS per 1/2 cup (100g)	LOW-FAT, NATURAL	WHOLEMILK, NATURAL	LIVE NATURAL
Calories	56	79	115
Protein (g)	5	6	6
Fat (g)	1	3	9
Calcium (mg)	190	200	150
Magnesium (mg)	19	19	12
Phosphorus (mg)	160	170	130
Vitamin B₁ (mg)	0.1	0.1	0.1
Vitamin B₂ (mg)	0.3	0.3	0.4
Vitamin B₆ (mg)	0.1	0.1	0.1
Vitamin B₁₂ (mcg)	0.2	0.2	0.2

MILK SUBSTITUTE

Yogurt is a good source of calcium, and supplies some protein and amino acids. It is a useful milk substitute for people who are not able to digest large amounts of the milk sugar lactose. When milk is made into yogurt, the bacteria produce lactase, which breaks down lactose.

★ HOW MUCH TO EAT

- A 2/3-cup serving of natural yogurt provides nearly 14 percent of an adult's daily requirement of phosphorus, which is 1g.
- 1 3/4 cups of natural yogurt provides the same amount of calcium as about 4 cups of milk.

CHOOSING & STORING

- Buy yogurt made from whole milk for children under five.
- Choose fat-reduced yogurts for older children and adults because these types are most beneficial to their health.
- Store yogurt in the refrigerator and eat by the "best before" date.

COOKING & EATING

- Use as a snack, on breakfast cereals, served with fruit, or as a topping for desserts.
- Stir into mashed potato as a low-fat replacement for butter.
- Use in dips and savory sauces.

HEALING PROPERTIES

✍ TRADITIONAL USES

Yogurt has long been credited with a range of therapeutic benefits, many of which involve the health of the large intestine and the relief of gastrointestinal upsets. Historical records state that yogurt was used to cure a recurrent intestinal disorder afflicting Francis I of France back in the 16th century. At the beginning of the 1900s, the Russian researcher Metchnikow won the Nobel prize for his investigations into why people in some parts of Eastern Europe live particularly active lives and stay in good health well into their nineties and beyond. He concluded that this phenomenon was attributable to the yogurt in their diet.

✤ SPECIFIC BENEFITS

High Cholesterol

Daily consumption of 1 cup of live yogurt that contains the bacteria *Lactobacillus acidophilus* has been shown to reduce total cholesterol by more than three percent and low-density lipoprotein (LDL) cholesterol (*see page 25*) by more than four percent. It is thought that the bacteria bind to the cholesterol in the intestine and reduce its absorption. Every one percent reduction in cholesterol is associated with an estimated two to three percent reduction in the risk of heart disease. Some scientists suggest that a daily intake of live yogurt may decrease the risk of heart disease by seven to ten percent.

Diarrhea

It has been shown that bacteria called *Lactobacillus* GG, which are added to some yogurts, are not digested, and colonize the walls of the large intestine. These bacteria fight harmful bacteria, including *Clostridium difficile*, which can cause diarrhea after a course of antibiotics. In human tests, *Lactobacillus* GG stopped diarrhea in people who had been ill with it for several months. As long as 25 years ago, doctors in the US showed in a study of 75 infants hospitalized with diarrhea, that those who were given only yogurt as a treatment recovered twice as quickly as those treated conventionally with a mix of neomycin, kaolin, and pectin.

Constipation

Increasing the amount of fiber in the diet is known to speed up the passage of stools. Research in France has shown that yogurt containing *Bifidus* bacteria has a similar effect on the large intestine to fiber. It therefore provides a good alternative for people who find it difficult or unpalatable to eat a high-fiber diet.

Irritable Bowel Syndrome

A regular intake of live yogurt can help to relieve some of the symptoms of irritable bowel syndrome (IBS). The yogurt encourages the intestines to increase their number of probiotic, or "friendly," bacteria, and helps to prevent the growth of harmful bacteria.

SEE ALSO CONSTIPATION, PAGE 175; DIARRHEA, PAGE 176; HIGH CHOLESTEROL, PAGE 154; IBS, PAGE 173

EGGS

Hen's eggs are the most common eggs to be eaten, but others are also available, including duck, goose, and quail eggs. These vary in size, color, and flavor. In recent years, there has been some concern that eggs raise cholesterol, but in most cases this is largely unfounded, because cholesterol in foods does not have a significant effect on the level of cholesterol in the blood.

KEY BENEFITS

- PROVIDE VITAMIN D TO HELP THE BODY TO ABSORB CALCIUM
- MAY IMPROVE MALE FERTILITY
- MAY PREVENT DAMAGE TO BLOOD VESSELS
- HELP TO KEEP NERVES IN WORKING ORDER

FOOD PROFILE

KEY NUTRIENTS *per 2 medium sized eggs (100g)*	HEN EGG	DUCK EGG
Calories	147	163
Protein (g)	13	14
Fat (g)	11	12
Saturated fat (g)	3	3
Monounsaturated fat (g)	5	5
Polyunsaturated fat (g)	1	2
Calcium (mg)	57	63
Iron (mg)	2	3
Vitamin D (mcg)	2	5
Vitamin B₁₂ (mcg)	3	5

HEN EGG

Color of yolk is due to carotenoids in bird's diet

GOOSE EGG

DUCK EGG

HIGH PROTEIN VALUE
Eggs contain a full complement of the eight essential amino acid protein building blocks. These are required for the growth and development of children and teenagers, and also help to keep adults in good health.

★ HOW MUCH TO EAT
- Eating three to four eggs a week, especially in the winter months, may help improve calcium absorption and possibly reduce the risk of osteoporosis.
- One egg supplies 8 percent of vitamin B₁₂.

CHOOSING & STORING
- Check the "use-by" date.
- Look for well-shaped eggs free from blemishes and cracks.
- Store in the refrigerator with the pointed ends facing down.

COOKING & EATING
- Boil or hard boil, poach, bake, fry, scramble, or pickle.
- Make into omelettes, soufflés, and pancakes.
- In cooking, make use of an egg's ability to thicken sauces, bind ingredients, coat foods, and glaze baked foods.

HEALING PROPERTIES

🗐 TRADITIONAL USES
Eggs have traditionally been a symbol of fertility in many cultures. In China, eggs are believed to be "warming," and are given to nourish the elderly and the weak. They are said to help cure diarrhea and prevent miscarriages, and are sometimes given to women who are carrying particularly active babies in their wombs. Eggs are thought to add moisture to the body and are often used to alleviate dry throats and eyes.

✛ SPECIFIC BENEFITS
Low Vitamin D Levels
Eggs are one of the few dietary sources of vitamin D, which the body needs to absorb calcium to create and maintain strong bones. Most of the body's vitamin D is made under the skin through the action of sunlight. The body can store it, and most people make enough during the summer to last the winter. Children up to three years old, who have not built up reserves, need an extra 7mcg a day, people over 65 need 10mcg, and pregnant women need 10mcg in the last three months of gestation. People who do not get enough exposure to the sun also need extra vitamin D. The intakes can be improved by including more eggs in the diet.

Male Infertility
Research has revealed that men require a good intake of selenium to ensure high sperm quality and quantity.

Intakes in Western Europe are falling, partly due to the use in bread of European soft flours, which are low in selenium, rather than American hard flours, which are relatively rich in this mineral. One egg supplies ten percent of an adult's recommended daily intake of selenium, and can contribute significantly to overall intakes when eaten regularly as part of a healthy, balanced diet.

Heart Disease
Eggs contain both selenium and vitamin E, two nutrients that are known to have antioxidant properties, which may reduce the risk of damage to blood vessels and therefore the likelihood of heart disease developing.

Nerve Damage
Eggs are useful sources of vitamin B₁₂, which is needed for the correct formation of the protective coating around nerves. A lack of B₁₂ can lead to irreversible nerve damage. Pregnant women who have a low intake of vitamin B₁₂ risk damaging their child's nervous system. Eggs also contain vitamin B₆ and folate, which are both necessary for healthy nerves.

CAUTION
Eggs can contain *Salmonella* bacteria, so they should not be eaten raw. People who may be particularly at risk, such as pregnant women, the elderly, and young children, should eat only well-cooked eggs.

SEE ALSO HEART DISEASE, PAGE 152; INFERTILITY IN MEN, PAGE 227

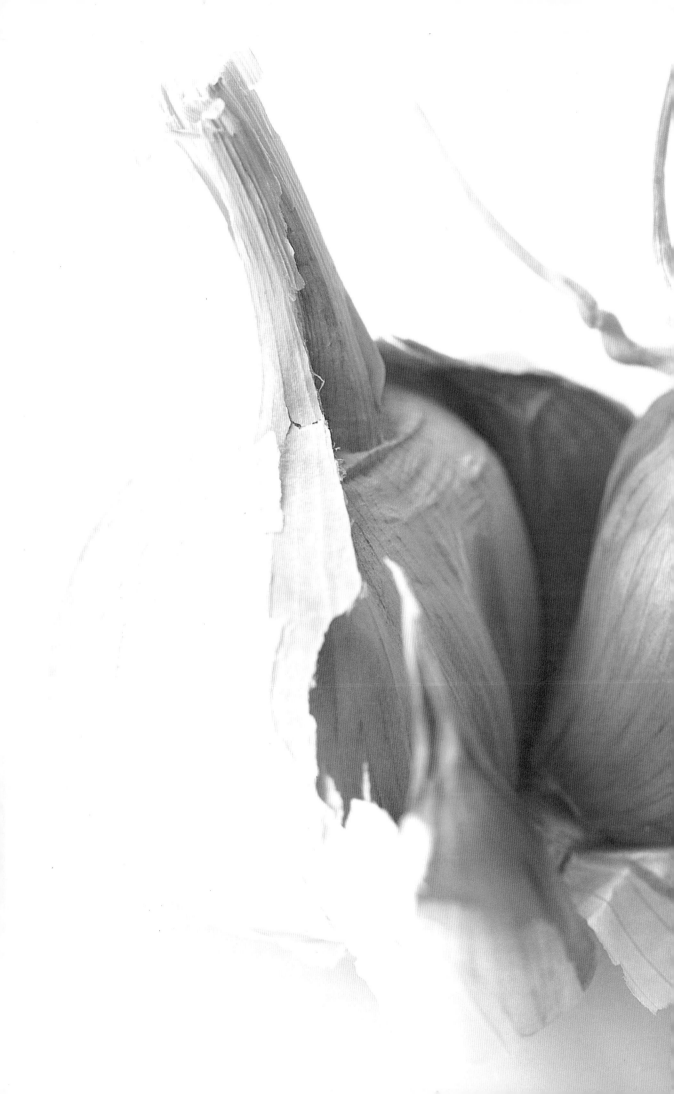

Life stages
& nutrition

It is now understood that our bodies
have different nutritional requirements
at different stages of life. It is increasingly
recognized that in many cases these
nutritional needs can be met through
dietary modification, while in other cases
modest supplementation with specific
nutrients may be of benefit.
This section outlines the dietary needs
for each of the main life-stages: infancy,
childhood, adolescence, adulthood, and
later life, with specific information
for men and women.

FOODS FOR LIFE

A BALANCED DIET IS an important foundation for health at all ages. From the age of five on, the definition of a balanced diet is one that takes most of its energy from carbohydrates – mainly complex carbohydrates rather than sugars – and which also includes several servings of protein a day and at least five servings of fruits and vegetables. Fats should provide the fewest calories of the major nutrient groups. During the first five years of life, again later on in life, and at certain stages in between, there are times when both males and females may need to alter the balance of major food groups in their diets and pay particular attention to specific nutrients.

THE IMPORTANCE OF ESSENTIAL FATS

While a diet that is relatively low in fat is generally recommended, it is nonetheless important throughout life to include adequate amounts of essential fats in the diet. These are found in oily fish, nuts, seeds, and vegetable oils. Until the age of five, children require greater amounts of total fats than adults. Putting infants and young children on a low-fat diet plan could stunt their growth. Adequate amounts of essential fats during infancy are also important, since they are needed for the development of the brain and the correct functioning of the eyes. Women who are pregnant or breast-feeding also need to take particular care to ensure adequate intakes of these essential fats, especially if pregnancies follow in quick succession, which may reduce the body's stock of nutrients.

VITAMINS & MINERALS

A well-balanced diet should provide enough energy to maintain the body and its activities. Sources of energy in foods come from carbohydrates, proteins, and fats. The diet should also contain sufficient vitamins and minerals, as well as plenty of protective phytonutrients, which are found in plants. At certain times in life, people need to pay special attention to these three nutrient groups, to promote optimum nutrition and reduce the risk of disease, or to build up stocks of nutrients that will be needed in later life. Adolescents should ensure that calcium intakes are high enough to maximize bone density, since the accumulation of calcium in the bones stops after the age of 20. Elderly people need to ensure that they have enough vitamin D to allow calcium absorption in order to protect against osteoporosis. People who may be susceptible to certain diseases, for example if heart disease or breast cancer is prevalent in their families, may

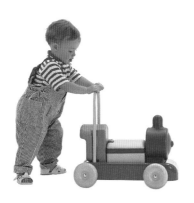

HEALTH FOR BABIES

Babies have special nutritional needs and should not be fed the same foods as the rest of the family. Breast milk is the ideal food for young babies, although some nutritional supplements, such as vitamins A, C, and D, may be necessary if the mother's diet is not adequate.

HEALTH FOR CHILDREN

Children grow rapidly and need whole-milk dairy products rather than low-fat varieties, particularly up to the age of five. Foods that are high in protein are more important than carbohydrates for this age group. A high intake of vitamin D is also necessary for growing bones.

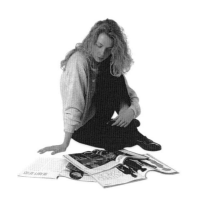

HEALTH FOR ADOLESCENTS

Adolescents need high-energy foods, which are necessary to fuel growth. Calcium is also very important at this stage, and a high intake of dairy products or other calcium-rich foods is advisable. Junk foods may exacerbate common adolescent problems, such as acne.

wish to alter their diet in order to reduce their chances of developing that condition. In the case of heart disease or breast cancer, this could be done by consuming more folate-rich foods, such as broccoli, or estrogen-rich foods, such as soybeans.

GROWTH & AGING

Growth is controlled by hormones and has four basic phases, during which time a person's nutritional requirements will alter. Children's weight, for example, can triple in the first year of life, and extra nutrients are needed to fuel this rapid growth. Then, until adolescence, growth rates slow down and are characterized by spurts and plateaus, which are often reflected in the child's changing appetite. Adolescence sees the next sustained burst in growth, and the diet will need to supply increased nutrient levels for a healthy transition into adulthood. The growth pattern tails off during adulthood and later, with old age, noticeable reductions in size and stature can be observed.

DIFFERENCES BETWEEN MEN & WOMEN

As a rule, men have higher energy requirements than women throughout life. At certain stages, variations in dietary requirements related to gender may widen, and extra care will need to be taken to make up any shortfalls. Teenage girls who experience heavy menstrual flows and women who have several pregnancies in quick succession, especially if they are vegetarian, need to be pariculary vigilant about iron intakes. Women planning a pregnancy need to increase folic acid intakes to help reduce the risk of giving birth to a baby with spina bifida or other defects of the spine. Boys and men may also need to alter their diets to meet their specific requirements. Many males in certain regions of the world have low intakes of the mineral selenium, which should be increased to reduce the risk of fertility problems and, possibly, the risk of cancer.

Men are generally at greater risk of developing heart disease than women, and they therefore need to take care to limit the amount of saturated fats in their diets in order to keep cholesterol levels down. Men also need good intakes of folate in foods or folic acid supplements in order to reduce the risk of raising levels of homocysteine in the blood. High levels of this substance can increase the risk of heart disease.

Increased intakes of some plant substances can benefit both men and women. For example, plant estrogens, which are found in soybeans, flax seeds, and alfalfa sprouts, are believed to lower the incidence of both prostate and breast cancer.

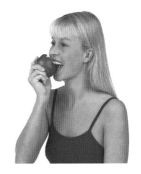

HEALTH FOR WOMEN

Women's nutritional needs will vary depending on their age, their menstrual cycle, and if they are pregnant or breastfeeding. At certain stages, it is wise to boost sources of various nutrients in the diet, such as iron, since these are likely to become depleted.

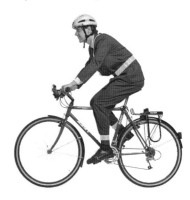

HEALTH FOR MEN

Regular exercise and a balanced diet that keeps fatty and fried foods to a minimum can have a strong influence on men's health. Many problems, such as heart disease, prostate cancer, and low fertility, can be avoided, or the risks lessened, by following these recommendations.

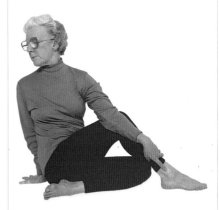

HEALTH FOR THE ELDERLY

Many health problems that are common in elderly people can be avoided by eating healthily and exercising regularly throughout life. Older people need to maintain these habits, and may also need dietary supplements of minerals such as vitamin C and zinc, which aid healing.

133

BABIES & NUTRITION

BREAST MILK IS THE IDEAL food for babies. It contains the correct proportion of nutrients required by a growing infant as well as key factors to help boost the baby's immune system, such as macrophages, lymphocytes, and antibodies, which protect a newborn child against both viral and bacterial infection. It has been shown that babies who are breast-fed for at least 13 weeks develop fewer diseases of the digestive tract and that this protection continues once breastfeeding has stopped. For mothers unable or unwilling to breast-feed, there are infant formulas available in powder and ready-to-feed liquid form. Although not giving the same immunological protection, these formulas are generally a nutritional match for breast milk. In spite of improvements to formulas, breastfeeding is encouraged because it provides other long-term benefits for a growing child.

THE FIRST FEW MONTHS

MOTHER'S DIET

When breastfeeding, it is important that a nursing mother's diet is varied and nutritious. Additional calcium is needed at this time: The usual daily requirement of 700mg should be boosted by 550mg. This is especially important for adolescent mothers, whose own growing bodies are still accumulating calcium to maximize bone density. Calcium-rich foods include milk, cheese, yogurt, and other dairy products, and tofu, legumes, sesame seeds and tahini, nuts, oily fish canned with their bones, and green leafy vegetables. Ten micrograms of vitamin D should be taken daily in supplement form to improve calcium absorption and ensure that calcium levels in breast milk are adequate. Oily fish, nuts, and seeds should be consumed regularly to boost the essential fats in breast milk and help the infant's brain and eyes to develop correctly.

VITAMIN SUPPLEMENTS

If a mother's diet is nutritionally balanced, a breast-fed infant should receive all the nourishment that he or she requires. Often, however, this does not happen, since the mother's diet does not contain the vitamins and minerals essential for an infant's development. If this is the case, the following daily supplements are advisable for breast-fed children until at least two years of age, and preferably until five years of age. In order to ensure that all of a child's dietary needs are covered, vitamins A, C, D, and K should be added to the diet in supplement form from about six months. Vitamins A, C, and D are available in the small quantities required at this stage in specially formulated infant drops. Ready infant formulas are fortified with vitamins and minerals, so additional vitamin supplements are not necessary.

FORMULAS

Modern formulas are a great improvement on their forerunners. While breastfeeding is always encouraged as the preferable method of feeding infants, these products offer an alternative for those who cannot breastfeed or choose not to do so. Based on cow's milk, the protein, carbohydrate, and fat contents are altered to match the quantities found in human milk. They also now contain long-chain essential fatty acids that are known to be essential for the development of the brain and sight in the infant. These substances occur naturally in the breast milk of women eating a diet containing oily fish, plant oils, nuts, seeds, fruits, and vegetables. Most babies require a daily intake of $^2/_3$ cup (150ml) of milk per 2lbs (1kg) of body weight. Intakes of milk that are below this level result in the infant being underfed. When making up powdered infant formulas, it is essential to follow the manufacturer's instructions exactly. Formulas that are overconcentrated can damage a baby's kidneys, while formulas that are inadequately concentrated can lead to poor growth.

DAILY CALORIE INTAKE

For the first three months, an infant's calorie intake is satisfied by milk. As weaning starts and progresses, other sources of energy become important.

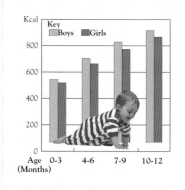

Kcal
Key: Boys, Girls

Age (Months): 0-3, 4-6, 7-9, 10-12

SOY FORMULAS

Soy-based formula milks are available for babies who are not breastfeeding and who cannot tolerate cow's milk formulas due to lactose intolerance. However, it is not advisable to use a soy formula without first consulting a doctor or nutritionist for advice.

WHEN TO WEAN A BABY

By the time a baby is four to six months old, its body systems have matured well enough for the baby to cope with the introduction of some solid foods to supplement the milk diet. Solids supply the extra energy required to meet the baby's increasing demands and satisfy the child's need to try out new tastes and textures. Delaying weaning beyond six months may lead to inadequate intakes of energy, protein, and a variety of vitamins and minerals.

KEY FOODS

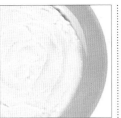

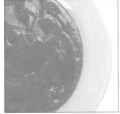

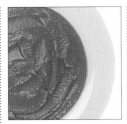

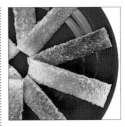

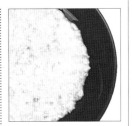

BABY RICE
Baby rice products can be mixed to a smooth consistency with water or baby milk formula. Rice cereal is bland, unlikely to cause allergic reaction, and usually very well tolerated by infants.

PURÉED FRUITS
Apples, pears, peaches, and apricots can be peeled and lightly cooked without sugar, then puréed. Fruit canned in natural juices may be used. Try different fruits to introduce new flavors.

PURÉED VEGETABLES
Carrots, cauliflower, rutabagas, potatoes, parsnips, and zucchini can be boiled without salt, then puréed. If one food is rejected, try another. Babies, like everyone else, have taste preferences.

TOAST
By six months of age, finger foods such as toast are suitable for babies. Wholewheat bread and toast can be introduced from six to seven months. Low-salt breads are available in supermarkets.

WHITE FISH
White fish is a source of protein that babies find easy to digest. A bland-tasting fish such as cod can be poached in milk, baked, or steamed. Always flake the fish and then strain it.

WEANING A BABY

WEANING FOODS

Foods need to be bland and without added sugar and salt. They should have a thin, smooth consistency so that the child's sucking reflex enables it to remove food from a spoon. At about four months, a baby can move food from the front to the back of the mouth, and swallow it. First-stage weaning foods can either be bought, or made by liquidizing or straining small amounts of suitable food. A vegetarian diet can be healthy for a baby, especially if eggs are included to supply essential nutrients. If parents or siblings have allergies to foods, such as cow's milk, wheat, or eggs, avoid introducing them into the diet until a baby is over six months old. Only whole cow's milk should be used until the age of two. Many mothers prefer to use formula milks until the age of one as they are fortified with vitamins and minerals and are more nutritious than cow's milk. It is essential that babies be supervised at all times when feeding to reduce the risk of choking. If one particular solid is rejected, another should be offered. If difficulties with feeding should arise, it may help to consult a speech therapist because the child may be having problems with mouth or tongue control.

INFANT DRINKS

There are many fruit-based infant drinks available that have no added sugar, but they are acidic and can damage the enamel of new teeth. Water is arguably the most suitable drink to quench a baby's thirst.

HOW MUCH TO FEED A BABY

AGE	PROGRESSION	FOODS	DRINKS
4 months	First 1–2 weeks	1 teaspoon of baby cereal mixed with formula milk to a runny consistency at one meal per day.	Maintain all milk formulas.
	Next 2 weeks	2 teaspoons of baby cereal mixed with formula milk to a smooth paste at two meals per day.	Maintain all milk formulas.
5 months	Next 4 weeks	Thicker cereals plus fruit and vegetable purées cooked without sugar or salt. Suitable fruits and vegetables include eating apples, apricots, peaches, pears, carrots, potatoes, parsnips, cauliflower, and zucchini. Ready-made weaning foods are available for this age group.	Maintain milk formulas and introduce extra fluids, such as cooled, boiled water.
6–8 months	Next 2–4 months	Minced or mashed foods and finger foods, such as pieces of toast, bananas, cooked carrots, and cooked cold meats. Always supervise a baby while these foods are being eaten.	Start reducing the number and quantity of milk formulas; give fluids such as cooled, boiled water.
8–10 months	Next 4–6 months	Mashed foods, white fish without bones, tuna, pasta, and chopped soft fruits.	Maintain a minimum of $2^1/_2$ cups (0.6 liters) of milk a day.
1 year	Next 6 months	Chopped-up family meals. At this stage, babies can start feeding themselves. Only give harder foods, such as chunks of raw apple and carrot, once a baby has learned to chew well. Never leave a baby alone with food, in case of choking.	Maintain $2^1/_2$ cups (0.6 liters) of milk a day.

CHILDREN & NUTRITION

HALF OF THE ENERGY in a baby's milk-based diet comes from fat. Between the time of weaning and five years of age, the contribution that fat makes to total calorie intake should be reduced gradually to 35 percent. Parents and caregivers are strongly advised against imposing an overly strict eating regime on small children. During this period of growth they need a varied diet. Overemphasizing starchy wholegrain foods and giving too many vegetables and fruits may displace energy-rich foods and protein foods by overfilling the child's relatively small stomach. On the other hand, eating large amounts of refined, sugary, and fatty foods could predispose a young child to poor habits in the long run and may compromise nutritional intake during these vital years. The key to good nutrition for children is to introduce plenty of new flavors and textures and, in this way, encourage children to enjoy foods that are inherently good for them.

FEEDING THE UNDER-FIVES

LAYING THE FOUNDATIONS

It is important to introduce as wide a variety of foods as possible. This helps to prevent nutritional imbalance and to establish the acceptance of a good range of textures and flavors, thus avoiding fussy eating habits. Occasional erratic eating patterns should not be too great a concern since children compensate for small intakes at some meals with larger intakes at others. Steady growth indicates that they are consuming adequate amounts. Increases of weight should average around $4^1/_2$ lbs (2 kg) per year from one to four years of age. If growth falls below this, it is worth discussing the possible causes with a doctor.

AVOIDING OBESITY

Children under five are dependent on others for providing the type and quantity of foods that they eat. So it is the responsibility of the parent or caregiver if a child starts to put on too much weight. Excessive amounts of candy, cookies, potato chips, and sugary drinks can lead to weight gain and should be avoided. Even at this early stage, exercise and active lifestyles need to be encouraged.

IRON DEFICIENCY

Late weaning, the early use of cow's milk rather than formulas, and a diet lacking in meats, fish, or other iron sources such as green vegetables, fortified cereals, and breads may contribute to iron deficiency and anemia. This makes children prone to infections, causes fatigue, and can adversely affect development. Parents with children on vegetarian diets need to take particular care. Foods containing vitamin C should be given with iron-rich plant foods to improve absorption of the iron.

FOOD REFUSAL

Refusing food is a powerful weapon used by toddlers against many an unsuspecting adult. If a child is growing normally, then bouts of tantrums concerning food are unlikely to cause any serious long-term nutritional problems. However, if growth or weight gain appear to be adversely affected, seek advice from a specialist.

PREVENTING CONSTIPATION

A number of simple measures can be taken to combat constipation. Foods such as baked beans, whole-grain cereals, lentil and ham soup or pea and ham soup, favorite fruits, and warmed fruit juice taken first thing in the morning can help. Make sure that a child drinks plenty of water throughout the day. A lack of fluids may be partly responsible for the problem.

DIARRHEA

It is not uncommon for otherwise healthy toddlers to have diarrhea, or pass very soft stools eight or more times a day. Often the root of the problem is that the stomach is still not fully developed, and a child will usually grow out of this by the age of four. Growth should be checked and, if on target, parents and caregivers need to ensure that the child is drinking plenty of fluids to avoid dehydration. They should also take care not to overfeed whole-grain cereals, wholewheat bread and pasta, and brown rice.

HOW MUCH TO FEED A CHILD

AGE	FOOD TYPES	AMOUNTS PER DAY
1–2 years	Milk (whole)	Three cups of milk a day plus milk on cereals.
2 years	Milk (low-fat)	Three cups of milk a day plus milk on cereals.
1 year	Sugary foods and drinks	Minimum amounts and only at mealtimes in order to help reduce risk of dental decay.
1–5 years	High-fiber foods	Moderate amounts since these foods are filling and may reduce nutrient intake.
	Low-fat foods	Moderate amounts since what is needed at this stage is plenty of energy-rich foods for proper growth and development.
Over 5 years	Low-sugar, low-fat, and high-fiber foods	More of these foods can be introduced gradually, but should not be relied on for most nutrients.

KEY FOODS

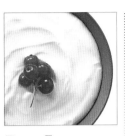

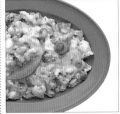

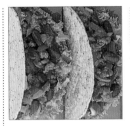

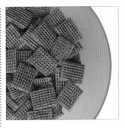

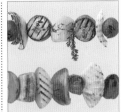

DAIRY FOODS
A small yogurt, $^3/_4$ cup (200ml) of milk, and $^1/_4$ cup (28g) of cheddar cheese together provide more than the 550mg of daily calcium that a ten-year-old needs for strong bones and teeth.

FISH, NUTS & SEEDS
These foods help the development of both sight and hearing and may prevent hyperactivity and dyslexia. Oily fish also supply iron and vitamin D, which is needed for calcium absorption.

LEAN RED MEATS
The best source of easily absorbed iron, meats help to prevent anemia and improve the body's ability to utilize plant sources of iron in the diet. Meats also supply vitamin B_{12}, needed for healthy nerves.

FORTIFIED CEREALS
Breakfast cereals provide fiber, and when fortified with iron and vitamins, they can contribute 15 percent or more of the recommended daily requirements of essential micronutrients.

FRUITS & VEGETABLES
These supply a range of protective vitamins, phytonutrients, and minerals. They also add texture, flavor, and a wide variety of color to the diet, thus stimulating an interest in food.

FEEDING THE OVER-FIVES

STARTING THE DAY
It is very important that children eat before leaving home for school. Skipping breakfast has been shown to lead to poor concentration and memory. Problem-solving ability is also reduced, and verbal reasoning and mathematical skills may also be affected. Cereal, toast, and fruit juice make an excellent start to the day by supplying energy, protein, and a wide range of vitamins and minerals.

PACKED LUNCHES
By the age of five it is appropriate for children to follow a healthy diet along the lines of those recommended for adults. Packed lunches for school need to provide a balance of nutrients. Some kind of protein in the form of cheese, meat, fish, or poultry should be included. Eggs, yogurt, legumes, nuts, and seeds are also good sources of protein. Carbohydrates can be provided in the form of bread, rice, or pasta. Some fruits and vegetables should also be included. Fruit juices make suitable drinks. Try to ensure that similar, vitamin-rich foods are offered by the child's other carers.

VEGETARIAN CHILDREN
Children can be brought up as vegetarians and be healthy. The key is providing alternatives to milk, such as soy milk with extra calcium. Iron requirements must be met through the careful inclusion of iron-rich foods. To ensure that all needs are being met, it is advisable to give a specially formulated children's vitamin and mineral supplement daily. Protein needs can be met by combining nuts, seeds, legumes, tofu, and soy milk with cereals and grains.

FOOD ADDITIVES
Many additives have been passed as safe for use in foods and drinks. A child's consumption of these can be minimized by limiting the number of processed foods in the diet.

TEETH
In order to protect a child's teeth, sugary and acidic foods should be consumed only at mealtimes. This helps to reduce the risk of tooth decay and tooth erosion. A poor diet during childhood adversely affects both first and second teeth. Acquiring the habit of chewing sugar-free gum after meals can help to reduce the risk of decay.

HYPERACTIVITY
Often starting at about the age of six and affecting more boys than girls, hyperactivity is distressing for the child, parents, and caregivers. A short attention span, impulsive behavior, and explosive outbursts may affect both home and school life. Learning difficulties, anxiety, and aggression are common symptoms. Great thirst is a common physical problem. Many hyperactive children benefit from a diet that is free of colorings and additives and supplemented by evening primrose oil, which supplies essential fatty acids needed for brain development. To avoid the risk of nutritional deficiencies, always seek advice from a qualified nutritionist before putting any child on a self-styled exclusion diet (*see page 247*).

FIGHTING INFECTIONS
High intakes of fruits and vegetables, including onions and garlic, may help to reduce the risk of infections in children. These foods can be given as wholefoods, as fruit and vegetable juices, or in dishes such as pizza and spaghetti with tomato sauce, to

DAILY CALORIE INTAKE
In considering how well a child's energy needs are being met, the key factor is whether he or she is growing at the rate expected. A doctor can advise on this.

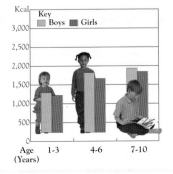

Kcal

Key
■ Boys ■ Girls

3,000
2,500
2,000
1,500
1,000
500
0

Age   1-3   4-6   7-10
(Years)

ADOLESCENTS & NUTRITION

THE FINAL AND PROFOUND growth spurt that takes place during adolescence brings with it specific nutritional requirements. Teenagers need adequate energy to support their growth in height, while teenage girls have an increased need of iron, especially once menstruation starts. Both sexes require extra vitamin D and calcium to allow the bones to reach maximum length and strength. These specific needs come at a time when dietary habits can be at their worst. Social and emotional pressures often adversely affect eating habits, leading to poor meal patterns, excessive snacking, and reliance on fast foods. As well as compromising vitamin and mineral intakes, these habits can make it hard to balance energy intakes. Teenagers may also restrict food intakes in order to maintain their preadolescent figures, and thus risk developing eating disorders.

HEALTH ISSUES

MINERAL INTAKES

A lack of calcium can be a particular problem for teenagers, especially if dairy products are not part of the diet. Calcium from these foods must be replaced by other good dietary sources because the bones establish their full density by the age of 20.

Many teenagers have inadequate calcium intakes. Calcium-rich foods that they might enjoy include milk shakes, yogurt, cheese, cereals with milk, baked beans, bread, ice cream, peanuts, and roasted sesame seeds. Calcium-enriched foods, such as cereal bars and orange juice, are now also available.

Increasingly, inadequate iron intake is becoming a problem for some teenage girls, especially for vegetarians. Iron needs increase with the onset of menstruation. The problem is made worse both by dieting to prevent weight gain and by early pregnancies. Suitable iron-rich foods include burgers that are 100 percent beef, oily fish, eggs, baked beans, fortified cereals, lentils, peanuts, dried apricots, and wholewheat bread. Foods rich in vitamin C, such as oranges and other citrus fruits, black currants, strawberries and other berries, potatoes, sweet potatoes, and peas, should be eaten with iron-rich foods to enhance iron absorption.

VITAMIN DEFICIENCIES

Levels of vitamin D may be low, especially during the winter, and if exposure to the sun in summer is limited. Vitamin D is essential for calcium absorption. Foods rich in vitamin D include mackerel, herrings and sardines, some yogurts, butter, and fortified margarines. A daily supplement of 10mcg may be advisable. Fortified breakfast cereals, eggs, and whole milk also supply vitamin D.

Vitamin C may be lacking in diets that contain few fresh fruits and vegetables. Fruit juices and drinks can be a useful way to improve intakes. In recent years, cases of scurvy caused by vitamin C deficiency have been identified in teenagers who rely on junk foods.

JUNK FOODS AND MISSED MEALS

Research has shown that adolescents snack regularly throughout the day. They tend to overindulge in potato chips, sweets, and canned drinks. Such foods are high in energy but relatively low in nutrients. In the long run, the prevalence and popularity of such foods highlights a nutritional paradox in the West: Namely, that in the midst of nutritional plenty, there is malnutrition.

A survey taken in the UK has shown that 18 percent of girls and 12 percent of boys aged 15 to 16 skip breakfast, replacing it with candy, chocolate, potato chips, and carbonated drinks. Breakfast can make an important contribution to daily vitamin and mineral intakes, especially if it includes a fortified cereal with milk. A nutritious, well-balanced breakfast can improve learning abilities and energy levels.

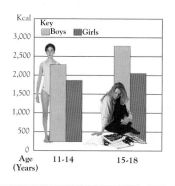

DAILY CALORIE INTAKE

Very active, athletic adolescents may require greater amounts of energy. Specific requirements for individuals vary according to height and build.

Key: Boys / Girls

(Bar chart — Kcal vs Age (Years), with values 0, 500, 1,000, 1,500, 2,000, 2,500, 3,000; ages 11–14 and 15–18)

LOOKING GOOD

Having clear skin is a priority for many adolescents. While there is no proof that chocolate and other candy cause pimples, there is good evidence to show that a diet rich in the essential fats found in nuts and seeds and oily fish contributes to a healthy, well-hydrated skin. The vitamin E in nuts, seeds, avocados, and green vegetables, and vitamin A found as beta carotene in orange, red, yellow, and green fruits and vegetables are also beneficial. Poor dietary habits can be reflected in the quality of skin and hair. Good dental health is also important. Avoiding sugary and acidic foods between meals can help to reduce the risk of tooth decay. Research shows that chewing sugar-free gum containing xylitol between and after meals can improve dental health and help to keep the breath fresh.

KEY FOODS

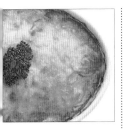 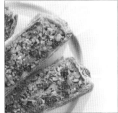 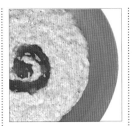 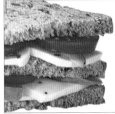 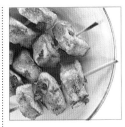

DAIRY FOODS	NUTS	FORTIFIED CEREALS	BREADS	MEATS & POULTRY
Milk, yogurt, and cheese supply the calcium that is needed for building bones in these critical growth years. There are reduced-fat versions, which limit the fat intake but without compromising on calcium.	Nuts supply not only energy but also protein, essential fats, calcium, and iron. Nuts do not promote tooth decay. As a sandwich filling, peanut butter is both convenient to use and nutritious.	Eaten with milk, these cereals are extremely nutritious. Vegetarians in particular should try to eat cereals fortified with iron, and drink fruit juices in order to build and maintain iron reserves.	Breads are a convenient source of carbohydrates, B vitamins, iron, and calcium. Eaten with a chunk of cheese or ham with tomato or peanut butter, they make a well-balanced meal or snack.	These are both excellent sources of protein and iron. Lean cuts of red meat are both low in fat and rich in zinc and selenium, two minerals that are important for the sexual maturity of adolescent boys.

THREATS TO ADOLESCENT HEALTH

EATING DISORDERS

The distribution of fat on the mature female body is at variance with the current fashionable look to have slim hips and thighs. Social and personal pressures brought on by this conflict can often trigger eating disorders in teenage girls, leading to bulimia and anorexia nervosa (*see page 181*). Such eating disorders need to be recognized and treated appropriately. Holistic approaches to healing, which attempt to address any underlying emotional problems, may be more appropriate than simply trying to reestablish the normal body weight through refeeding programs. Though for many years associated mainly with teenage girls, an increasing number of teenage boys are also falling prey to eating disorders such as anorexia, often triggered by stress (*see page 231*). The warning signs include weight loss or lack of growth, refusal or reluctance to eat at home, and eating unusual food combinations.

STRESS & INFECTIONS

Coping with the stresses of growing up, as well as those imposed by modern school life, makes demands upon the adolescent body's inner reserves. A varied diet that is rich in starchy carbohydrate foods supplies a range of B vitamins needed for healthy nerves, while plenty of fruits and vegetables supply vitamins and minerals to boost the immune system, thereby helping to fight infections.

ALCOHOL & DRUGS

The consumption of alcohol and recreational drugs can seriously compromise nutritional health, particularly if consumption is excessive and becomes a serious habit. Taking appropriate care of nutritional health is not behavior that is commonly associated with people who have problems with alcoholism or with drug or substance abuse. The risk of harming the body through such neglect is particularly high during the formative adolescent years. Addiction and inadequate nutrition at this stage of life are likely to have lasting adverse effects on development and growth. Alcohol and drug abuse therefore need to be identified and help sought promptly.

HOW MUCH TO EAT

CEREALS 5–11 SERVINGS DAILY	FRUITS & VEGETABLES 5 SERVINGS DAILY	MILK PRODUCTS 3 SERVINGS DAILY	MEATS & ALTERNATIVES 2 SERVINGS
1 slice of wheat bread 2 slices of rye bread $1/2$ cup (40g) breakfast cereal 2 cups (180g) boiled potatoes $1^3/4$ cups (150g) rice 2 cups (230g) pasta $1/2$ cup (40g) oatmeal	1 cup (200ml) fruit juices 1 cup (200ml) vegetable soup $3/4$ cup (80g) vegetables Salad vegetables in sandwiches and as garnish Tomatoes, peppers, and mushrooms on pizzas Onions and tomatoes in sauces	1 cup (200ml) milk $3/8$ cup (40g) cheese $2/3$ cup (150ml) yogurt 1 cup (200ml) soy milk fortified with calcium $3/4$ cup (190ml) custard	$1/4$lb (120g) lean meat $4^1/2$oz (130g) chicken breast $4^1/2$oz (130g) turkey $1/4$lb (120g) whire fish 3oz (90g) oily fish $1/2$ cup (50g) nuts $1/3$ cup (50g) legumes
SUPPLY	SUPPLY	SUPPLY	SUPPLY
Protein B vitamins Vitamin D and iron (in fortified cereals) Fiber	Vitamin C Carotenes Folate/Folic acid Potassium and iron Phytonutrients Fiber	Calcium Protein Vitamins A and D Magnesium	Protein Iron B vitamins Zinc Essential fats

WOMEN & NUTRITION

ONCE PHYSICAL AND SEXUAL maturity have been reached during adolescence, a woman's size, strength, and general health have to be maintained. This can be difficult given the wide variety of physical, psychological, social, and environmental pressures encountered throughout life. Of all the nutrition-related issues affecting women, body weight often assumes a high priority. Sensible eating patterns throughout adult life, combined with regular physical activity, can help a woman maintain a weight with which she feels comfortable. This strategy may help in reducing the risk of psychological problems, heart disease, and breast cancer. Regular intakes of soy-based foods may also discourage breast cancer, while eating plenty of foods rich in antioxidants may help to delay both the visible and the invisible signs of aging.

HEALTH ISSUES

WEIGHT FLUCTUATION
For many women, life-changing events such as pregnancy, child rearing, and menopause can affect their weight and how they see their own bodies. Good nutrition and a realistic attitude play important roles in helping to maintain a sensible body weight. Metabolism gradually slows down after the age of 30. Maintaining muscle mass by means of regular exercise helps to limit this process and to control weight if combined with a diet rich in fruits and vegetables; slowly digested carbohydrates, such as pasta; lean proteins, such as chicken, pork, and fish; and low-fat dairy products.

IRON DEFICIENCY
Iron deficiency is now a widespread problem. A woman should have 500mg of iron stored in her body, yet many women have just 150mg and some have none at all. In the UK for example, average intakes are about 11mg per day, compared with a recommended daily intake of 15mg. Iron is needed for the transportation of oxygen in blood. A lack of it leads to iron-deficiency anemia (*see page 160*), causing poor concentration, fatigue, irritability, and hair loss. Heavy menstrual blood loss and pregnancies in quick succession deplete reserves of iron even further.

LOW BONE DENSITY
Low bone density is a common problem after menopause. As levels of the hormone estrogen fall at this time of life, calcium levels in the bones also decrease. This reduces bone strength, making women prone to osteoporosis (*see page 199*) and fractures after menopause. It is essential to maintain good supplies of both calcium and vitamin D throughout life. Diets rich in dairy products or soy substitutes enriched with calcium, fish canned with their bones, legumes, sesame seeds, and tofu provide calcium. Vitamin D is found in eggs, oily fish like herrings and mackerel, and fortified breakfast cereals, and is also made in the skin on exposure to sunlight. Meats, fish, and foods rich in vitamin C help the body to absorb iron. Tea, coffee, and large quantities of dairy products, when taken at the same time as iron-rich foods, lower absorption of iron.

MAINTAINING LOOKS
Eating a wide variety of fruits, vegetables, and whole-grain cereals supplies an array of vitamins, minerals, and phytonutrients that seem to play key roles in keeping the skin, eyes, gums, nails, and hair in good condition. Regular daily intakes may help to combat the physical signs of aging. Plant estrogens, such as the isoflavones, behave in the body like human estrogen. Six to eight hours after foods rich in isoflavones are eaten, blood levels of isoflavones peak, before being excreted in the urine. So dietary intakes must be regular to maintain good plant estrogen levels. Isoflavones are similar to the human estrogen, estradiol. They can latch onto estrogen receptors in the breast, but do not make breast cells replicate, so they may reduce the risk of breast cancer. Studies reveal that isoflavones depress cholesterol levels by ten percent and reduce vaginal dryness and hot flashes associated with menopause.

HOW MUCH TO EAT

FOOD	EXAMPLES OF SERVING SIZES	SERVINGS PER DAY
Breads, cereals, and potatoes	1 slice of bread, 3 tbsp breakfast cereal, 1 tbsp cooked rice or pasta, 1 small potato (100gm)	5–11
Fruits and vegetables	2 tbsp vegetables, small salad, 3oz (80g) of fruit, $^1/_2$ cup (100ml) fruit juice	5+
Meats and meat alternatives	2–3oz (55–85g) lean skinless meat, oily fish, or poultry. 4–5oz (110–140g) white fish or eggs, $1^1/_3$ cups (300g) cooked beans	3
Fats	1 tsp butter or margarine, 1 tsp oil, 1 tsp mayonnaise, 2 tsp reduced-fat spread	1–2
Refined foods	Small portions of fatty foods, $1^1/_2$oz candy, 2 cookies, 1 slice of cake	1–2

KEY FOODS

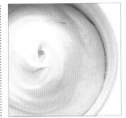

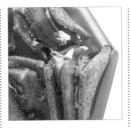

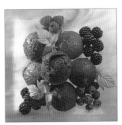

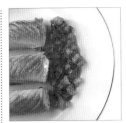

SOY

Soy and soy products such as soy milk, soy yogurt, and tofu supply quantities of plant estrogens that may reduce the risk of heart disease and breast cancer. Soy products that have been enriched with calcium are the most appropriate ones to select.

DAIRY FOODS

Skim milk, low-fat yogurt, and reduced-fat cheeses provide calcium and may help to reduce the risk of osteoporosis after menopause. Since calcium is in the watery part of milk, removing fat from milk does not reduce its calcium content.

WHOLEWHEAT

Rich in insoluble fiber, wholewheat breads and cereals are low-fat sources of energy that may help to reduce the risk not only of breast cancer, but also of colonic cancer by adding to the bulk and weight of stools and speeding their passage through the colon.

BERRIES

Rich in phytonutrients, black- and blueberries may help to strengthen collagen. Collagen is the protein network that gives skin its structure and plumpness. A diet rich in these antioxidants may help to delay the visible signs of skin aging.

FISH, NUTS & SEEDS

Oily fish, nuts, and seeds contain essential fatty acids needed to keep the cells well hydrated. A lack of essential fats can lead to skin dryness. Oily fish also provides a form of iron that is easily absorbed by the body and enhances iron absorption.

PLANNING A DIET FOR LIFE

DELAYING AGING

Antioxidant nutrients, such as vitamins C and E and beta carotene, as well as the phytonutrients found in many fruits, vegetables, and drinks such as tea appear to help to delay aging. There is evidence that these foods may also slow down age-related damage to the eyes, improve the strength of the collagen under the skin, and reduce the risk of heart disease (*see page 152*). Some foods may also help to relieve some symptoms of menopause (*see page 223*). Diets that are rich in plant estrogens, which are found, for example, in soy and flaxseeds, have been linked to a reduction in hot flashes and vaginal dryness.

PREVENTING DISEASE

Manipulating the diet has been shown to reduce women's health problems. Regular consumption of cranberry juice, for example, can prevent and relieve the urinary infection cystitis (*see page 190*). Removing sugar and yeast from the diet can prevent yeast infections, while cutting out wheat-based foods and dairy products can combat irritable bowel syndrome (*see page 173*). Adding essential fatty acids to the diet in the form of oily fish, nuts, seeds, and supplements of evening primrose oil can help to alleviate a number of problems, such as the breast discomfort associated with the menstrual cycle and also some premenstrual symptoms, including low moods and irritability (*see page 222*).

A long-term diet that is both low in fat and alcohol and rich in the plant estrogens that are found in soybeans, soy-based foods such as tofu, and whole-grain cereals may help reduce the risk of breast cancer (*see page 214*). Nutritionists recommend a diet that is low in saturated fats but rich in fruits and vegetables packed with antioxidants, and high in folic acid. Regular exercise is also useful in helping to stabilize weight and prevent osteoporosis (*see page 198*).

FOODS TO AVOID

Fried foods, meat products, potato chips, cookies, cakes, and chocolate tend to be rich in fats. Fats have more calories per ounce than protein and carbohydrates foods, and high intakes are therefore likely to lead to weight gain. Reducing foods that are high in fats may help women who are trying to control their weight. Refined and sugary foods rapidly raise blood sugar levels and may lead to cravings. Sugary foods are often high in fat, which can adversely affect appetite control. Alcohol should only be taken in moderation since regular intakes are associated with an increased risk of breast cancer.

DAILY CALORIE INTAKE

A woman's daily calorie requirements are less affected by her age than by whether she is pregnant or breastfeeding.

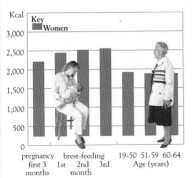

Kcal

Key
Women

3,000
2,500
2,000
1,500
1,000
500
0

pregnancy brest-feeding   19-50 51-59 60-64
first 3   1st 2nd 3rd   Age (years)
months   month

PLANT ESTROGENS

Of the four plant estrogen groups, the most important to the human diet are the isoflavones and the lignans.

PLANT ESTROGEN	SOURCE
Isoflavones	Soybeans, tofu, soy milk, chickpeas, cherries
Lignans	Wheat, bran, rye, oatmeal, barley
Coumestrans	Green beans, sprouts, split peas, alfalfa, soy
Resorcylic acid lactones	Oats, rye, sesame

MEN & NUTRITION

IT IS WIDELY PERCEIVED that a man can help to reduce his risk of heart disease by making certain changes to his diet. Reducing the total amount of fat and saturated fat and maintaining the correct weight for height are fundamental to this protective process. It is increasingly being recognized that many health problems in men – from diabetes to impotence – may be affected by regular food intakes. High blood pressure can be lowered by achieving and maintaining the correct body weight. Evidence is emerging that the risk of heart disease may also be reduced by increasing intakes of the B vitamin folic acid. New research has revealed that the risk of prostate disease and infertility may also be linked to a man's lifelong dietary habits, and it is generally accepted that a diet rich in insoluble fiber may lessen the risk of colonic cancer.

HEALTH ISSUES

HEART DISEASE

Before the age of about 50, men are more likely to develop heart disease (*see page 152*) than women. Risk factors for heart disease are many, and include lifestyle and emotional factors as well as diet. Nutrition can play a big role in offering protection from this disease, which is a major cause of death in middle-aged men. Maintaining the correct body weight can help to keep blood pressure down, while a diet that is low in saturated fats, and rich in antioxidants from fruits and vegetables, and fish oils from oily fish can help to reduce the risk of clogged and blocked arteries.

Recent research has indicated that a diet supplying good amounts of folate or folic acid can reduce blood levels of homocysteine. It is now believed that excess levels of this substance are just as likely to be responsible for heart disease as high levels of cholesterol.

PROSTATE PROBLEMS

Cancer of the prostate appears to have a higher incidence in the West than in China or Japan. It is possible that the Eastern diet, which is rich in plant estrogens, may help to protect against this cancer (*see page 214*). Levels of plant estrogen in the blood of Japanese men have been found to be 110 times higher than in the blood of men who eat Western-style diets. Soybeans and soy products are the main sources of plant estrogens. These foods should be consumed on a regular basis in dishes based on textured vegetable protein, soy milk and soy yogurt, tofu, berries, and wholewheat bread.

Supplements of saw palmetto, rye pollen, and golden rod have been used successfully to relieve symptoms of benign prostatic hyperplasia. This is the noncancerous swelling of the prostate gland, and leads to urinary problems that can otherwise only be treated with drugs or surgery.

FERTILITY

Male fertility (*see page 225*) is affected by the supply of vitamins and minerals in the diet. Sperm activity and viability seem to be directly related to the available amounts of vitamins C and E as well as the minerals selenium and zinc. It is therefore important that men choose foods from as wide a range as possible, including red meats and fish, whole-grain cereals, and plenty of fruits and vegetables.

STRESS

The pressures on men to perform in so many areas of life, including work and in their family and personal relationships, can lead to high levels of stress (*see page 231*). The nervous system may be fortified by ensuring regular intakes of B vitamins, which are found in milk, meats, and vegetables, and folate in cereals.

WEIGHT & LIFESTYLE

The speed at which calories are burned by the body is determined by metabolic rate. Factors that affect metabolic rate include height, weight, genetic tendencies, and, very importantly, the amount of lean body tissue or muscle. The burning up of calories is also affected by levels of activity. Those men who do plenty of exercise or manual work may need as many as 2,500 calories more than the average recommended daily intake. Men who lead a sedentary lifestyle may need less than the recommended intake in order to maintain body weight.

HOW MUCH TO EAT

FOOD	EXAMPLES OF SERVING SIZES	SERVINGS PER DAY
Breads, cereals, and potatoes	1 slice of bread, 3 tbsp breakfast cereal, 1 tbsp cooked rice or pasta, 1 small potato (100g)	5–11
Fruits and vegetables	2 tbsp vegetables, small salad, 3oz (80g) fruit, $1/_2$ cup (100ml) fruit juice	5+
Meats and meat alternatives	2–3oz (55–85g) lean skinless meat, oily fish, or poultry, 4–5oz (110–140g) white fish or eggs, $1^1/_3$ cups (200g) cooked beans	3
Fats	1 tsp butter or margarine, 1 tsp oil, 1 tsp mayonnaise, 2 tsp reduced-fat spread	1–2
Refined foods	$1^1/_2$oz candy, 2 cookies, 1 slice of cake	1–2

KEY FOODS

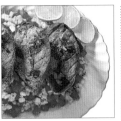 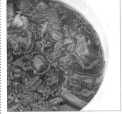 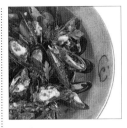 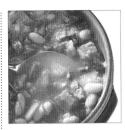 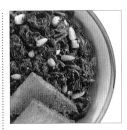

OILY FISH
Salmon, mackerel, tuna, pilchards, and sardines are rich in essential fatty acids that appear to reduce the risk of blood clots and so lower the risk of heart disease. They are also an excellent source of protein, which is needed for the maintenance of body tissues, especially muscle.

GARLIC & ONIONS
Garlic and the onion family, for example, chives, all contain plant nutrients, known as phytonutrients, that help to reduce cholesterol and lower the risk of heart disease. They are also known to have antibacterial and antiviral properties and may reduce the risk of infections.

SEAFOOD
Shellfish are excellent sources of zinc needed for sperm production, and also supply a low-fat source of protein. Although some, such as shrimp, contain cholesterol, this is mostly excreted from the body and therefore does not raise cholesterol levels.

LEGUMES
Foods such as baked beans, red kidney beans, and lentils supply the body with soluble fiber. Also found in oats, soluble fiber helps to reduce cholesterol levels, reducing the risk of heart disease. Legumes are also sources of both protein and carbohydrates.

GREEN VEGETABLES
These supply folate, the B vitamin believed to reduce homocysteine levels in the blood. In excess, homocysteine seems to clog arteries and increase the risk of heart disease. Green vegetables also provide the valuable antioxidants vitamin C and beta carotene.

CONTROLLING WEIGHT

UNDERSTANDING WEIGHT GAIN
A man's metabolic rate is highest at the age of 27. After this it falls each year, with a drop of 12 percent likely between this age and 47. A fall in metabolic rate means that fewer calories are needed to maintain the same body weight. Exercise increases and maintains muscle mass and can help to reduce this fall in metabolic rate.

It is important for a man to maintain a suitable weight for his height. The pattern of weight distribution in men tends to lead to fat deposition around the abdomen. This in turn puts particular strain on the heart and internal organs. A man should aim for a diet in which no more than 35 percent of the calories comes from fat; for a man consuming 2,500 calories per day, this is a total daily allowance of about 90g of fat. Men who wish to lose weight may safely reduce their daily fat intake to 50g. Regular aerobic and strength-training exercise, combined with sensible eating habits, form the basis of a long-term strategy for successful weight management.

BUILDING MUSCLE
Body weight can be increased by augmenting fat reserves or muscle mass. Extra fat and extra muscle both appear the same on the scales, but their appearance on the body is very different. Lean muscle is built through strength or resistance training, which stimulates the growth of muscle fibers. The correct diet is crucial for this process. It is realistic to expect an increase in muscle of 1–2lbs (0.5–1kg) a month. It takes 2,500 calories to build 1lb (0.5kg) of muscle. People who gain muscle slowly should increase food intake by 500 calories a day; those who gain muscle rapidly may only need to increase daily food intake by 300 calories. About 1.4–1.7g of protein per pound (kg) of body weight are needed to support a strength-training program. Extra protein needs are usually met by the normal diet. About 65 percent of the calories consumed need to be carbohydrates, and it is recommended that the day's food be divided into five or six meals and snacks so that food is eaten every two or three hours.

EXERCISE
A diet rich in cereals, fruits, and vegetables, and thus carbohydrates, is important for all men. For those who get regular exercise, it is even more important that the diet have a high proportion of carbohydrates, which fuel working muscles.

FOODS TO AVOID
Men typically gain excess fat around the abdomen, and thereby develop a "beer gut." This fat accumulation increases the risk of heart disease and imposes a strain on the back, affecting posture. Many foods can increase the risk of male middle-age spread, including fried foods, such as fish and chips, fast foods, meat products, and rich desserts. Regular eating habits can contribute to a steady weight gain; for example, eating bread and butter with meals or including a dessert as part of all meals, putting butter on cooked vegetables or in sauces, adding mayonnaise and dressings to meat, fish, and salads, and drinking alcohol on a regular basis.

DAILY CALORIE INTAKE
These vary with size and activity level. A large, active man may need up to 3,000 more calories than a small, inactive man.

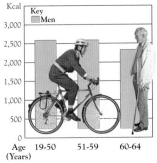

Key: Men

Age (Years): 19-50, 51-59, 60-64

THE ELDERLY & NUTRITION

T HE CONCEPT OF "ELDERLY" has changed over the decades as lifespans extend. Current thinking divides older members of society into the young-old, aged from 65 to 74, the older-old, aged from 75 to 84, and the oldest-old, aged 85 years and upward. Gerontology, the study of the aging process, recognizes that the process both affects nutritional status and is affected by the nutritional composition of the diet. It is now believed that good nutrition throughout life may help to reduce the risk of certain cancers and heart disease, and lessen the risk of age-related damage to the eyes, bones, muscles, and brain. While a healthy balanced diet remains central to good nutrition among the elderly population, the smaller amounts of food consumed and less efficient digestive processes may help to increase the acceptability of nutrient supplementation.

HEALTH ISSUES

AGING

Rates of aging are affected by genetics, traumas encountered throughout life, and nutritional history. The aging process changes the way that certain vitamins are absorbed. For example, if less acid is produced in the stomach, the absorption of vitamin B_1 is reduced, and vitamin B_{12} absorption may be affected. A reduction in the amount of digestive juices and a slowing down of movement in the digestive tract can reduce the body's absorption and utilization of various nutrients.

A dry mouth is due to a severe reduction in saliva flow and affects about one elderly person in five. A lack of saliva means that the initial digestion of starches that takes place in the mouth does not occur, which makes swallowing difficult. This, combined with a dulling of the sense of smell, which reduces the ability to taste foods, can lead to a decline in their enjoyment and consumption, resulting in a reduction in intakes of all nutrients.

Aging leads to a reduction in lean muscle and organs. As a result there is a decrease in resting metabolic rate – the rate at which energy is burned by the body (*see page 146*) – and therefore a reduced energy need. Since the micronutrient needs either remain unchanged or may increase, the overall quality of the diet must be high. If the decline in muscle mass is combined with a decrease in activity but no adjustment to the quantities of food eaten, weight gain may occur and the risk of diabetes and heart disease increase.

MENTAL AGILITY

It is known that dehydration through an inadequate intake of fluids can contribute to confusion in older people. A lack of potassium has a similar effect. Although many older people prefer to limit their fluid intakes in order to avoid frequent urination, it is important that fluid levels are kept up throughout the day to reduce the likelihood of dehydration. Bananas and other fruits, fruit and vegetable juices, and all vegetables are good sources of potassium and should be included in the diet daily.

KEEPING ACTIVE

Maintaining levels of physical activity in old age is extremely important. Exercised muscles provide both stability and strength. Resting metabolic rates are maintained by exercised muscles, and their strength also helps to prevent falls and bone fractures. Exercise can also improve mental well-being. All these factors can help elderly people to maintain their independence, and can affect their chances of living well and enjoying life into old age.

HOW MUCH TO EAT

FOODS	SERVING SIZE	SERVINGS PER DAY
Breads, cereals, and potatoes	2 slices of bread, 1 medium-sized potato, 1 cup (150g) pasta, $1/4$ cup (30g) cereal	at least 1 at each meal
Meats, fish, poultry, eggs, cheese, legumes	3–4oz (80–100g) meat, fish, or poultry, 1 large egg, 4oz (100g) cheese or legumes	1 serving at two meals per day
Carrots, broccoli, and other vegetables	3oz (80g)	2–3 per day
Apples, bananas, and other fruits	3oz (80g)	2–3 per day
Milk, yogurt, rice pudding, and custard	$1^1/4$–$2^1/2$ cups (0.3–0.6 liters)	Each day
Butter and spreads	small amounts	

DAILY CALORIE INTAKE

Calorie intake requirements fall as people age. Between ages 65 and 75 there is a daily reduction of about 230 calories for men, and about 90 calories for women.

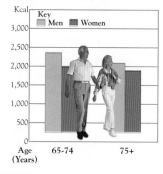

KEY FOODS

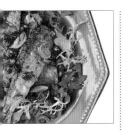 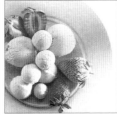 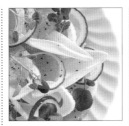 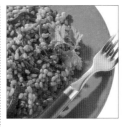 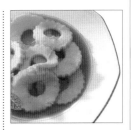

SARDINES
These are a good source of protein and supply omega-3 essential fatty acids, which help to protect against heart disease and inflammation. Canned sardines are an excellent source of bone-strengthening calcium.

DAIRY FOODS
Milk products, such as cheese, yogurt, and ice cream, are excellent sources of calcium. Whole-milk versions contain vitamin A, which helps to keep the lining of the respiratory and digestive tracts in good condition.

ORANGES
Oranges are rich in vitamin C, and eating them is an easy way to get this key antioxidant. Regular, high intakes help to keep the immune system strong, and may help to prevent cataracts and glaucoma.

WHOLEGRAINS
Eating whole-grain cereals, brown rice, and wholewheat bread and pasta is a good way to increase intakes of soluble fiber. Fiber, if combined with adequate water intakes, helps to treat and prevent constipation.

APPLES
Apples contain soluble fiber, which helps to keep cholesterol and blood sugar levels down. Apples are rich in potassium, which helps to maintain normal blood pressure, and sorbitol, which helps to prevent constipation.

FIGHTING DISEASE

HEALING & IMMUNITY
Vitamin C, found in vegetables and fruits, and zinc, available in meat and fish, are important for wound repair and a strong immune system. Diets rich in these nutrients, or supplemented by them, are advisable to heal wounds and fight infection, especially after surgery.

NUTRITION AND DRUGS
Nutrient absorption can be affected by prescription drugs, some of which may impair appetite, digestion, and saliva production. For example, the anticonvulsant phenytoin can reduce absorption of vitamin D and folate. Biguanides, used to treat diabetes, can destroy vitamin B_2 and folate, and drugs known as thiazide diuretics and loop diuretics can cause potassium, magnesium, and zinc deficiencies. Though these effects are recognized, often little is done to help the elderly overcome them.

ANTIOXIDANT PROTECTION
One branch of biomedical research is focusing on how damage to cells by free radicals affects aging. Good intakes of antioxidant nutrients such as vitamins C and E, the mineral selenium, and phytonutrients such as carotenoids and bioflavonoids may help to reduce the risk of conditions such as cataracts, glaucoma, arthritis, and even mental degeneration.

INFLAMMATORY CONDITIONS
Elderly people in particular may benefit from eating oily fish, such as sardines, pilchards, tuna, herrings, and kippers. These supply essential fats, which are known to lessen the inflammatory processes in the body and may alleviate such medical problems as rheumatoid arthritis.

KEEPING BONES HEALTHY
Osteoporosis results from the long-term decline in bone mass and leads to fractures, most often of the femur and the vertebrae. Adequate calcium intake is therefore important for older age groups, to help with the maintenance of bone density. Osteomalacia, or adult rickets, results from too little vitamin D, which is needed for calcium absorption. People who get little exposure to sunlight often have a vitamin D deficiency. Dietary sources include oily fish, eggs, some cereals, and cod liver oil. Adults over 65 years of age are advised to maintain a dietary intake of 10mcg of vitamin D a day.

SUPPLEMENTARY BENEFITS

VITAMIN E Powerful antioxidant able to protect against free-radical damage and possibly reduce heart disease.
Suggested daily intake: 100mg

BETA CAROTENE May help to reduce the risk of cataracts.
Suggested daily intake: 15mg

BILBERRY EXTRACTS Seem to help maintain vision, improve the function of arteries and veins, and possibly improve memory.
Suggested daily intake: 200mg

SELENIUM Antioxidant properties may reduce the risk of heart disease as well as some cancers.
Suggested daily intake: 50–200mg

ZINC Needed for a strong immune system to help fight infections.
Suggested daily intake: 15mg

COENZYME Q10 Appears to stimulate heart muscle cells.
Suggested daily intake: 30mg

GINGKO BILOBA May improve blood circulation to limbs and all organs, including the brain and heart.
Suggested daily intake: 40mg

FISH OIL Appears to keep the blood thin and reduces the risk of heart disease and stroke.
Suggested daily intake: 1g

EVENING PRIMROSE OIL When combined with fish oils, may improve symptoms of rheumatoid arthritis.
Suggested daily intake: 3g

GARLIC Known to fight infections and may help to reduce the risk of heart disease.
Suggested daily intake: 10g

ASSESSING YOUR HEALTH NEEDS

AS AN INDIVIDUAL, each person has specific, individual nutritional needs that are shaped by his or her age, gender, lifestyle, activity levels, and state of health. In addition, a person has a unique set of biochemical processes at work in the body that determine how food is broken down and nutrients absorbed. When assessing nutritional needs, it is necessary to take as much of this information as possible into account. An accurate assessment of dietary needs is not always easily achieved, but a broad overview may be enough to tailor the diet to meet general requirements. The overall aim should be to keep the body healthy and to ensure that the correct body weight is maintained, and the best way to do this is with a balanced diet. Health professionals can provide specialized dietary advice if necessary.

UNDERSTANDING YOUR NEEDS

BEING AWARE OF YOUR DIET
It can be easy to disregard the role the diet plays in keeping the body healthy. A balanced, regular intake of foods from a variety of food groups is needed in order to maintain a healthy weight. Keeping the weight within a certain range is not the only reason for eating. The nutrients in foods have special health-giving qualities. A deficiency in the diet can produce conditions such as depression or irritability, as well as physical problems such as anemia. It is the tendency of many people in the West not to see food in terms of its healing properties, but simply as something to stave off hunger. By becoming aware of the range of functions that food has in the body, it is possible to adjust the diet as necessary to maintain good health.

KEEPING A FOOD DIARY
Making a note of everything you eat over a number of days can provide a good insight into overall dietary balance, and will highlight areas that may need adjustment. Make a detailed record of all the foods and drinks that you consume every day over the course of a week. Fill in the time at which you ate each meal or snack. Note how many servings of the following foods you eat: fruits and vegetables, and carbohydrates such as breads, pasta, potatoes, and rice. Also note if the starchy foods were 100 percent wholewheat or whole-grain, and record how much sweet or salty snack foods and fried foods you ate, and if you had any alcoholic drinks.

Then read the guidelines for a balanced diet (*see page 10*) and see how well your diet compares. If you are not eating a wide enough range of foods from the different food groups, you may not be ingesting all of the essential nutrients that your body needs.

HOW HEALTHY IS YOUR DIET?

The checklist below will help you to find out if your diet is balanced. Check the box if you can answer "yes" to the question. If you check more than eight boxes, your diet is fairly good. Fewer than that and your diet could be improved.

Do you eat five or more servings of fruits and vegetables each day? ❑

Do you choose a wide variety of fresh or frozen fruits and vegetables? ❑

Do you include some carbohydrates, such as rice or pasta, in most meals? ❑

Do you choose whole-grain cereals, rice, and pasta, as often as possible? ❑

Do you vary your diet and have a few meat-free days each week? ❑

Do you discard all of the fat on meats and the skin on poultry? ❑

Do you try to avoid processed meats such as sausages, pies, and burgers? ❑

Do you bake or grill most of your food rather than fry it? ❑

Do you use vegetable oils for cooking wherever possible instead of lard? ❑

Do you use butter and margarine as sparingly as possible? ❑

Do you tend to choose lowfat rather than whole-milk dairy products? ❑

Do you restrict your intake of cakes, cookies, candy, and salty snacks? ❑

ASSESSING CALORIE INTAKES

The body uses food as a source of energy, and the amount of energy used by the body is measured in calories.

Metabolic rates
The number of calories that the body uses over 24 hours when totally at rest is known as the Resting Metabolic Rate or RMR. You can work out your RMR using the following equation:

Calculating your RMR (1kg = 2.2lb)
• 18–30 yrs: (weight kg x 14.7) + 496
• 31–60 yrs: (weight kg x 8.7) + 829

Calculating calorie needs
To estimate your total calorie needs for the day you need to take into account activity levels. Choose a figure from those below based on the amount of regular exercise that you do. Sedentary people should multiply their RMR by 1.4. If you are moderately active, multiply your RMR by 1.7. For those who are very active, multiply RMR by 2.0. For example, a 45-year-old woman who weighs 60kg, has an office job, and does little physical exercise will calculate her RMR and calorie needs as following:
• 60 x 8.7 + 829 = 1,351 RMR
• 1,351 x 1.4 = 1,891.4 calories per day.

EFFECTS OF FOOD PROCESSING

CHECKING YOUR WEIGHT

These tables will help to give you an idea of whether your weight-to-height ratio is within the healthy range. Choose the appropriate table, then pick your height from the list on the left-hand side. Run your finger across and find your weight.

The colored bars indicate whether you are overweight, underweight, or average for your height. If your weight is more than 20 percent above the normal range, you are considered obese, which may endanger your health.

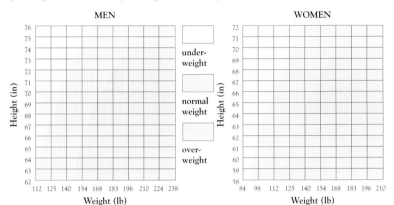

influencing factors, such as age, body shape, genetic, and metabolic make-up, vary from person to person. The tables (left) can help you to work out if your weight is "healthy."

NUTRITION AT DIFFERENT AGES

People have special dietary requirements at different ages. For example, children under five years of age need to eat whole-milk dairy products, which are essential for growth and development. Extra calcium and vitamin D are needed by adolescents to ensure that their bones have the best chance of reaching maximum density by the age of 20. Elderly people need high intakes of vitamin D, which helps to improve calcium absorption, in order to maintain bone health.

FOOD & METABOLISM

Metabolism is the name for all the chemical processes that occur in the body. One result of metabolic processes is the production of energy, which comes from the burning of energy sources (calories) in food.

The metabolic rate is the energy required to maintain the body's basic functions, such as breathing and blood circulation. This rate is controlled by hormones, and it increases in response to factors such as fear and exertion.

These hormones influence the rate at which cellular processes are carried out. A person may have a naturally slow metabolic rate, which is likely to be caused by a deficiency in one of the types of hormone that control this process. This means that the body burns energy less efficiently. A person with a slow metabolic rate who gains weight easily may find that eating smaller meals more frequently helps to speed up their metabolism.

A slow metabolic rate may also be brought about by dieting or not eating enough. The metabolic rate slows down in order to preserve energy, which may cause a person to gain weight. For this reason, it is advisable to avoid skipping meals.

BODY WEIGHT

With an increasing trend toward less active lifestyles and diets that tend to be rich in fat, many people struggle to avoid gaining excess body fat. Being honest with yourself in assessing your weight is the first step toward getting the balance right. There is no ideal weight, since

NUTRITIONAL DEFICIENCIES

The effects of a poor diet can sometimes be seen clearly in the physical condition of different parts of the body. The chart below describes some problem areas and suggests the nutritional deficiencies that may be responsible.

SIGNS OF NUTRITIONAL DEFICIENCIES

PROBLEM AREA	PHYSICAL CONDITION	NUTRIENT DEFICIENCY
Skin	Dry, flaky, scaly skin Broken veins Pale skin Thick patches of skin	Vitamins A, E, essential fatty acids Vitamin C, anthocyanidins Iron Niacin
Eyes	Poor sight in darkness Dull eyes Pale conjunctiva membranes Redness of skin around eyes	Beta carotene Vitamin A and beta carotene Iron Vitamin B_2
Mouth	Cracked fissures around sides of mouth	Vitamin B_2
Teeth	Decayed teeth	Fluoride, phosphorus
Gums	Gingivitis	Vitamin A, B_2, niacin
Tongue	Sore tongue	Iron, folic acid
Hair	Changes in condition, such as dry, dull, fine, or brittle hair; changes in hair color, or hair that falls out easily	Protein, general calorie intakes
General	Fatigue, lack of energy Forgetfulness Irritability	Iron, vitamin C, carbohydrates Potassium Vitamin B_6

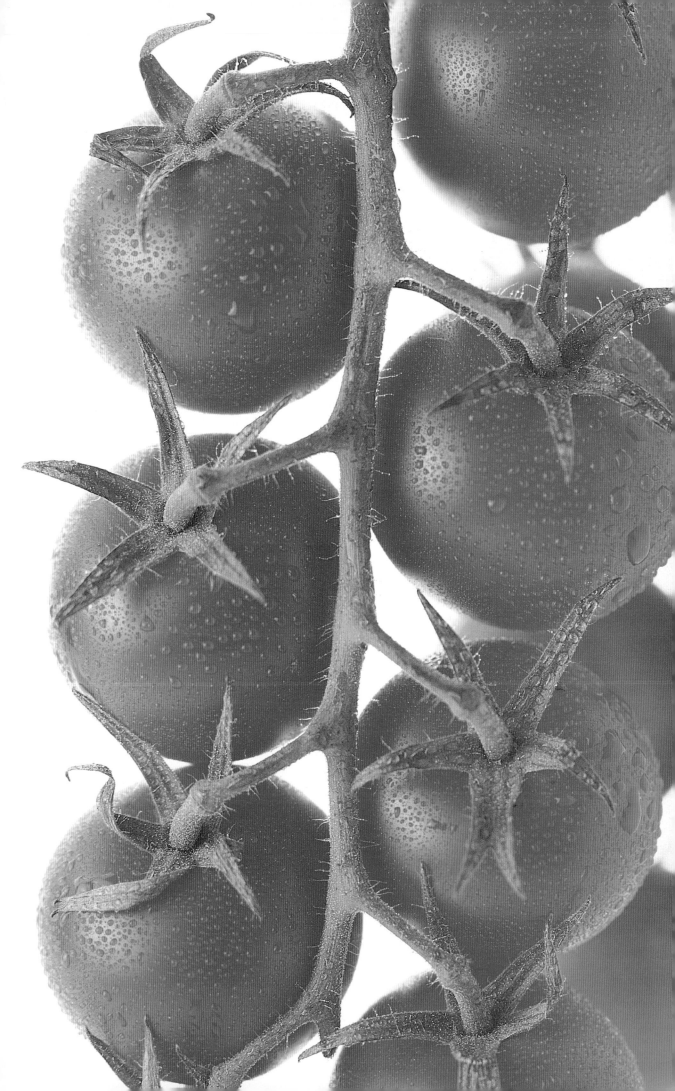

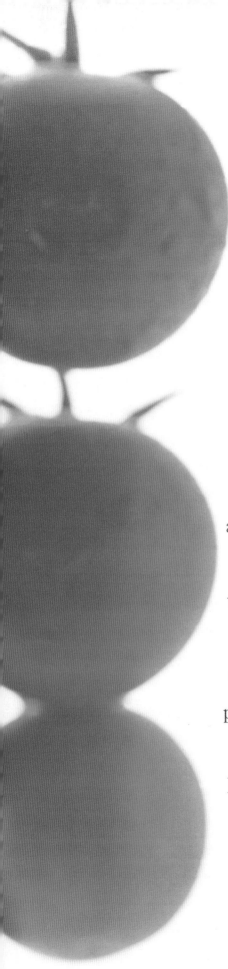

Treating ailments

Foods have long been used to treat human ailments. Scientists are now corroborating many of the ideas of ancient healers, and have identified links between the foods that people eat and their states of health. This section covers 80 common ailments, outlining their symptoms, conventional treatments, and possible causes. Beneficial foods are listed, as well as those that are best avoided. It is essential that a doctor or nutritionist be consulted before dietary changes are made to treat health problems.

HEART & CIRCULATION

BEATING CONTINUOUSLY and automatically, the heart pumps blood through the arteries of the circulatory system. This intricate system, which is approximately 90,000 miles long, carries blood to the lungs to receive oxygen, transports oxygen around the body, and removes waste matter produced by the body. A highly sophisticated transportation network, it ensures that every cell receives oxygen and essential nutrients.

DIET & THE HEART

Research shows that there is a direct link between heart disease and diet. Studies indicate that vegetarians and people who eat fish regularly tend to have lower blood pressure than meat-eaters, and have a reduced risk of heart disease. Overconsumption of foods rich in saturated animal fats can raise cholesterol levels – one cause of coronary heart disease. In some countries in the West, this illness accounts for 25 percent of all deaths, and associated strokes account for a further 12 percent.

A HEALTHY HEART

Eating healthily is fundamental to circulatory well-being. Limiting intakes of saturated fats and alcohol is very important, as is ensuring high intakes of fresh fruits, vegetables, and oily fish. Regular exercise is strongly advisable, while smoking and carrying excess weight should be avoided at all costs.

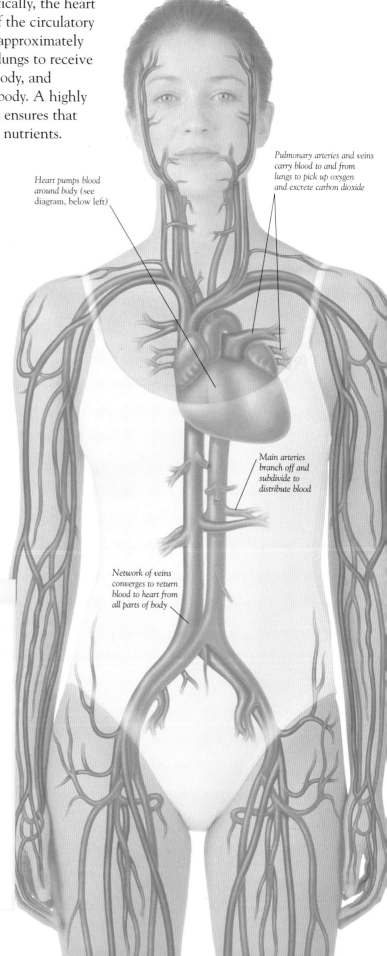

Heart pumps blood around body (see diagram, below left)

Pulmonary arteries and veins carry blood to and from lungs to pick up oxygen and excrete carbon dioxide

Main arteries branch off and subdivide to distribute blood

Network of veins converges to return blood to heart from all parts of body

HOW THE HEART WORKS

The heart is a powerful muscle that functions as two coordinated pumps. One sends blood to the lungs to pick up oxygen, while the other pumps oxygenated blood to the body tissues. Four valved chambers control the flow of blood.

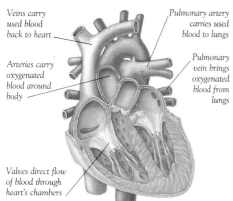

Veins carry used blood back to heart

Arteries carry oxygenated blood around body

Pulmonary artery carries used blood to lungs

Pulmonary vein brings oxygenated blood from lungs

Valves direct flow of blood through heart's chambers

TOP HEALING FOODS

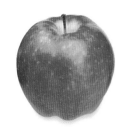

APPLES   PAGE 74

Benefits Antioxidants present in the skins of apples may help to reduce levels of LDL cholesterol (*see page 25*).
Useful for Those with high levels of blood cholesterol.
Nutrients Vitamin C, potassium.

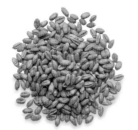

WHEAT   PAGE 97

Benefits Good for the heart and circulation in general. Also may reduce levels of LDL cholesterol (*see page 25*).
Useful for Those affected by stress and high cholesterol.
Nutrients Vitamins B and E.

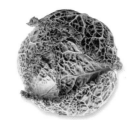

CABBAGE   PAGE 47

Benefits The dark outer leaves contain antioxidants.
Useful for Cardiovascular disease and stroke. Also may relieve high blood pressure.
Nutrients Vitamins B and C, beta carotene, potassium.

OILY FISH   PAGE 118

Benefits Can reduce the risk of blood clots forming and the risk of plaque formation in the arteries.
Useful for The heart and circulation in general.
Nutrients Vitamins D and E, iron, omega-3 fatty acids.

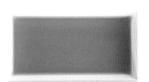

OLIVE OIL   PAGE 106

Benefits Extra virgin oil lowers levels of LDL cholesterol and raises levels of beneficial HDL cholesterol (*see page 25*).
Useful for Cardiovascular disease and blood clotting.
Nutrients Monounsaturated fats.

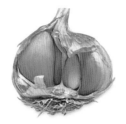

GARLIC   PAGE 66

Benefits Lowers cholesterol levels and is thought to "thin" the blood.
Useful for Lowering blood pressure and cholesterol levels, and preventing blood clots.
Nutrients Allicin, potassium.

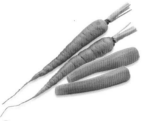

CARROTS   PAGE 56

Benefits Good supplier of carotenoids, which help to provide protection against free-radical damage.
Useful for Smokers who are at risk of heart disease.
Nutrients Beta carotene.

OATS   PAGE 95

Benefits Good for the health of the arteries. Also reduces harmful levels of cholesterol.
Useful for Moderating high levels of cholesterol and stress.
Nutrients Vitamin E, zinc, carbohydrates.

OTHER BENEFICIAL FOODS

BEETS   PAGE 57

Benefits Contains folate, which may help to reduce risk of heart disease by reducing homocysteine.
Useful for Lowering blood pressure and cholesterol levels.
Nutrients Folate, vitamin C.

SWEET POTATOES   PAGE 55

Benefits The orange flesh contains high levels of antioxidants.
Useful for Cardiovascular disease and stroke.
Nutrients Vitamins C and E, beta carotene.

PARSLEY   PAGE 109

Benefits Helps the body to get rid of excess sodium; protects against free-radical damage.
Useful for High blood pressure.
Nutrients Iron, carotenes, high levels of vitamin C.

WALNUTS   PAGE 102

Benefits May help reduce harmful levels of cholesterol.
Useful for High cholesterol levels and arteriosclerosis.
Nutrients Vitamin E, omega-3 fatty acids.

FOODS TO AVOID

SATURATED FATS

Foods containing saturated fats can raise levels of low-density lipoprotein (LDL) cholesterol (*see page 25*) in the body. A raised level of LDL is a risk factor in stroke, heart disease, and arteriosclerosis. Intakes of visible fat on meats, animal-based fats, and meat products such as pâtés should be reduced.

EGGS

As eggs are a source of cholesterol and saturated fat, people with high cholesterol may need to restrict intakes.

SODIUM (SALT)

Excessive sodium intakes in the diet are thought to raise blood pressure; cardiologists usually recommend minimum intakes. It is inadvisable to add sodium (as salt) to food during or after cooking. Foods rich in sodium, such as salty snacks, soups, pies, and ready-made meals, should be avoided.

SUGAR

Foods rich in sugar, such as cakes, cookies, and candy, should be kept to a minimum. Large quantities of these foods, which are also high in fat, can lead to weight gain and elevated cholesterol levels.

CAFFEINE

Caffeine, found in tea, coffee, and some carbonated drinks, stimulates the cardiovascular system, and may cause abnormal heart rhythms, palpitations, and high blood pressure. Boiled filtered coffee has been associated with elevated cholesterol. It is recommended that intakes of caffeine-rich drinks should be limited to no more than two cups a day.

TRANS FATS

During the digestive process of turning oils into solid fats, substances known as trans fats are formed, and these are known to elevate cholesterol levels. Because white cooking fats contain the largest amounts of trans fats, people with heart and circulatory problems should avoid pastries, cakes, and cookies made with these fats.

HEART DISEASE

KEY FOODS

VEGETABLES
pages 42–71

OILY FISH
page 118

OATS
page 95

LEGUMES
pages 58–60

FRUITS
pages 74–75

OILS
page 106

NUTS &
SEEDS
pages 100–105

CORONARY HEART DISEASE represents a group of disorders that includes angina and acute myocardial infarction (heart attack). The process leading to heart disease involves the gradual buildup of fatty deposits, or plaques, known as atheroma, on the inner lining of artery walls, restricting blood flow through the arteries, and this is known as atherosclerosis. A blood clot may form on the surface of the plaques which, if it is big enough, may block the blood flow to the surrounding cells. If the affected area of the heart is large enough, it can result in death.

✪ SYMPTOMS
There are usually no obvious symptoms until the damage to the arteries is serious enough to restrict blood flow to the heart, causing the pain of angina. Complete blockage of an artery supplying the heart may result in a sudden, fatal heart attack.

✚ CONVENTIONAL TREATMENT
The condition known as atherosclerosis may be prevented by reducing blood pressure, eating a low-fat diet, losing excess weight, and giving up smoking. Some people may be offered drugs to decrease their blood cholesterol levels.

✔ BENEFICIAL FOODS
Brussels sprouts, spinach, kale, asparagus, black-eyed peas, broccoli, cabbage, green beans, peas, cauliflower, chickpeas, kidney beans, and yeast extract supply the B vitamin folate, and many breakfast cereals and breads are fortified with folic acid, the version added to foods. There is a growing belief that the folate found naturally in foods, and folic acid in fortified foods, can lower a substance called homocysteine in the blood and help to reduce atherosclerosis. Homocysteine is thought to directly damage artery walls, which leads to the development of atherosclerotic plaques. It is estimated that increasing intakes of folic acid by 100mcg a day could prevent seven percent of coronary-related deaths in men and five percent in women.

Mackerel, salmon, and other oily fish contain the active fatty acids eicosapentaenoic acid (EPA) and docosahexaenoic acid (DHA). Populations that consume large amounts of oily fish have been observed to have a lower incidence of coronary heart disease than those who eat very little fish. It is thought that these fatty acids reduce a substance called arachidonic acid in the blood platelets, which lowers the risk of having blood clots and raised levels of blood triglycerides (fats). This may reduce the stickiness of the blood and

the likelihood of clotting. Eating oily fish at least three times a week is strongly advised for those with a history of coronary heart disease and for those wishing to take preventive measures.

Oats, legumes, apples, and pears are rich in soluble fiber, which is believed to help reduce cholesterol levels. Garlic has a similar effect. High blood cholesterol, particularly low-density lipoprotein (LDL) cholesterol, is believed to be a major risk factor in the development of atherosclerosis. Regular consumption of such foods may help to reduce LDL cholesterol.

Olive oil, rapeseed oil, nuts, and seeds contain monounsaturated fatty acids, which appear to help reduce LDL cholesterol levels.

Fruits and vegetables contain antioxidant vitamins, minerals, and phytonutrients, which may stop the damage to artery walls caused by free radicals. At least five servings of these foods should be eaten each day. A glass of fruit or vegetable juice counts as a serving.

✖ FOODS TO AVOID
Meat products, whole-milk dairy products, butter, and lard are all rich in saturated fats, which can increase levels of LDL cholesterol. These foods must be kept to a minimum.

Cakes and cookies often contain saturated fats or fats rich in trans fatty acids. Both types of fat are capable of increasing LDL cholesterol levels.

Ready-made meals and soups, take-out meals, salty snacks, meat products, luncheon meats, bacon, and sauces are rich in sodium. High sodium intakes are related to increases in blood pressure, a major factor in the risk of developing heart disease. A reduction in sodium in foods, and in table salt at mealtimes, helps reduce blood pressure.

✪ OTHER MEASURES
❑ Smokers are advised to give up the habit, since nicotine increases heart rate, blood pressure, and the demand of heart tissue for oxygen. The carbon monoxide produced by smoking decreases the blood's ability to carry oxygen. Carbon monoxide is a source of free radicals, which can set off the damage to artery walls.

❑ Relaxation is important in order to reduce stress levels, which increase the production of adrenaline and other substances that cause cholesterol production.

See Also Angina, page 158; High Blood Pressure, page 155; Obesity, page 178; Stress & Anxiety, page 231; Stroke, page 156; Thrombosis, page 157

EATING PLAN FOR HEART DISEASE

Choosing a diet that is low in saturated fat, contains regular amounts of fish oils and antioxidant vitamins, and helps to maintain a normal body weight can help to reduce the risk of heart disease. Below are some meals and snacks that may be useful for those with this condition.

BREAKFASTS	LIGHT MEALS	MAIN MEALS	SNACKS
Bowl of cooked cereal made with skim milk and topped with slices of fresh peach	*Walnut, cottage cheese, and peach salad with wholewheat roll*	*Broiled herring or mackerel with oven-baked vegetables*	*Bowl of fruit-and-fiber cereal with skim milk*
◆	*Apple and pear with low-fat cottage cheese*	*Baked apple topped with cinnamon and low-fat vanilla yogurt*	◆
Broiled tomatoes and mushrooms on two slices of wholewheat toast	◆	◆	*Banana and a small pack of sunflower seeds*
◆	*Tuna and pepper brown rice salad*	*Lentil and bean casserole with sweet baked potato*	◆
Toasted wholewheat muffin spread with reduced fat cream cheese and topped with smoked salmon	*Fresh berries*	*Stewed prunes with fat-free Greek yogurt*	*Low-fat plain yogurt with grated apple*
	◆	◆	
	Lean ham and tomato rye bread sandwich	*Pork, pepper, and baby corn stir-fried with brown rice*	
	Banana smoothie made with banana, low-fat yogurt, and pineapple	*Orange sections with lemon sorbet*	

FLUID RETENTION (EDEMA)

YOGURT
page 128

BANANAS
page 90

VEGETABLES
pages 42–71

POULTRY
page 124

FISH
pages 118–121

FLUID RETENTION, OR EDEMA, can be a symptom of a heart, liver, or kidney disorder. It can be caused by an allergy, and some women may experience premenstrual fluid retention each month. Fluid retention can also be a result of an inability to absorb protein from the digestive tract, and it can occur as a side effect of certain drugs, or as a result of prolonged immobility. This condition should always be checked by a doctor.

✪ SYMPTOMS Sudden weight gain is one of the most noticeable symptoms. The ankles, face, or eyes take on a general look of puffiness.

✚ CONVENTIONAL TREATMENT The type of treatment depends on the cause of the fluid retention. Treatment may include drugs and intravenous fluid and nutrient replacement.

✔ BENEFICIAL FOODS
Yogurt may reduce the number of histamine-producing bacteria present in the gut. Histamine can lead to localized fluid retention.
Bananas and other fruits and vegetables supply potassium, and about 1 lb (400g) (five servings) of these foods should be consumed every day. Potassium helps to relieve fluid retention.

Poultry, fresh fish, and meats are low-sodium sources of protein, and pasta, potatoes, oats, and rice are good low-sodium carbohydrates.
Coffee and tea contain caffeine, which has a diuretic effect. One cup each morning may help to clear excess fluid that can build up overnight.
Bilberries are rich in anthocyanidins, plant chemicals that may be able to strengthen blood vessel walls. Bilberry extracts taken in supplement form may also help fluid retention.

✖ FOODS TO AVOID
Bacon, luncheon meats, ready-made meals, canned foods, including vegetables, and many processed foods are high in added sodium, which may increase water retention.

❂ OTHER MEASURES
❑ Losing any excess body weight by decreasing calorie intake and increasing exercise may help to alleviate symptoms.
❑ A daily supplement of evening primrose oil may be useful for premenstrual fluid retention.

See Also Kidney Disorders, page 192; Premenstrual Syndrome, page 222; Proteins, page 20

HIGH CHOLESTEROL

KEY FOODS

LEAN MEATS
page 122

POULTRY
page 124

FISH
pages 118–121

LEGUMES
pages 58–60

WHOLE GRAINS
pages 92–99

FRUITS
pages 72–91

GARLIC
page 66

VEGETABLES
pages 42–71

OLIVE OIL
page 106

AS PEOPLE GROW OLDER, their cholesterol levels gradually rise, so that by middle age, most people have levels above the desirable concentration of 5.2 milligrams per liter of blood (5.2 mg/l). When levels exceed 6.5 mg/l, a person is said to have high cholesterol.

Cholesterol is transported around the body in the form of "lipoproteins," which are particles of cholesterol and other fats in a coating of proteins. The most important lipoproteins are high-density lipoprotein (HDL) cholesterol and low-density lipoprotein (LDL) cholesterol. High levels of HDL are desirable as they remove excess cholesterol from the cells and take it to the liver. High levels of LDL are undesirable, since they take cholesterol from the liver and carry it to the body tissues, where it seems to be involved with the buildup of fatty deposits, or atheroma, on artery walls, particularly around the heart and brain. Atheroma cause arteries to become narrow, reducing blood flow.

✪ SYMPTOMS
The constriction of arteries and other blood vessels can lead to atherosclerosis, which may cause angina, in which pain is felt in the left arm, shoulder, and neck on exertion. The effects of atherosclerosis may not become apparent until the blockage has become severe enough to reduce blood flow, causing sudden, and often fatal heart failure.

✚ CONVENTIONAL TREATMENT
This depends on the cause. If it is secondary to other conditions, such as obesity, alcoholism, or diabetes, these need to be treated. If an inherited factor is involved, the condition is usually treated with cholesterol-lowering drugs and diet.

✔ BENEFICIAL FOODS
Strict vegetarians tend to have much lower cholesterol levels than meat eaters, which is thought to be due to differences in saturated fat intakes. Reducing the total amount of fat in the diet, and helping people to achieve a normal body weight, are the main dietary methods employed to help reduce high levels of LDL cholesterol.

Lean meats, poultry, fish, nuts, and legumes are protein sources that contain less saturated fats than fatty red meats, sausages, and ready-made meals. Trimming fat from meat can reduce cholesterol concentration by almost nine percent when following a diet that supplies 35 percent of the total calories from fat.

Breads, potatoes, pasta, and rice should be eaten in increased amounts, since they allow the amount of fatty foods consumed to be reduced. People in the West typically obtain about 40 percent of their total calories from fats. Reducing fat intake to 30–35 percent is recommended by many medical practitioners, and some advise reducing it to ten percent.

Wholewheat breads, pasta, and brown rice contain insoluble fiber, which bulks up the stools and speeds their passage through the colon. Cholesterol in the colon can be reabsorbed back into the body. Bulky stools reduce this process.

Apples, pears, oats, and beans are rich in soluble fiber, which is believed to bind and lower LDL cholesterol. Incorporating oats and beans into the diet can lower cholesterol by more than 20 percent over the long term and can also raise levels of HDL cholesterol.

Garlic is believed to lower the risk of heart disease and seems to be helpful in reducing levels of LDL cholesterol while raising levels of HDL cholesterol.

Fruits and vegetables are low in fat but high in fiber. Filling up on these foods helps to reduce the amount of fat and total calories eaten. A diet rich in fruits and vegetables can help those who are overweight to achieve weight loss, which in turn helps to lower high LDL cholesterol.

Oily fish such as mackerel, sardines, and salmon should be eaten three times a week to increase omega-3 fatty acids. These reportedly increase HDL cholesterol while lowering LDL cholesterol.

Olive oil and rapeseed oil lower LDL blood cholesterol when used instead of saturated fats.

✖ FOODS TO AVOID
Butter, cream, cheese, fatty meats, and hard margarines all contain large amounts of saturated fats, which are associated with increasing levels of LDL cholesterol.

Cakes, cookies, pies, and pastries are all rich in fats, and are best eaten in strict moderation.

Coffee that has been percolated and boiled can, when consumed in large quantities, increase LDL cholesterol. Fresh, filtered coffee does not have this effect.

✪ OTHER MEASURES
❏ Smokers are advised to give up the habit because smoking may worsen this condition.
❏ Shedding excess weight, if overweight, helps to lower cholesterol levels.
❏ Eating little and often and "grazing" on a low-fat, high-fiber diet may lower cholesterol levels.

See Also Angina, page 158; Fats, page 22

HIGH BLOOD PRESSURE (HYPERTENSION)

AS THE HEART RESPONDS to the body's demands, the pressure of the blood flowing through the arteries rises and falls. Exercise, anxiety, and stress can all lead to a temporary rise in blood pressure. As people get older, their blood pressure usually rises naturally. Healthy people in their mid-twenties could expect to have a blood pressure reading of about 120/80. Most doctors consider treatment when blood pressure is persistently above 160/90. Approximately 15 percent of people have permanently high blood pressure, which is known as hypertension. In five percent of these individuals, this is due to conditions such as kidney disease, hormonal disorders, or pregnancy. For the rest, there is no obvious cause. In 70 percent of people with high blood pressure the condition runs in the family.

Obesity and excess weight are indisputably associated with high blood pressure. The condition is twice as common in young overweight individuals and 50 percent more prevalent in older obese people than in those of normal weight.

☻ SYMPTOMS
The majority of people have no symptoms, but inside the body high blood pressure can cause severe or chronic damage to various parts of the body. In the brain, this can be manifested by hemorrhaging of the blood vessels, causing stroke. In the eyes, hypertension can damage blood vessels and impair sight, and in the kidneys it can result in kidney failure. Symptoms may include headaches, chest pain, and shortness of breath.

✚ CONVENTIONAL TREATMENT
Cases that are borderline are often left untreated. Nondrug treatment includes reducing sodium in the diet, giving up smoking, taking regular exercise, and following relaxation strategies. Antihypertensive drugs may be prescribed.

✔ BENEFICIAL FOODS
It is generally accepted that people with high blood pressure need to reduce their intakes of sodium. Extra potassium and calcium may also help to lower blood pressure.

Bananas, apricots, figs, grapefruits, peaches, grapes, mangoes, and prunes are fruits rich in potassium, while potatoes, legumes, broccoli, zucchini, lettuce, mushrooms, and tomatoes are some of the highest vegetable sources. Fruits and vegetables are low in sodium and should be consumed in generous quantities. In studies comparing vegetarians with nonvegetarians, average blood pressures were found to be lower in vegetarians. Higher potassium intakes in vegetarians are thought to account in part for the differences in blood pressures, which have been found on average to be 126/77 in vegetarians and 147/88 in nonvegetarians.

Citrus fruits, berries, and green leafy vegetables are good sources of vitamin C. Low levels of this vitamin are associated with high blood pressure. Supplementation with vitamin C has been found to decrease blood pressures in people with both normal and high levels.

Meats and poultry that are fresh or frozen and cooked without sodium, stock cubes, or sauces are acceptable for those with high blood pressure. Meats can be flavored with herbs, spices, and fruits. Marjoram and rosemary go well with lamb, tarragon and dill with chicken, apples and cloves with pork, and oranges with liver.

Fish, fresh, frozen, or canned without brine — for example, tuna in water — is low in sodium and can be flavored with bay leaves, dill, red cayenne pepper, allspice, other herbs and spices, citrus fruits, and wine to avoid the need for using added salt and ready-made sauces.

Root vegetables such as potatoes, and oatmeal, rice, and pasta are low sodium carbohydrates that can be used as the basis of meals.

Sesame seeds, tofu, and green leafy vegetables supply low-sodium sources of calcium.

✖ FOODS TO AVOID
Bacon, ham, sausages, canned meats, burgers, and other meat products should be avoided due to their high levels of sodium. Vegetables canned in brine, baked beans, instant mashed potato, and salted potato chips are also high in sodium and should be avoided by those with hypertension.

Smoked and canned fish, and ready-made fish meals are high in sodium.

Sauces, soups, stock cubes, and soda water may raise blood pressure.

Alcohol consumption is linked with high blood pressure and can worsen this condition.

◔ OTHER MEASURES
❑ Weight reduction and weight maintenance are essential parts of any program that is designed to deal with hypertension.

❑ Smokers are advised to give up the habit, as smoking worsens high blood pressure.

See Also Stress & Anxiety, page 231; Obesity, page 178; Stroke, page 156

STROKE

KEY FOODS

FRUITS
pages 72–91

VEGETABLES
pages 42–71

LEGUMES
pages 58–60

NUTS &
SEEDS
pages 100–105

WHOLE GRAINS
pages 92–99

OILS
page 106

THE TERM "STROKE" describes damage to part of the brain that is caused when its blood supply is interrupted or when its blood vessel walls break down and blood seeps out. Stroke is the third most common cause of death in many countries in the West, and its incidence increases with age. Strokes are often associated with high blood pressure and are likely to occur while the person is involved in physical exertion.

✛ SYMPTOMS During the preceding few days before a stroke there may be headaches, drowsiness, and vertigo, and the eyesight may be affected. Sometimes symptoms build up over several weeks. After a stroke, one side of the body is often completely or partially paralyzed.

✚ CONVENTIONAL TREATMENT Many people are left with some form of paralysis or speech problem, and therapy may be required. The risk of another stroke may be reduced by anticoagulant drugs, and the reduction of high blood pressure through drugs, lifestyle, and diet.

✔ BENEFICIAL FOODS
There is, as yet, no strong evidence that diet conclusively affects the incidence and outcome of strokes, but many doctors agree that certain dietary steps may reduce high blood pressure and thus the risk of strokes. Atherosclerotic buildups in the blood vessels of the brain occur more rapidly in the presence of free radicals. Increasing daily intake of antioxidant nutrients may help to combat excessive, harmful amounts of these free radicals.
Fruits and vegetables, including juices and frozen vegetables, are rich in antioxidant vitamins, potassium, and phytonutrients, and low in sodium, and should be consumed frequently, with at least five servings a day. Studies in the UK have suggested that a high consumption of fruits and vegetables may be associated with a lower incidence of stroke. A Belgian study revealed that patients with high levels of vitamin A from vegetables rich in beta carotene recovered better from stroke, while a large study in the US also suggested that increased intakes of vitamin E had a protective effect. Avocados and green leafy vegetables are rich in vitamin E.
Legumes, tofu, nuts, seeds, and other vegetable protein could be eaten more often in order to reduce the amount of animal protein consumed. This may be advisable in the light of studies in the West that reveal generally lower rates of stroke in vegetarians than in meat-eaters.
Oily fish such as salmon and mackerel seem to improve blood flow. Eating oily fish at least twice a week may offer protection against stroke.
Bread, rice, pasta, potatoes, and breakfast cereals are low in fat but high in slow releasing energy, which helps to keep people feeling full for longer. Consuming a diet in which 55 percent of calories come from these foods with 30 percent or less from fat helps with weight control.
Nuts, seeds, and flax oil supply linoleic acid. In Finnish tests, middle-aged male stroke victims seemed to have lower levels of this essential fatty acid than men who had not had strokes.
Brazil nuts are one of the richest food sources of selenium. It is suggested that low intakes of this mineral are associated with an increased risk of stroke. Eating three nuts a day improves intakes.

✖ FOODS TO AVOID
Salty foods should be avoided in order to help reduce high blood pressure. Intake of ready-made meals with added sodium, meat products, vegetables canned in brine, and smoked foods should be restricted.

◔ OTHER MEASURES
❏ Drinking alcohol in modest amounts may reduce the risk of stroke. Intakes of about $1/4$–$1/2$ cup per week have been associated with a 40–60 percent reduction in the risk of stroke.
❏ Conversely, heavy drinking can lead to sudden increases in blood pressure, which can result in stroke. Heavy drinkers who consume more than $1^1/4$ cups of alcohol per week are four times more likely to have a stroke than nondrinkers.
❏ Smokers are advised to give up the habit.

See Also High Blood Pressure, page 155

CASE HISTORY

Peter Marrick, 68, had a mild stroke during an operation on his prostate gland. As a result, he lost the hearing in one ear and found it difficult to speak. In order to lessen the risk of having another stroke, Peter gave up eating salty foods, and began to watch his weight closely. All the old favorites, such as smoked bacon, sausages, and ready-made meals were eliminated from Peter's diet. He now rarely eats convenience foods and he incorporates more herbs and spices into meals so that cutting back on his sodium intake does not make dishes taste bland. One year after having had a stroke, Peter's hearing is almost back to normal and his speech has improved.

THROMBOSIS

KEY FOODS

OILY FISH
page 118

LEGUMES
pages 58–60

WHOLE GRAINS
pages 92–99

CITRUS
FRUITS
pages 86–88

BRASSICAS
pages 44–47

CAYENNE
PEPPER
page 113

SEEDS
pages 103–105

BERRIES
pages 82–85

A BLOOD CLOT, OR THROMBUS, forms within a blood vessel as a result of damage to the blood vessel wall, for example through attack by free radicals, infection, or trauma. This in turn leads to the formation of atherosclerotic buildup. The damaged area acts like a magnet to platelets flowing past in the blood. These platelets stick to the site, creating a blood clot that can grow large enough to block the blood vessel.

✪ SYMPTOMS The first sign of thrombosis is usually when the blood clot causes a blockage that is severe enough to cause an acute incident such as a heart attack or stroke.

✚ CONVENTIONAL TREATMENT In many cases of thrombosis, anticoagulant drugs are given to discourage clotting, or thrombolytic drugs are given to break down clots that have already formed. The drugs most often used in the West are heparin and warfarin.

✔ BENEFICIAL FOODS
For those being treated with drugs for thrombosis, it is essential to seek advice from a doctor before making any changes to the diet.
Oily fish, such as salmon, mackerel, and sardines, contain two main fatty acids known as eicosapentaenoic acid (EPA) and docosahexaenoic acid (DHA), which have a similar blood thinning action to aspirin. Long-term studies from the US, Sweden, and the Netherlands have shown that eating oily fish two to three times per week can have profound effects on improving blood flow and can lower the risk of blood clot formation. Increasing the consumption of oily fish is one of the well-known ways of "thinning the blood" through diet.
Soybeans and soy products contain the antioxidant known as genistein. As well as seeming to interfere with cancer formation, genistein appears to stop the rapid growth of smooth muscle cells which, when left uncontrolled, promote the formation of blood clots. Bean curd or tofu, soy milk, and textured vegetable protein all supply genistein.
Legumes, including lentils and soybeans, contain coumarins, which are Nature's own blood thinners (chemically, the blood thinning drug warfarin is, in fact, a coumarin). Legumes can be used in stews, soups, casseroles, and dahls.
Wholewheat breads, brown pasta, and whole-grain breakfast cereals are rich in coumarins.
Citrus fruits, broccoli, cauliflower, squashes, parsley, flax seeds, pineapples, and green tea are full of warfarin-like coumarins. Foods that are rich in coumarins should be eaten on a regular basis.
Cayenne pepper is known by herbalists to stimulate the circulatory system and can be included in spicy dishes and dips.
Flaxseeds are a rich source of the omega-6 fatty acids, which are converted into prostaglandin E1 in the body. This hormonelike substance dilates the blood vessels and helps to prevent the formation of blood clots.
Sunflower, sesame, and pumpkin seeds supply omega-3 fatty acids. Four tablespoons of flaxseeds can be ground with two tablespoons each of sesame, sunflower, and pumpkin seeds, and stored in an airtight jar in the refrigerator. This mixture can be sprinkled over breakfast cereals and yogurts to ensure a good anti-inflammatory mix of omega-6 and omega-3 fatty acids.
Berries, and citrus fruits such as oranges, which are rich in vitamin C and phytonutrients, help to maintain elasticity of the blood vessels. These foods should be consumed regularly.
Seek medical advice before taking these steps.

✖ FOODS TO AVOID
Butter, cream, and lard are rich in saturated fats, which increase the tendency of the blood to clot. These should be kept to a minimum in the diet.
Coconut cream, oil, and shredded coconut are rich in saturated fats and need to be avoided. Coconut milk can be used in cooking, however, since it is low in both total and saturated fats.
Whole milk and yogurts should be replaced by low-fat dairy products in order to reduce the intake of saturated fats.
Fatty meats and meat products such as beef burgers, pies, and sausages need to be limited. Any visible fat surrounding bacon strips and lamb or pork chops should be discarded.
Cakes, pies, and pastries should be kept to a minimum. Store-bought products tend to use the cheapest fats available, which are often the highly saturated varieties.

❷ OTHER MEASURES
❑ Excess body weight should be lost, since this automatically increases the risk of blood clots.
❑ Regular exercise ensures good blood flow. Seek medical advice before increasing exercise.
❑ Smokers are advised to give up the habit, as smoking increases the risk of thrombosis.

See Also Heart Disease, page 152; Obesity, page 178; Stroke, see opposite

KEY FOODS

EGGS
page 129

LOW FAT DAIRY PRODUCTS
pages 126–128

LEGUMES
pages 58–60

WHOLE GRAINS
pages 92–99

GREEN VEGETABLES
pages 44–51

CITRUS FRUITS
pages 86–88

BERRIES
pages 82–85

ANGINA

THE CONDITION known as angina is characterized by a pain in the chest brought on by exertion and relieved by rest. Angina is commonly caused by narrowed coronary arteries which supply blood, and therefore oxygen, to the heart muscle. The narrowing is usually the result of fatty deposits, or atheroma, building up in the artery walls. While enough blood may be able to flow through the arteries to the heart when a person is resting, it may be inadequate when they are exercising.

SYMPTOMS The pain experienced with angina is often described as a tightness in the chest. It is brought on by exertion, and is worse during cold weather, or when exercising after a meal. Pain may also occur in the left arm, wrists, and hands. In severe cases, angina is sparked by gentle activities, such as walking.

CONVENTIONAL TREATMENT Drugs such as nitrates, beta-blockers, and calcium channel blockers are given to relieve or prevent symptoms. Heart bypass surgery may be performed. In certain cases, an operation known as angioplasty is carried out to clear the arteries.

BENEFICIAL FOODS
Scientists have discovered that by taking a very low-fat and low-cholesterol approach to angina, symptoms can be reversed. Some experts advise restricting fat to ten percent of the total calories, most of which should be polyunsaturated or monounsaturated. About 70–75 percent of the calories should come from carbohydrates and 15–20 percent from protein. A daily intake of just 5mg of cholesterol is also recommended. This diet, combined with giving up smoking, and taking up relaxation techniques and exercise, has been shown to result in an average reduction in angina of 91 percent.
Egg whites contain no fat or cholesterol, yet supply all the essential building blocks of protein, known as amino acids. Egg whites are among the few animal-derived foods recommended for angina.
Skim milk and virtually fat-free yogurts and fromage frais supply good quality complete protein without containing saturated fats.
Legumes such as soybeans, fagioli, and kidney beans provide soluble fiber, which helps to reduce the absorption of cholesterol. These foods should be eaten in combination with a cereal such as wholewheat bread, brown rice, or pasta. The combination of amino acids in these two food groups creates a complete protein, providing all the essential amino acids in a low-fat package.

Oats and oat bran contain soluble fiber, which helps to lower cholesterol levels in the blood, decreasing the risk of atherosclerosis.
Whole-grain foods, green leafy vegetables, and breakfast cereals fortified with folic acid may play a role in reducing blocked arteries by decreasing the levels of homocysteine in the blood. High homocysteine is believed to damage artery walls, where cholesterol then deposits itself.
Citrus fruits and berries are rich in vitamin C, which may help to reverse atherosclerosis.
Seaweed contains omega-3 fatty acids and is recommended as a low-fat alternative to oily fish for those following a very low-fat diet. Omega-3 fatty acids are thought to help thin the blood and lower cholesterol.

FOODS TO AVOID
Coconuts, cocoa products, and large quantities of nuts and seeds are not advisable, since they contain significant amounts of fat.
Coffee, colas, and cocoa contain caffeine, which can make angina worse. Decaffeinated versions of these drinks are suitable alternatives.
Fatty meats, butter, margarine, and oils are to be avoided by those experiencing angina.

OTHER MEASURES
❏ Smokers are advised to give up the habit. The nicotine in cigarettes constricts the blood vessels to the heart and increases the risk of blockages.
❏ Losing excess weight, if overweight, helps to reduce the extra pressure on the heart.
❏ Regular exercise and some form of relaxation can help in the process of reversing angina.

See Also Fats, page 22; Heart Disease, page 152

VARICOSE VEINS

KEY FOODS

WHOLE GRAINS
pages 92–99

GREEN VEGETABLES
pages 44–51

CITRUS FRUITS
pages 86–88

BILBERRIES
page 83

NUTS & SEEDS
pages 100–105

OILY FISH
page 118

THIS CONDITION IS characterized by bulbous protrusions of veins beneath the skin, particularly in the lower leg. In each vein there are valves controlling blood flow. Varicose veins occur when these valves become inefficient and fail to work properly. This may be due to pressure inside the digestive tract, for example as a result of constipation. Some varicose veins are deeply embedded in the leg and are not visible. Varicose veins can lead to a decrease in the supply of nutrients to the skin and muscles, which can become gangrenous and ulcerated as a result.

In the West, the treatment of varicose veins uses much medical time and expense. The incidence of varicose veins is much lower in less developed countries, a fact that some scientists believe could be related to dietary habits. People living in less developed countries tend to eat more dietary fiber than those living in the West.

✪ SYMPTOMS Varicose veins may cause mild symptoms, such as aching and slightly swollen ankles. The protruding veins may be unsightly. Sometimes there are no symptoms.

✚ CONVENTIONAL TREATMENT The treatment can involve wearing tight-fitting supportive stockings, and sitting with the legs raised above the level of the heart, to relieve symptoms. Varicose veins are frequently operated on in order to relieve the problem.

✔ BENEFICIAL FOODS

Constipation is thought to increase pressure on the veins in the legs, leading to the formation of varicose veins. A fiber-rich diet decreases constipation and helps to prevent varicose veins. **Whole-grain breakfast cereals**, wholewheat breads and rolls, brown pasta, and rice are recommended to help bulk up the stools and prevent constipation. Cereals rich in insoluble fiber bulk up the stools and bind water. The resulting larger, softer stool is much easier to pass, leading to less straining and less pressure on the leg veins. On increasing fiber intake in the diet, water intake should also increase, to at least six cup or glasses a day.

Green leafy vegetables and cruciferous vegetables such as broccoli and brussels sprouts help to bulk up the stools with the insoluble fiber that they supply. Increased fiber intakes are particularly important during pregnancy, when high levels of the hormone progesterone slow down contractions of the large intestine, making the occurrence of constipation more likely.

CASE HISTORY

Nick O'Neill, aged 43, developed varicose veins as a result of prolonged periods of sitting at his desk, lack of regular exercise, and excess weight. An operation was performed to remove the varicose veins, after which Nick became determined to prevent a recurrence of the condition. Nick's doctor advised a diet of 1,500 calories a day, combined with regular exercise to help him shed excess weight. Nick followed the low fat diet for three months, combined with daily walks, and lost 29lbs. He has now progressed to include running in his weekly routine, and makes the time to take short breaks at work and walk around to keep his circulation going. So far, the varicose veins have not returned.

Citrus fruits such as oranges and grapefruits, and raspberries, black currants, strawberries, peppers, and green leafy vegetables all supply vitamin C. This vitamin is vital for maintaining the strength of collagen, the material that helps to support vein walls. A lack of vitamin C in the diet leads to the breakdown of small veins, which may worsen varicose veins.

Bilberry extract contains antioxidants called anthocyanidins, which have been shown to decrease the leakage of tiny blood vessels in people with varicose veins. The anthocyanidins seem to be able to help mend the damaged connective tissues in the walls of the veins that make the veins bulge and protrude. Eating bilberries may have similar effects.

Nuts, seeds, and oily fish contain essential fatty acids and eating some of these foods each day helps to strengthen the walls of veins.

✖ FOODS TO AVOID

Butter, margarine, oils, cakes, cookies, pies, candies, and pastries are all rich in fat and supply considerable amounts of calories, which increase the likelihood of weight gain and the development of varicose veins.

⊘ OTHER MEASURES

❑ Losing excess weight is crucial for those who are overweight. Strain on the veins, which is caused by carrying too much body fat, is associated with an increased risk of developing this condition.
❑ Regular exercise helps to burn off calories.

See Also Constipation, page 175; Fiber, page 14; Hemorrhoids, page 175; Plant Nutrients, page 34

ANEMIA

KEY FOODS

RED MEATS
page 122

OILY FISH
page 118

SHELLFISH
page 120

LEGUMES
pages 58–60

FIGS
page 80

**NUTS &
SEEDS**
pages 100–105

FRUITS
pages 72–91

VEGETABLES
pages 42–71

THERE ARE SEVERAL FORMS of anemia, the most common of which is iron deficiency. This affects about eight percent of people in the West. Iron deficiency anemia is usually caused by a lack of iron in the diet, an increased demand for iron, or excessive blood loss. Iron is needed by the blood for the formation of hemoglobin, the pigment that carries oxygen in the blood. Hemoglobin collects oxygen from the lungs, then transports it to all the cells in the body. When the iron reserves in the liver are depleted, hemoglobin levels fall, and delivery of oxygen to cells decreases. It is recommended that people have at least 500mg of stored iron. Many women in the West have only 150mg, and 20–30 percent have none at all.

✪ SYMPTOMS

Iron deficiency anemia causes fatigue, a lack of energy, weakness, an inability to concentrate, breathlessness, and palpitations. It impairs the memory, and causes pain thresholds to decrease. The body's temperature control may also be affected due to disruption of the thyroid gland, and the immune system may lose some of its strength. The nails can become brittle, the tongue smooth and shiny, and cracks may appear at the sides of the mouth. During pregnancy, a lack of iron in the diet may affect the development of the fetus's brain.

✚ CONVENTIONAL TREATMENT

Since there are several different types of anemia, it is essential to seek medical advice before taking any kind of treatment, including food supplements. Often a course of iron tablets is all that is required, but some kinds of anemia do not need treatment, and taking extra iron may even make the anemia worse. A blood test should be carried out before any advice is given. Pregnant women often need to take iron and folic acid supplements.

✔ BENEFICIAL FOODS

Red meats and poultry contain what is known as "hem" iron, which is much more easily absorbed by the body than the "non-hem" iron obtained from vegetables and other plant sources. On average, the body absorbs ten percent of the iron obtained from the diet, but with hem iron the level of absorption increases to 30 percent.
Oily fish, such as salmon, mackerel, tuna, pilchards, and sardines, supply hem iron.
Fish and shellfish increase iron absorption from plant sources and are particularly useful for elderly people, who become a third less efficient at absorbing iron once over the age of about 70.
Baked beans and other legumes supply non-hem

iron. Haricot beans, red kidney beans, and lentils supply about 5mg of non-hem iron per serving.
Fortified breakfast cereals and breads provide up to 11mg of iron per serving and also supply vitamins B_{12} and folic acid, which help to prevent certain types of anemia.
Figs, dried apricots, and nuts and seeds supply useful amounts of iron.
Fruits and vegetables contain vitamin C, which enhances the absorption of non-hem iron. It is suggested that 25mg of vitamin C should be consumed at every meal. Sauerkraut is rich in citric acid, which also promotes iron absorption.

✖ FOODS TO AVOID

Tea and coffee contain phenolic compounds, which prevent iron absorption. The tannins in tea have a similar effect.
Milk, cheese, and other dairy products are rich in calcium, which decreases the amount of iron available to the body. Avoid consuming dairy foods with iron rich meals.
Soy protein, phytates in whole grains, and oxalic acid in rhubarb all inhibit iron absorption.

⊘ OTHER MEASURES

❑ To enhance iron absorption, foods and drinks that inhibit its absorption should not be eaten or drunk at the same time as iron rich foods.
❑ Vegetarians are advised to cook acidic foods, such as tomato-based chili, soups, and sauces, in cast-iron cookware, since the acid causes some of the iron from the pan to leach out into the food. The acid also improves iron absorption.

See Also Fatigue, page 235; Minerals, page 30; Women & Nutrition, page 140

EATING PLAN FOR ANEMIA

Try to consume iron rich foods such as meat and fish daily and eat them with foods that are rich in vitamin C, such as green leafy vegetables.

Vegetarians are particularly at risk from iron deficiency anemia, so lentils, beans, and other legumes should be eaten on a regular basis.

BREAKFASTS	LIGHT MEALS	MAIN MEALS	SNACKS
Whole-grain cereal fortified with iron	*Baked beans on toast*	*Paella with shellfish and chicken*	*Dried fruits*
Wholewheat toast and peanut butter	*Fresh fruit salad*	*Raspberry sorbet*	◆
Orange juice	◆	◆	*Orange juice*
◆	*Pita bread with hummus and crudité*	*Spaghetti bolognese with green salad*	◆
Fruit salad with prunes, dried apricots, figs, and sesame seeds	*Satsuma*	*Strawberries or seasonal fruits*	*Sunflower seeds*
◆	◆	◆	◆
Poached egg on toast with sliced tomatoes	*Roast beef sandwich*	*Pork stir-fry with cashew nuts*	*Unsalted peanuts*
	Apple	*Caramelized oranges*	◆
			Iron-fortified breakfast cereal

RAYNAUD'S DISEASE

KEY FOODS

OILY FISH
page 118

CITRUS FRUITS
pages 86–88

BERRIES
pages 82–85

DAIRY PRODUCTS
pages 126–128

GINGER
page 114

PEOPLE WHO HAVE AN exaggerated response to the cold may be displaying a symptom of this circulatory disorder. Normally, the small blood vessels in the fingers and toes contract when there is a drop in temperature. These contractions decrease blood flow, leading to Raynaud's disease.

✪ SYMPTOMS Typically there is numbness, tingling, and a burning sensation in the fingers or toes. Symptoms may be accompanied by pain, and the sensitivity to cold can be disabling.

✚ CONVENTIONAL TREATMENT A drug called nifedipine is used to dilate the arteries. A synthetic form of prostaglandin E1 has also been used effectively to treat this condition.

✔ BENEFICIAL FOODS
No studies have been carried out to reveal how specific foods affect Raynaud's, but certain dietary habits may help to lessen the symptoms. Eating nutritious snacks between meals helps to maintain blood sugar levels and prevent hypoglycemia, which can otherwise lead to cold extremities and worsen symptoms of Raynaud's Disease. A diet high in protein, low in carbohydrate, and free of caffeine may also help.
Oily fish, such as mackerel and salmon, contain fatty acids known as eicosapentaenoic acid (EPA) and docosahexaenoic acid (DHA). These help in the production of prostaglandins, which are involved in dilating blood vessels.
Citrus fruits, berries, and fruit juices are rich in vitamin C. People with Raynaud's have been found to have low levels of this vitamin.
Dairy products and cereals are good sources of magnesium, which has been found to decrease in people with Raynaud's in the winter months. Increased intakes may lessen symptoms.
Ginger stimulates the circulation. Add $^1/_3$oz of ginger to $2^1/_2$ cups of water and simmer for an hour. Strain the liquid, then drink hot or cold.

✖ FOODS TO AVOID
Frozen foods and cold drinks can worsen symptoms if handled by those with Raynaud's.

◷ OTHER MEASURES
❑ Smokers are advised to give up the habit, since smoking worsens symptoms of this condition.
❑ Regular exercise may improve the circulation and help to lessen symptoms.
❑ Evening primrose oil and flax oil are rich in gamma linolenic acid (GLA), which is thought to have a positive effect on circulation.

See Also Heart & Circulation, page 150

SKIN

VARYING IN THICKNESS from .06 to .16 inches in different areas of the body, skin is one of the largest organs of the body. It is self-repairing and highly sensitive to heat, light, and touch, with numerous nerve endings and blood vessels within its inner layer. The appearance of the skin can vary according to the state of a person's health and mind, and may reveal signs of a wide range of disorders.

DIET & THE SKIN

Research into skin conditions indicates that diet plays a major role in the maintenance of healthy skin. Certain substances in foods protect skin from damage by the sun's rays, while psoriasis may be alleviated by increasing dietary intakes of essential fatty acids. On the other hand, vitamin deficiencies may result in dry skin and poor wound healing, while food intolerances may lead to eczema, requiring the offending food to be removed from the diet.

CARING FOR THE SKIN

Skin must be kept clean and treated with respect. Regular brushing of the skin improves circulation. Moisturizing can help to protect the skin against pollution, dirt, and dehydration. Using sunscreens and keeping the skin covered in strong sunlight reduces the risk of developing skin cancer, especially in fair-skinned people.

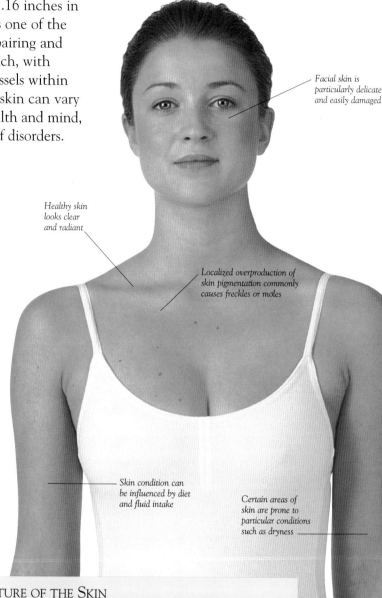

Facial skin is particularly delicate and easily damaged

Healthy skin looks clear and radiant

Localized overproduction of skin pigmentation commonly causes freckles or moles

Skin condition can be influenced by diet and fluid intake

Certain areas of skin are prone to particular conditions such as dryness

STRUCTURE OF THE SKIN

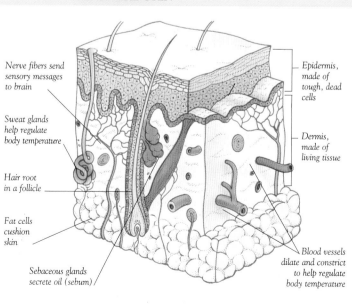

Skin consists of two main layers: a thin, waterproof outer layer, called the epidermis, and a fibrous, elastic inner layer called the dermis. The dermis contains thousands of sweat glands, sebaceous glands, blood vessels, muscle tissue, nerve fibers, fat cells, and hairs, each embedded in a follicle. Skin contains a brown or black pigment called melanin, which protects the skin against the harmful effects of ultraviolet rays. The amount of melanin present in the skin is determined by race and by exposure to sunlight.

Nerve fibers send sensory messages to brain

Sweat glands help regulate body temperature

Hair root in a follicle

Fat cells cushion skin

Sebaceous glands secrete oil (sebum)

Epidermis, made of tough, dead cells

Dermis, made of living tissue

Blood vessels dilate and constrict to help regulate body temperature

TOP HEALING FOODS

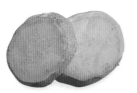

AVOCADOS
PAGE 51

Benefits Contain nutrients that help to maintain skin structure and help wounds to heal.
Useful for Acne, sun damage, wound healing, and herpes.
Nutrients Vitamin E and mono-unsaturated oils.

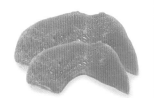

RED MEATS
PAGE 122

Benefits Contain nutrients that may help to reduce inflammation, promote wound healing, and enable skin to renew itself.
Useful for Wound healing, burns, anemic skin.
Nutrients Zinc, protein, iron.

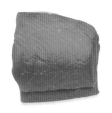

SUNFLOWER SEEDS
PAGE 104

Benefits May help to improve skin that is rough, dry, or flaky, and to keep skin watertight.
Useful for Eczema, dry patches, and generally dehydrated skin.
Nutrients Zinc, protein, omega-6 essential fatty acids, vitamin E.

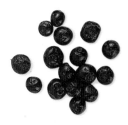

CITRUS FRUITS
PAGE 86

Benefits Repairing grazes and cuts and maintaining the structure of collagen, the protein responsible for smooth, plump-looking skin.
Useful for Damaged skin, aging and sagging skin, and wrinkles.
Nutrients Vitamin C.

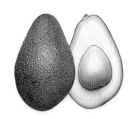

SWEET POTATOES
PAGE 55

Benefits Useful for aiding wound healing, helping scars to fade, and protecting against sun damage.
Useful for Acne and cuts, and preventing sun damage.
Nutrients Beta carotene, vitamins C and E.

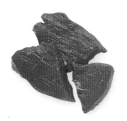

TURKEY
PAGE 124

Benefits Contains an amino acid that may reduce viral growth. Its low allergenicity is good for those on exclusion diets.
Useful for Wound healing, burns, eczema, and herpes.
Nutrients The amino acid lysine.

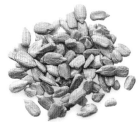

OILY FISH
PAGE 118

Benefits Contains fatty acids that decrease inflammation and improve the skin's watertightness.
Useful for Some forms of dry skin, psoriasis, and inflammation.
Nutrients The omega-3 fatty acids EPA and DHA.

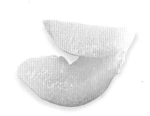

BILBERRIES
PAGE 83

Benefits Very rich in a group of strong antioxidants, which help to strengthen blood capillaries and collagen fibers.
Useful for Aging and sun-damaged skin.
Nutrients Anthocyanidins.

OTHER BENEFICIAL FOODS

FLAX SEEDS
PAGE 105

Benefits Helps skin to stay smooth and retain moisture. May help to reduce inflammation.
Useful for Dry skin and psoriasis.
Nutrients Omega-3 and -6 essential fatty acids, vitamin E.

CARROTS
PAGE 56

Benefits May give protection from the sun's ultraviolet rays and help reduce the appearance of scars.
Useful for Acne, cuts and grazes, and sun damage.
Nutrients Beta carotene.

OYSTERS
PAGE 120

Benefits May help to bolster the efficiency of the immune system and reduce viral infections.
Useful for Herpes, and possibly some cases of psoriasis.
Nutrients Zinc.

LIVER
PAGE 123

Benefits Contains nutrients that help to promote skin regeneration.
Useful for Psoriasis, wound healing, scar reduction in acne.
Nutrients Vitamin A.

FOODS TO AVOID

DAIRY PRODUCTS

People with eczema may benefit by excluding milk and other dairy products from their diet. Most cheese, cream, butter, yogurt, chocolate, and other foods containing milk products should not be eaten.

ALCOHOL

Alcoholic drinks have a diuretic effect on the body and can lead to dehydration. Since good water balance in the body is needed in order to maintain the skin's flexibility and resilience, the effects of dehydration quickly become apparent. Skin takes on a dry appearance, and may even look rough and cracked.

SEAWEEDS

Seaweed is a particularly rich source of iodine, a substance that is thought by some dermatologists to worsen skin conditions such as acne. There are several types of edible seaweed, such as nori and carrageen, and these should be avoided, as should foods that are made from seaweed, such as laver bread.

COFFEE

The caffeine present in coffee has a diuretic effect on the body. Drinking large amounts of coffee on a regular basis may bring about dehydration, which is manifested as dry, inflexible skin.

EGGS

There is some evidence that excluding eggs and egg-based foods from the diet may help to alleviate the symptoms of eczema. Foods containing egg yolk, egg white, egg albumin, and lecithin should all be avoided as far as possible.

CHOCOLATE

There are several foods that are commonly believed to have a detrimental effect on the condition of skin. Chocolate, for example, is suspected by many professionals of being a potential factor in the development of acne, particularly if eaten regularly. There is, however, no scientific evidence to corroborate this popular belief.

ACNE

KEY FOODS

SHELLFISH
page 120

RED MEATS
page 122

CARROTS
page 56

WHOLE GRAINS
pages 92–99

SEEDS
pages 103–105

BERRIES
pages 82–85

CITRUS FRUITS
pages 86–88

AVOCADOS
page 51

GARLIC & ONIONS
pages 66–67

EGGS
page 129

THE DISTRESSING SKIN condition known as acne affects 35–40 percent of teenagers, and boys experience more problems than girls. The main cause of acne is an increased excretion of oily sebum, or grease, by the sebaceous glands in the skin, a blockage of the sebum duct, and bacterial growth. The male prevalence of acne during the teenage years is reversed in later life, when it is not unusual for women in their late twenties and thirties to be affected by acne. The precise cause of the condition is not known. Some doctors in the West rule out diet, the use of cosmetics, and lack of personal hygiene as possible causes.

SYMPTOMS

Acne ranges from mild to severe. Most people with acne have clusters of angry red pimples, often with pus, usually on the face and also possibly on the shoulders and back. The distended areas may include whiteheads and blackheads. After the inflammation has subsided, pigmented areas are left. It is the combination of these symptoms that leads to the overall appearance of acne. Scarring, both physical and psychological, is the most severe consequence. In some variants of the disorder, such as *Acne fulminans*, there may be explosive outbreaks of acne accompanied by fever and aching joints.

CONVENTIONAL TREATMENT

Topical treatments such as benzoyl peroxide, a bleach, are mostly antimicrobial. Antibiotic creams such as erythromycin may also be applied. Oral antibiotics, including tetracyclines, are often prescribed for three months or more. Oral retinoid (vitamin A) treatment is also popular. The drug isoretinoin shrinks the sebaceous glands in the skin and helps to reduce the blocking of the glands. It may also have anti-inflammatory effects. Women on oral retinoid therapy must avoid becoming pregnant, as the high doses of vitamin A affect the growth of the embryo.

BENEFICIAL FOODS

Few dermatologists in the West believe that diet can influence acne in any way, yet there are qualified nutritionists and alternative health practitioners who have had success with a dietary approach. Preliminary findings suggest that exclusion diets (*see page 245*) may be beneficial.
Oysters are the richest known dietary source of zinc. Other shellfish, red meats, and whole-grain breads and cereals are also good sources of this mineral. It has been suggested that a lack of zinc in the diet can play a role in skin inflammation, wound healing, and the form

CASE STUDY

At the age of 30, Caroline Johnston was diagnosed with late onset acne. Her dermatologist prescribed oral retinoid, or "vitamin A" treatment. This meant that she would have to avoid becoming pregnant for at least a year after the treatment in order to allow the very high intakes of vitamin A to work their way out of her system. Caroline decided to find out if there were any alternatives, and consulted an allergy expert, who recommended that she cut out wheat and dairy foods. This helped the condition a little. She was then advised to cut out foods that contained yeast as well, which led to an improvement in her condition.

and course that any outbreak of acne takes.
Liver contains exceptionally high levels of vitamin A, which helps to minimize scarring.
Carrots and sweet potatoes supply beta carotene, which is converted to vitamin A. Good intakes of beta carotene may be beneficial for acne.
Whole-grain breakfast cereals, breads, and pasta supply chromium, which is thought to help reduce infections of the skin.
Flaxseeds, sesame, pumpkin, and sunflower seeds contain essential fatty acids that are needed by the skin for wound healing. These seeds can be ground together, stored in a refrigerator, and then sprinkled over cereals, soups, stews, yogurt, and fruits.
Berries, citrus fruits, peppers, and papaya are rich in vitamin C, which is needed for a healthy immune system, to fight bacterial infections.
Avocados and wheatgerm supply vitamin E, which assists the skin's structure and healing.
Garlic, onions, and eggs contain sulfur, which is thought by optimum nutritionists (*see page 13*) to help the skin, in particular to relieve acne.

FOODS TO AVOID

Seaweed supplies large amounts of iodine, which can make acne worse in some cases.

OTHER MEASURES

❑ Evening primrose oil supplements contain gamma linoleic acid, which helps to build new skin and keep it waterproof and supple.
❑ Some herbalists recommend rubbing tea tree oil, liquidized cabbage leaves, and raw garlic on to areas of skin affected by acne.
❑ Supplements of zinc may be beneficial.

See Also Adolescents & Nutrition, page 138

ECZEMA

KEY FOODS

MEATS
page 122

RICE
page 94

BRASSICAS
pages 44–47

ATOPIC ECZEMA IS A COMMON inflammatory skin disease that affects about ten percent of children in the developed world. It is commonly found on the cheeks, scalp, elbow creases, backs of knees, neck, and hands. Severe childhood eczema can persist into adulthood. Atopic eczema often occurs in people who have asthma and hayfever.

✪ SYMPTOMS In most people, chronic itching is the main symptom, often leading to damaged skin, bleeding, and infection.

✚ CONVENTIONAL TREATMENT
Emollient creams are given to keep the skin moist and supple, and weak steroidal creams are prescribed to reduce inflammation. Infections are treated with antiseptic creams or antibiotics.

✔ BENEFICIAL FOODS
The Few Foods Exclusion Diet (*see page 245*) should be followed for six weeks under the guidance of a doctor and a registered dietician. Other foods can then be introduced one at a time. On an exclusion diet, wheat and dairy products are not allowed.

Lamb, turkey, and rabbit are low-allergenic sources of protein and can be eaten regularly. **Rice, rice-based breakfast cereals, potatoes,** sago, and sago flour are suitable carbohydrates. **Carrots, cauliflower, broccoli,** brussels sprouts, celery, lettuce, and stewed apples are acceptable. **Milk substitute** containing the correct nutrients is essential for any child on this restricted diet. **Water and tea without milk** are suitable drinks. **Sugar, molasses, and syrup** are suitable sweeteners.

✖ FOODS TO AVOID
Eggs, milk, cheese, and other dairy products can worsen symptoms of eczema. This includes skim milk powder, non-fat milk solids, caseinates, whey, lactalbumin, and lactose.

⊘ OTHER MEASURES
❏ Evening primrose oil supplements may improve the condition in both adults and children.
❏ Cotton sheets and clothing are recommended and biological laundry detergents best avoided.

See Also Children & Nutrition, page 136

HERPES

KEY FOODS

CITRUS FRUITS
pages 86–88

BERRIES
pages 82–85

SHELLFISH
page 120

WHOLE GRAINS
pages 92–99

THE VIRUS KNOWN as *herpes simplex* causes cold sores, usually around the lips or nose, and genital outbreaks of painful, infectious, fluid-filled blisters. Herpes is difficult to control and the virus can lie dormant in nerve endings for months or years before suddenly flaring up again.

✪ SYMPTOMS A mild tingling is the first sign that an episode of herpes is about to start. This occurs around the mouth or, in the case of genital herpes, around the vagina in women and in the groin, penis, and scrotum in men. Muscles may begin to ache and lymph glands around local lymph nodes may feel tender. Blisters associated with herpes can be painful for several days.

✚ CONVENTIONAL TREATMENT Antiviral drugs, available in tablet and cream form, are the most common treatment for herpes.

✔ BENEFICIAL FOODS
Citrus fruits and berries are some of the richest sources of vitamin C, which is important for healing sores. Increasing intakes of vitamin C to 1,000mg a day may prevent recurrent outbreaks.

Oysters and other shellfish, wholewheat breads, cereals, and red meat are good sources of zinc, which is needed for skin healing. Zinc may suppress recurrent herpes eruptions when taken in conjunction with vitamin C.
Berries, other fruits, and vegetables supply bioflavonoids. Taken in supplement form, these nutrients have been found to help speed up the recovery from genital herpes in women.
Fish, meat, and chicken are rich in the amino acid lysine, which may reduce herpes outbreaks.

✖ FOODS TO AVOID
Nuts, seeds, and chocolate contain the amino acid known as arginine. The herpes virus thrives in an environment that is rich in arginine.

⊘ OTHER MEASURES
❏ Low levels of the amino acid lysine are linked with an increased risk of herpes recurring. Taken in supplement form, this amino acid may help to reduce the frequency and severity of symptoms.

See Also Minerals, page 30; Vitamins, page 26

PSORIASIS

KEY FOODS

OILY FISH
page 118

CARROTS
page 56

NUTS &
SEEDS
pages 100–105

WHOLE GRAINS
pages 92–99

BRASSICAS
pages 44–47

SHELLFISH
page 120

THIS DISTRESSING INFLAMMATORY skin condition usually starts between the ages of 15 and 25. Outbreaks of chronic psoriasis are often associated with anxiety and stress, and can be chronic or sporadic. Illness, surgery, some drugs, viral and bacterial throat infections, cuts, and contact with poison ivy have also been known to spark the disease. Psoriasis that is associated with arthritis is known as psoriatic arthritis.

✪ SYMPTOMS
Psoriasis is characterized by patches of thick, red skin, often covered by silvery white scales, on the legs, knees, arms, elbows, scalp, ears, and back. These can be uncomfortable and embarrassing. Scalp psoriasis is a cause of dandruff, which is often itchy and involves the shedding of scales and skin debris.

✚ CONVENTIONAL TREATMENT
The treatment depends on the type and severity of the condition. It includes ultraviolet light therapy, ointments and lotions, steroidal creams and, in the case of psoriatic arthritis, non-steroidal anti-inflammatory drugs.

✔ BENEFICIAL FOODS
Oily fish such as salmon, sardines, and mackerel all contain the omega-3 fatty acid known as eicosapentanoic acid (EPA). Studies have found that people with chronic psoriasis who consumed 5oz of oily fish a day were able to reduce the use of steroidal creams without experiencing a decline in their condition. This effect seems to be due to the conversion of EPA in the body into anti-inflammatory substances including leucotrienes 3 and 5, which dampen down the factors that can trigger this disease.

Carrots, apricots, mangoes, and green leafy vegetables are high in beta carotene, which the body converts into vitamin A, essential for healthy skin. Research has revealed that people who eat large amounts of these foods have less risk of psoriasis than those who have low intakes. This could be due to the vitamin C, beta carotene, and other antioxidants present, which improve the strength of the immune system.

Flaxseeds are a valuable source of omega-3 fatty acids and they may have a similar effect to oily fish. Sunflower and sesame seeds also supply these fatty acids. A selection of seeds can be ground together, stored in an airtight container in the refrigerator, and sprinkled over breakfast cereals, yogurt, or other foods.

Brazil nuts are a rich source of selenium, needed for the production of the enzyme glutathione

CASE STUDY
Lucy Perez, aged 44, developed chronic psoriasis in her late twenties, after getting married. Her condition was treated with steroidal creams, which helped to keep the symptoms under control for most of the time. She also received tanning bed treatment. Lucy decided to alter her diet and began to eat 5oz of oily fish each day. This was consumed in various ways: as baked or broiled salmon, in fish cakes, and as tuna fish salads. Due to the increased amounts of omega-3 fatty acids, Lucy was able to wean herself from the steroidal creams and onto emollient creams over an eight-week period. As a result, some of the psoriatic areas healed, while others improved, becoming less red and itchy.

peroxidase. This enzyme stops the formation of certain leucotrienes, which may worsen psoriasis. **Breakfast cereals, breads,** and yeast extracts that are fortified with folic acid may help to correct a deficiency of this vitamin, which has been observed in some people with psoriasis.

Broccoli, cabbage, and other green leafy vegetables supply folate, the natural form of the vitamin folic acid.

Shellfish and whole-grain foods are rich in zinc, which is lost through the skin. Zinc loss is thought to be high in those with psoriasis.

✖ FOODS TO AVOID
Red meats and dairy products should be eaten in moderation, since they contain arachadonic acid, a natural inflammatory substance that is believed to make psoriasis sores red and swollen.

Alcohol may be a trigger factor in psoriasis. In tests, alcohol consumption in people who developed psoriasis was twice that of control groups without the disease.

⊘ OTHER MEASURES
❏ Several studies have indicated that excess weight is associated with an increased risk of psoriasis. Excess weight should be lost in order to reduce this extra stress factor.

❏ A diet that includes an ounce of protein a day and very little fat has produced dramatic reductions in, or disappearance of, skin lesions in people with psoriasis within just two to three months.

❏ Herbalists advise an infusion of yellow dock or figwort. Alternatively, take a decoction of bittersweet.

See Also Stress & Anxiety, page 231

BURNS

KEY FOODS

POULTRY
page 124

MILK
page 126

BERRIES
pages 82–85

SHELLFISH
page 120

A SEVERE BURN CAUSES the body to produce the most pronounced response to stress that it is able to make. As protein and fat is broken down to help mend the burned areas, the body's rate of metabolism rises dramatically, and weight loss of up to 3.3lbs a day might occur. For serious burns, specialized treatment and full nutritional support in a hospital are essential. For minor burns, a well-balanced eating plan at home can speed recovery.

✪ SYMPTOMS Minor burns cause pain, redness, and swelling. More severe burns may be accompanied by shock, the burned area may be open, and the skin below may be exposed.

✚ CONVENTIONAL TREATMENT Small burns and scalds can be treated at home by immersion in cold water, or by the application of cold, wet towels for at least ten minutes, or until the pain is relieved. The area should be covered loosely with a clean, dry dressing. No lotions, oils, ice-cold water, or fluffy dressings should be applied. If the pain persists, or if there are signs of infection, medical help should be sought. Electrical burns must be treated by a doctor.

✔ BENEFICIAL FOODS
Turkey, chicken, eggs, and milk help to replace the protein used up during the healing process.
Berries, citrus fruits, papaya, and peppers supply vitamin C, needed for collagen and new skin.
Avocados and wheat germ are rich sources of vitamin E, which helps wound healing.
Oysters and other shellfish and red meat supply zinc, which speeds up the healing process.
Carrots, sweet potatoes, and red peppers supply beta carotene which, when converted to vitamin A, helps to minimize scarring.
Oily fish, and flax, sunflower, pumpkin, and sesame seeds all provide fatty acids.

✘ FOODS TO AVOID
Candies, cakes, cookies, and low-nutrient foods.
Alcohol and coffee, which encourage fluid loss.

◔ OTHER MEASURES
❑ At least six to eight glasses of water are needed every day in order to maintain fluid balance.

See Also Minerals, page 30; Vitamins, page 26

WOUND HEALING

KEY FOODS

MEATS
page 122

DAIRY
PRODUCTS
pages 126–128

OILY FISH
page 118

EGGS
page 129

PINEAPPLES
page 78

POOR NUTRITION CAN significantly delay the healing of cuts and other wounds, and in some cases, such as bedsores, an inadequate diet can actually cause new wounds to develop. Those who are well nourished prior to sustaining a wound or before surgery tend to recover more quickly than those on diets low in nutrients.

✪ SYMPTOMS The symptoms of wound healing vary according to the cause and the outcome of the individual wound.

✚ CONVENTIONAL TREATMENT Wounds are treated with a variety of dressing and drugs, according to their position in or on the body.

✔ BENEFICIAL FOODS
Meats, poultry, dairy products, and fish are excellent sources of protein, needed for the formation of antibodies to combat infection.
Liver and egg yolks supply vitamin A, and carrots and sweet potatoes provide beta carotene, which is converted into vitamin A. This vitamin stimulates the immune system, which can become depleted in injured people.

Oysters and red meat contain the mineral zinc, which can become depleted when the skin is damaged. Zinc deficiency delays the healing of wounds. An increased intake of these foods may help to speed up skin repair.
Red meat, nuts, and seeds provide iron, needed for DNA synthesis and the regeneration of cells.
Citrus fruits, berries, and green leafy vegetables are rich in vitamin C, which is essential for collagen. Wound healing directly uses vitamin C.
Pineapples supply bromelain, which has been shown to improve wound healing.
Oily fish, and sunflower, flax, and sesame seeds provide essential fats needed for new cell walls.

✘ FOODS TO AVOID
Cakes, cookies, candies and other low-nutrient foods since they do not assist the healing process.

◔ OTHER MEASURES
❑ Postoperative supplements of vitamin A, taken for seven days, can strengthen new tissue.

See Also Proteins, page 20; Vitamins, page 26

DIGESTIVE SYSTEM

FOODS HAVE TO BE DIGESTED before the body can absorb and use the nutrients they contain. The digestive tract is essentially a long tube, surrounded by muscles, which assumes different shapes and roles as it winds its way through the body. Within the digestive system, the liver, gallbladder, pancreas, and other organs have particular functions, such as enzyme production. Digestion involves the nervous system and is ultimately controlled by the brain.

DIET & DIGESTION

Dietary manipulation has been used to treat digestive disorders for centuries. Ayurvedic medicine in India traditionally uses a yogurt-based drink to aid digestion, and Chinese medicine prescribes flax seeds to treat constipation. Recent research in the West has shown that diseases of and imbalances in the digestive system can be treated or prevented by dietary manipulation. A fiber-rich diet, for example, may relieve symptoms of constipation or an irritable bowel, and help to prevent colon cancer.

EATING FOR HEALTH

Diets rich in whole-grain foods, fruits, and vegetables are recommended for the maintenance of digestive health. The sizes of servings and frequency of meals are also important in keeping the digestive system in shape.

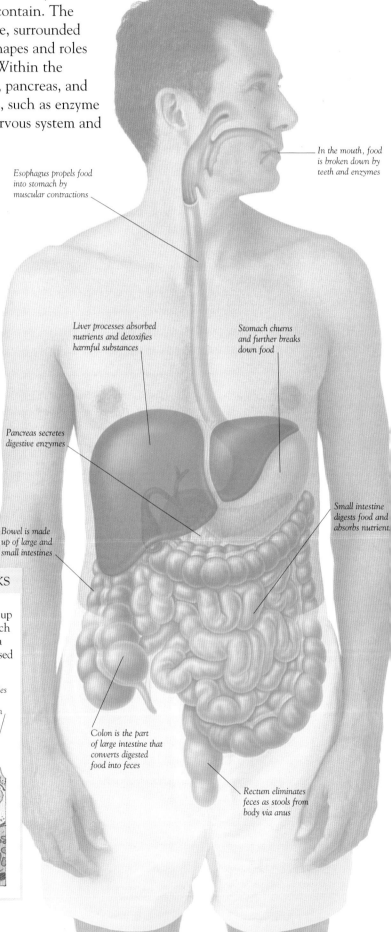

In the mouth, food is broken down by teeth and enzymes

Esophagus propels food into stomach by muscular contractions

Liver processes absorbed nutrients and detoxifies harmful substances

Stomach churns and further breaks down food

Pancreas secretes digestive enzymes

Small intestine digests food and absorbs nutrient.

Bowel is made up of large and small intestines

Colon is the part of large intestine that converts digested food into feces

Rectum eliminates feces as stools from body via anus

HOW THE SMALL INTESTINE WORKS

The inner wall of the small intestine is made up of millions of tiny projections, called villi. Each villus has its own blood supply. Villi provide a vast surface area through which nutrients released by digestion can pass into the bloodstream.

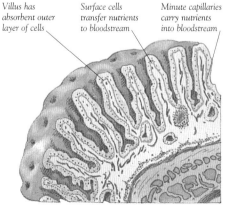

Villus has absorbent outer layer of cells

Surface cells transfer nutrients to bloodstream

Minute capillaries carry nutrients into bloodstream

TOP HEALING FOODS

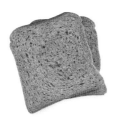

WHOLEWHEAT BREAD PAGE 98

Benefits Rich in insoluble fiber, it increases the bulk of stools and so eases their passage along the colon.
Useful for Those with irritable bowel syndrome, hemorrhoids, and constipation.
Nutrients Carbohydrates.

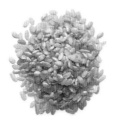

WHOLE GRAINS PAGE 92

Benefits Supply insoluble fiber, which improves stool texture.
Useful for Those with IBS, hemorrhoids, constipation, diverticulitis, and gallstones.
Nutrients Carbohydrates, protein, B vitamins.

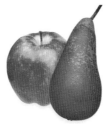

APPLES & PEARS PAGES 74-75

Benefits Contain soluble fiber and sorbitol, a sweetener with laxative properties.
Useful for Lowering the levels of cholesterol in the body and in the treatment of gallstones.
Nutrients Carbohydrate.

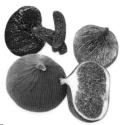

FIGS PAGE 80

Benefits Contain natural, gentle laxatives to ease and increase the frequency of bowel movements.
Useful for Constipation, diverticulitis, and hemorrhoids.
Nutrients When dried, iron, potassium, calcium.

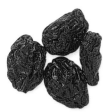

PRUNES PAGE 79

Benefits Their gentle laxative property, due to the presence of hydroxyphenylisatin, helps to move stools along the colon.
Useful for Constipation.
Nutrients Beta carotene, calcium, potassium, selenium.

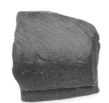

TUNA PAGE 119

Benefits Contains omega-3 fatty acids that reduce inflammation.
Useful for May improve the symptoms of inflammatory bowel conditions such as diverticulitis and Crohn's disease.
Nutrients Vitamin D.

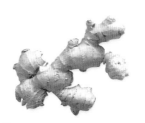

GINGER PAGE 114

Benefits May help to relieve symptoms of nausea associated with morning and travel sickness.
Useful for Nausea.
Nutrients Vary depending on its form, for example as ginger ale or in cookies.

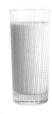

SOY MILK PAGE 60

Benefits Alternative to dairy milk, since it does not contain the sugar lactose.
Useful for Those whose lactose intolerance gives them flatulence.
Nutrients Added calcium and protein.

OTHER BENEFICIAL FOODS

CARROTS PAGE 56

Benefits Rich source of beta carotene, which may aid the healing of damaged tissue in the lining of the stomach.
Useful for Peptic ulcers.
Nutrients Beta carotene.

TROUT PAGE 118

Benefits Excellent source of easily digested protein.
Useful for Diverticulitis, nausea, and recovery of the digestive system from illness generally.
Nutrients Protein, calcium.

BANANAS PAGE 90

Benefits Rich in potassium.
Useful for Rebalancing electrolytes following diarrhea, especially that related to IBS.
Nutrients Carbohydrate, magnesium, potassium.

APRICOTS PAGE 76

Benefits Contain the sugar alcohol sorbitol, which is slowly absorbed from the digestive system and helps loosen stools.
Useful for Constipation.
Nutrients Vitamin C.

FOODS TO AVOID

CARBONATED DRINKS

Carbonated drinks introduce extra air into the digestive system, causing bloating and gas in the upper digestive tract. This may lead to discomfort, making clothes feel tight and causing pain in the chest. Plain water and juices are healthier options.

DAIRY PRODUCTS

People who are unable to tolerate the milk sugar lactose should avoid, or strictly limit, dairy products, such as milk, yogurt, and cheese. Lactose that has not been digested moves into the colon, where bacteria use it as a food source, and in so doing create large volumes of gas.

LEGUMES

Many legumes contain raffinose and stacchyose. Both are carbohydrates that move largely undigested into the colon, where they are food for gas-producing bacteria.

WHOLE-GRAIN FOODS

While fiber-rich grains are effective in the treatment of some digestive disorders, insoluble fiber may actually exacerbate other disorders and may therefore need to be avoided. For those with diarrhea and certain irritable bowel disorders, a diet that is low in whole-grain foods may be advisable.

CERTAIN VEGETABLES

Jerusalem artichokes contain inulin, a carbohydrate that cannot be digested and which commonly causes uncomfortable gas. Many people are unable to digest onions or green peppers, while others have difficulty with turnips and rutabagas.

SNACK FOODS

Some other foods, both sweet and salty, should be avoided to alleviate symptoms of disorders such as peptic ulcers, heartburn, liver disease, gallstones, hemorrhoids, and obesity. Digestion can be assisted by avoiding or limiting fried foods, animal fats, red meats, sugar, salt, pastries, white bread, alcohol, and caffeine.

MEATS
page 122

FISH
pages 118–121

POULTRY
page 124

DAIRY
PRODUCTS
pages 126–128

WHOLE GRAINS
pages 92–99

HEARTBURN

WHEN LARGE AMOUNTS of acidic stomach contents are regurgitated past the stomach's valve and up into the gullet, heartburn occurs. Small amounts of acid reflux are normal and harmless, since constantly swallowing saliva quickly washes it back into the stomach. However, if the amount of refluxed material is greater than normal and persists over a period of time, this can result in debilitating heartburn, which affects the enjoyment of food. It can lead to inflammation, bleeding, narrowing of the gullet, anemia, and, in some cases, results in cancer.

✪ SYMPTOMS Heartburn is usually described as a burning sensation in the chest and upper abdomen. It is hardly surprising that heartburn is painful, since it is associated with the production of gastric acid. The stomach wall secretes hydrochloric acid to help kill bacteria that enter the body via food and drink. The stomach lining is coated with a thick layer of mucus to protect it from this acid. The throat and mouth have no such protection, hence the pain associated with refluxed material. If reflux is regurgitated into the mouth, it also creates an unpleasant acidic taste.

✚ CONVENTIONAL TREATMENT Most people treat heartburn with over-the-counter or prescribed antacid preparations. These usually contain sodium, aluminum, calcium, and magnesium. Prolonged use of antacids can lead to a mineral imbalance.

✔ BENEFICIAL FOODS
Lean meats, fish, poultry, and low fat dairy products are all rich in protein and appear to enhance the tone of the valve at the top of the stomach. Making sure that all meals and snacks contain some protein may help to tighten the valve over time and diminish the problem.
Whole-grain cereals, wholewheat breads, and brown rice are rich in insoluble fiber. This fiber bulks up the stools and prevents constipation, which may otherwise cause a buildup of pressure in the colon. This pressure can move up into the stomach and force the stomach valve to open. If this happens, heartburn occurs. It is important when increasing intakes of whole-grain foods to increase fluid intake to six to eight cups a day, in order to keep the stools soft. Increasing fiber without extra fluid can make the stools hard.
Apple cider vinegar mixed with water and sipped during a meal can help those who are affected by heartburn. One tablespoon of apple cider vinegar should be mixed with a glass of water.

✘ FOODS TO AVOID
Fried foods, fatty meats, pies, cakes, cookies, margarine, butter, oils, and cream appear to weaken the stomach valve.
Peppermint taken as tea or as a sweet following a meal relaxes the smooth muscles in the stomach valve and encourages reflux.
Coffee, tea, and cola all contain caffeine, which encourages extra acid production and weakens the stomach valve.
Chocolate contains methylxanthines, which are related to caffeine and appear to have a valve-weakening effect. Those with reflux should avoid chocolate and chocolate drinks after meals.
Fruit and vegetable juices may irritate the lining of the throat if it has previously been damaged by chronic heartburn.
Onions and garlic may have adverse effects on stomach-valve tone.

✐ OTHER MEASURES
❑ Alcohol weakens the stomach valve and may increase heartburn.
❑ Large meals are best avoided, especially during pregnancy. The stomach is pushed out of position by the growing fetus, forcing the contents of the stomach up into the throat.
❑ Being overweight can cause the stomach to be pushed out of position, forcing the stomach contents up into the throat.
❑ Eat meals and snacks slowly and chew food well, preferably in a stress-free environment.
❑ Bending over or lying down after a meal tips the stomach contents and encourages reflux.

See Also Anemia, page 160; Constipation, page 175

KEY FOODS

CARROTS
page 56

CITRUS
FRUITS
pages 86–88

MEATS
page 122

FISH
pages 118–121

NUTS &
SEEDS
pages 100–105

PEPTIC ULCERS

GASTRIC AND DUODENAL ulcers, commonly known as peptic ulcers, are areas of erosion in the lining of the gastrointestinal tract. They occur when the balance between the digestive juices and the protective lining is disturbed. Ulcers may also be caused by the harmful effects of aspirin and the bacteria known as *Helicobacter pylori*.

⊗ SYMPTOMS
These can include mild discomfort, a burning pain in the upper abdomen, vomiting, and weight loss.

✛ CONVENTIONAL TREATMENT
The symptoms may disappear if treated with drugs that reduce the amount of acid and pepsin that is secreted by the stomach, and by antibiotic drugs.

✔ BENEFICIAL FOODS
Carrots, red peppers, and apricots are rich in beta carotene, which helps the gut wall to heal.
Citrus fruits and green leafy vegetables are rich in vitamin C, which may help avoid further damage.
Red meats, shellfish such as oysters, and wholegrain cereals help the healing process.
Oily fish, nuts, and seeds contain essential fatty acids that may protect the digestive tract.
Meats, milk, and potatoes contain vitamin B$_6$, which is low in some people who have ulcers.
Nuts, seeds, eggs, whole-grain cereals, avocados, and green leafy vegetables supply vitamin E, well known for its ability to heal body linings.

⊗ FOODS TO AVOID
Fried foods, alcohol, coffee, tea, and sodas may cause overproduction of acid in the stomach.
Pickles, black pepper, spices, chilies, and mustard irritate the lining of the stomach.
Milk temporarily neutralizes acid secretion, but this is followed by a rise in levels of acidity.
Salt and soy sauce, taken in large quantities, have been linked to an increased risk of ulcers.

⊘ OTHER MEASURES
❏ Eat regularly and avoid large meals, as they can increase acid production and the risk of ulcers.
❏ Smokers are advised to give up the habit, as it increases acid production.

See Also Digestive System, page 168

KEY FOODS

HERBS
page 108

WHOLE GRAINS
pages 92–99

HALITOSIS

BAD BREATH, OR HALITOSIS, can be due to poor dental hygiene, a decayed tooth, a buildup of tartar, infected gums, or an abscess. Halitosis may also be a sign of constipation or sinusitis. In some cases, halitosis is caused by a serious underlying condition, such as kidney or liver failure, or uncontrolled diabetes.

✛ CONVENTIONAL TREATMENT
Unless halitosis is caused by an underlying illness, it can usually be eliminated by adopting sensible eating habits and thorough oral hygiene. If the cause of halitosis is unknown and is not easily remedied, advice from a dentist or doctor may be required. Various commercial mouthwashes are available. These are effective at removing odors as well as killing off harmful bacteria.

✔ BENEFICIAL FOODS
Fresh parsley chewed after a meal can reduce odors from foods that have just been eaten. Chewing fresh thyme, mint, and tarragon may have a similar effect.
Fresh dill, coriander, or cardamom seeds chewed after a meal can help to prevent halitosis.
Whole-grain breads, rice, and pasta eaten on a regular basis can help to prevent constipation, and may thereby help to improve halitosis.

⊗ FOODS TO AVOID
Candies, sweet drinks, cakes, and cookies should be avoided, since these may lead to an increase in dental decay and mouth disease.
Garlic, onions, and spicy foods can increase halitosis. Some people may wish to avoid them.

⊘ OTHER MEASURES
❏ Drink at least six to eight glasses of water a day to help avoid constipation and to keep the mouth moist. This reduces the severity of halitosis.
❏ Chewing sugar-free gum that contains the natural decay preventing substance xylitol after and between meals can improve dental hygiene.
❏ Brush the teeth regularly for good oral hygiene.
❏ Smokers are advised to give up the habit since it can make the breath smell worse.

See Also Gum Disease, page 206; Tooth Decay, page 207

KEY FOODS

DAIRY
PRODUCTS
pages 126–128

WHOLE GRAINS
pages 92–99

FRUITS
pages 72–91

VEGETABLES
pages 42–71

GALLSTONES

HARD LUMPS OF cholesterol, calcium, or bile that become crystallized in the gallbladder, or bile duct, are known as gallstones. These often go undetected until they grow large enough to cause discomfort. The condition is common in the West and affects twice as many women as men. Excess weight increases the risk of gallstones.

✪ SYMPTOMS The symptoms range from mild abdominal discomfort to severe pain and vomiting. After a meal of rich, fatty foods there may be bloating, flatulence, and discomfort. The stools may be yellow in color.

✚ CONVENTIONAL TREATMENT This involves dietary advice to relieve symptoms and to prevent further gallstones. If symptoms are severe, surgery may be necessary to remove the stones or the whole gallbladder.

✔ BENEFICIAL FOODS
A low-fat, high-fiber diet rich in vegetables may help to prevent gallstones, which appear to be twice as likely in meat-eaters as in vegetarians. **Skimmed milk and low-fat yogurts** are good choices for those with gallstones.
Wholewheat breads, and wholewheat pasta and rice should be eaten instead of refined versions.
Apples, pears, oats, and legumes contain soluble fiber, which helps to decrease high cholesterol levels that could lead to gallstones.
Vegetable and fruit intakes should be increased.
Artichokes contain a substance called cynarin, which may help to reduce cholesterol levels.

✖ FOODS TO AVOID
Fried foods, pastry, and foods such as sausages and burgers, which are high in animal fats.
Full-fat dairy products, such as butter, cheese, and oils. Replace these with low-fat products.

⊘ OTHER MEASURES
❏ For those trying to lose weight, fasting should be avoided, since missing meals makes the gallbladder inactive. Breakfast is important, since the lack of food in the night increases the chance of cholesterol buildup in the gallbladder.

See Also Obesity, page 178

KEY FOODS

MEATS
page 122

FISH
pages 118–121

WHOLE GRAINS
pages 92–99

GREEN
VEGETABLES
pages 44–51

EGGS
page 129

INFLAMMATORY BOWEL DISEASE (IBD)

CHRONIC INFLAMMATORY DISORDERS of the bowel, such as Crohn's disease and ulcerative colitis, are known collectively as inflammatory bowel disease (IBD). Crohn's disease can affect any part of the intestinal tract, whereas ulcerative colitis is a disease that affects only the large intestine. The condition may be triggered by food intolerance.

✪ SYMPTOMS Crohn's disease leads to diarrhea, abdominal tenderness, weight loss, flatulence, fever, and anemia. Ulcerative colitis causes bloody diarrhea, cramps in the lower abdomen, weight loss, and often fever.

✚ CONVENTIONAL TREATMENT Pain-killers and anti-inflammatory drugs are usually prescribed. Dietary advice may be given. In severe cases, surgery may be required.

✔ BENEFICIAL FOODS
Meats, poultry, fish, and dairy foods supply high-value protein that can be easily digested by those who have lost weight during bouts of IBD.
Whole-grain breads, green vegetables, breakfast cereals, and yeast extracts fortified with folic acid help to correct folate deficiency, which can occur with IBD. Folic acid supplements may be needed.
Eggs and oily fish supply vitamin D, which can be low in people with IBD due to a deficiency in bile salts. Oily fish also contain essential fatty acids, which have anti-inflammatory effects.
Fruit juices, fruits, and vegetables supply potassium, which is lost through diarrhea.
Nuts, seeds, dairy products, and fortified soy products supply calcium, which may be poorly absorbed due to diarrhea.

✖ FOODS TO AVOID
Foods that some people with IBD find helpful, such as dairy products, whole grains, nuts, fruits, and shellfish, may actually worsen symptoms in others. Food intolerances are often transitory.
Whole-grain foods rich in insoluble fiber may trigger diarrhea in certain people.

⊘ OTHER MEASURES
❏ Supplements of fish oils may reduce symptoms.

See Also Nonallergic Food Intolerances, page 211

KEY FOODS

VEGETABLES
pages 42–71

FRUITS
pages 72–91

MEATS
page 122

OILS
page 106

IRRITABLE BOWEL SYNDROME (IBS)

THIS CONDITION IS ONE of the most common digestive disorders. The cause is poorly understood, but its effects may result from an abnormality in the part of the nervous system that controls the intestines. Irritable bowel syndrome (IBS) is commonly triggered by stress, food intolerance, abdominal operations, antibiotic drugs, and hormonal changes during the menstrual cycle.

✪ SYMPTOMS There may be abdominal pain, flatulence, bloating, and irregular bowel habits alternating between diarrhea and constipation. Pain may be relieved by passing stools or gas.

✚ CONVENTIONAL TREATMENT Drugs that reduce the time that it takes for the bowel contents to move through the bowel may help to relieve diarrhea, and antispasmodic drugs may relieve pain. Some IBS specialists believe that food intolerances lie at the heart of this problem, and recommend an exclusion diet (*see page 245*) when an intolerance is suspected.

✔ BENEFICIAL FOODS
Vegetables and fruits boost intakes of essential vitamins, minerals, and soluble fiber.
Fruit juices that contain *Lactobacillus plantarum* can help the colon to establish beneficial bacteria. This is useful for IBS if there is an intolerance to milk and dairy products.

Plain, lean meats and white fish supply a good-quality protein and are usually well tolerated by people with IBS who have food intolerances.
Olive oil and safflower oil are advisable in preference to other fats and oils.
Soy milk can be used instead of dairy products.

✖ FOODS TO AVOID
People with IBS are often intolerant to dairy products and cereals. The most poorly tolerated cereal is wheat. An exclusion diet may help.
Seek advice from a dietician.
Chickpeas, red kidney beans, lentils and peas, apples, grapes, and raisins can trigger symptoms.
Brussels sprouts, cauliflower, broccoli, and other brassicas may make symptoms worse.
Preserved meats, bacon, sausages, smoked fish, and shellfish can be excluded for 14 days to see if the symptoms improve.

⊘ OTHER MEASURES
❏ Stress is often associated with IBS. Lifestyle changes, psychotherapy, hypnotherapy, relaxation techniques, and exercise may help.
❏ Regular eating patterns are essential. It is also important to maintain a varied diet.
❏ Evening primrose oil supplements may be beneficial in menstrual-related IBS.

See Also Nonallergic Food Intolerances, page 211

EATING PLAN FOR IRRITABLE BOWEL SYNDROME

People with IBS are usually aware of the kinds of food that they can tolerate and those that worsen their symptoms. The following eating plans give a few suggestions for meals and snacks that are usually well tolerated and may be suitable for people who have this condition.

BREAKFASTS	LIGHT MEALS	MAIN MEALS	SNACKS
Cornflakes with chopped banana and skim milk or soy milk	*Baked potato with tuna*	*Salmon steak with green leaf salad*	*Rice cakes*
Glass of fruit juice	*Apple and pear*	*Orange sorbet*	*Rye crispbreads*
◆	◆	◆	
Poached egg on rye toast	*Ham sandwich with tomato and rye bread*	*Mushroom risotto with steamed zucchini and green beans*	*Oatcakes*
Glass of orange juice	*Soya yogurt*	*Fruit compote*	*Banana*
◆	◆	◆	◆
Live yogurt and fruit salad sprinkled with toasted, crushed almonds	*Rice cakes with hummus and salad*	*Roast lamb with baked potato and honey glazed carrots*	*Live yogurt*
	Large banana	*Peach and pear*	◆
			Wheat-free oatmeal squares

KEY FOODS

WHOLE GRAINS
pages 92–99

PRUNES & FIGS
pages 79–80

VEGETABLES
pages 42–71

FRUITS
pages 72–91

DIVERTICULITIS

THIS COMMON BOWEL disorder is usually a result of long-term constipation. A buildup of pressure in the bowel and straining to pass hard feces cause weak areas of the bowel wall to balloon outwards, forming pouchlike diverticulae. If these diverticulae become infected and inflamed, diverticulitis results. The first signs of this condition can be identified in 15 percent of people over the age of 50.

✪ SYMPTOMS
The symptoms of this condition include abdominal pain that is colicky and associated with nausea, flatulence, fever, and changed bowel habits. Diverticulitis may result in perforation, an abscess, or bleeding.

✚ CONVENTIONAL TREATMENT
Up until the 1960s, the treatment for diverticulitis was to rest the bowel by providing a diet free of fiber. It is now well established that lack of fiber is a main cause of the condition. Treatment for diverticulitis includes bed rest, pain relief, and antibiotics. Surgery may be necessary if there is an abscess, perforation, or severe bleeding.

✔ BENEFICIAL FOODS
Wholewheat breads, brown pasta, and wholegrain rice are more beneficial than the refined versions of these foods. The insoluble fiber present in whole grains helps to bulk up the stools and decreases pressure in the colon.

Prunes contain hydroxyphenylisatin, a substance that stimulates the smooth muscle of the colon wall and increases the speed of contractions in the colon, helping to prevent constipation.
Figs help to keep the bowels moving and are useful additions to the diet.
Vegetables and fruits of all types provide extra bulk and help to keep the contents of the colon moving, thereby preventing constipation.

✖ FOODS TO AVOID
Refined foods such as white breads, cakes, and cookies, since they supply little dietary fiber.
Red meats have been shown to lead to a higher incidence of diverticular disease, due to their apparent ability to weaken the wall of the colon.

❷ OTHER MEASURES
❑ At least six glasses of water are required each day. A diet rich in insoluble fiber without plenty of water causes hard, compacted stools.
❑ Regular physical activity, such as walking or swimming, helps to keep the colon moving.
❑ Diverticulitis seems to occur less frequently in vegetarians than in meat-eaters. This is attributed to their extra intake of fiber. Meat-eaters who are prone to diverticulitis may consider a more vegetarian-based eating plan.

See Also Flatulence, page 176; Nausea, page 180

EATING PLAN FOR DIVERTICULITIS

It is possible to improve constipation, and thereby diverticulitis, by making gradual changes to the diet. Choosing wholewheat breads, pasta, and breakfast cereals in preference to white, refined versions makes the most difference. It is important to increase daily fluid intake as well as fiber intake.

BREAKFASTS	LIGHT MEALS	MAIN MEALS	SNACKS
Bran flakes with chopped dates and skim milk	*Wholewheat pasta salad with flaked tuna fish and fresh corn*	*Cauliflower in cheese sauce with wholewheat bread*	*Dried figs and prunes*
Glass of orange juice	*Fresh plums or cherries*	*Ice cream with baked pear*	◆
◆	◆	◆	*Whole-grain crispbreads*
Ruby red grapefruit	*Rye bread with reduced-fat cream cheese and peach slices*	*Vegetable stir-fry with red peppers and cashews, and whole-grain rice*	◆
Toasted wholewheat muffin served with poached egg	*Fruit yogurt with banana*	*Prunes and yogurt*	*Wholewheat fruit scone or plain scone*
◆	◆	◆	◆
Bowl of muesli with strawberries and skimmed milk	*Granary turkey roll with tomato and lettuce*	*Cottage pie with baked potato and green beans*	*Wholewheat muffin with mashed banana*
Glass of apple juice	*Pineapple with fromage frais*	*Mango in meringue with fromage frais*	◆
			Slice of wholewheat bread

KEY FOODS

WHOLE GRAINS
pages 92–99

PRUNES & FIGS
pages 79–80

FRUITS
pages 72–91

VEGETABLES
pages 42–71

CONSTIPATION

IN GENERAL TERMS, constipation is the delayed movement of stools through the large intestine, which occurs because the stools are small, hard, dry, and difficult to pass. The condition has two main causes. Continually ignoring the signals that the body sends out when it is time to defecate can cause constipation, particularly in the elderly. The other main cause is eating a highly refined diet that contains very little fiber.

✚ SYMPTOMS
The overwhelming symptom of constipation is the discomfort and difficulty experienced on passing stools.

✚ CONVENTIONAL TREATMENT
Laxatives, lubricants, suppositories, and enemas are some of the medical interventions that doctors may use to relieve constipation.

✔ BENEFICIAL FOODS
If serious medical causes have been ruled out, dietary intervention is highly recommended. **Wholewheat breads, whole-grain** breakfast cereals, and pasta play a central role in a high-fiber diet.

Prunes directly stimulate the large intestine wall, triggering increased movement of the bowels.
Figs supply fiber and are well known as a natural remedy for constipation.
Apples, other fruits, and vegetables provide bulk and help to keep the contents of the colon moving, thereby preventing constipation.

✖ FOODS TO AVOID
Refined white cereal products and baked goods such as white bread are low in fiber.

⦶ OTHER MEASURES
❑ Drinking at least six glasses of water or other fluids is required every day to help prevent constipation.
❑ Psyllium husks infused in boiling water act as a bulking laxative that lubricates the bowel.
❑ Massaging the stomach gently can help to stimulate bowel function.
❑ Regular exercise such as swimming and walking can help to relieve this condition.

See Also Fiber, page 14

KEY FOODS

WHOLE GRAINS
pages 92–99

CITRUS FRUITS
pages 86–88

MEATS
page 122

OILY FISH
page 118

HEMORRHOIDS

SOMETIMES REFERRED TO as "piles," hemorrhoids are distended veins in the lining of the anus. This condition is common, and it is often attributed to a low fiber diet and an inadequate intake of fluid. Straining to pass small, hard stools increases the pressure in the abdomen, which slows the flow of blood in the veins around the anus. Repeated straining produces the distended veins known as piles.

✚ SYMPTOMS
Hemorrhoids can cause local pain and sometimes itching. Bright red blood on the surface of the stool may be observed.

✚ CONVENTIONAL TREATMENT
This condition may improve following dietary advice and sometimes with the use of various bulking agents to relieve constipation. For more severe cases, surgery may be recommended.

✔ BENEFICIAL FOODS
Wholewheat breads and pasta, brown rice, oats, legumes, and apples are rich in fiber, which bulks up the stools and helps to prevent constipation.
Citrus fruits, figs, prunes, berries, and legumes

should be eaten regularly if hemorrhoids are associated with bleeding.
Meats and oily fish are good suppliers of "hem" iron (*see page 160*), which improves absorption of iron from legumes and vegetables.

✖ FOODS TO AVOID
White rice, pasta, and breads need to be replaced with unrefined versions of these foods.
Cakes, cookies, pastries, candies, and chocolate provide very little fiber and are best avoided.

⦶ OTHER MEASURES
❑ Losing excess weight will relieve some of the internal strain on the colon and hemorrhoids.
❑ Avoid sitting or standing for long periods of time, since this can make symptoms worse.
❑ Do gentle exercise, such as swimming, and minimize heavy physical work.
❑ At least six glasses or cups of fluid are required each day. A diet rich in insoluble fiber but low in fluids has the effect of compacting stools.

See Also Fiber, page 14

DIARRHEA

KEY FOODS

BANANAS
page 90

RICE
page 94

YOGURT
page 128

THIS CONDITION IS A SYMPTOM of anxiety, bacterial, viral, or other infections, food intolerances, intestinal disease, hormonal disorders, or an excessive intake of sorbitol, fructose, or fiber. Severe diarrhea depletes the body's water, sodium, potassium, calcium, and magnesium levels. Long-term, it disturbs the absorption of essential nutrients.

✪ SYMPTOMS Accompanying symptoms of diarrhea can include drowsiness, irritability, muscle cramps, headaches, fever, and faintness.

✚ CONVENTIONAL TREATMENT Acute diarrhea usually clears up without treatment. When chronic diarrhea is due to an underlying disorder, treatment focuses on the primary illness.

✔ BENEFICIAL FOODS
Fruit and vegetable juices diluted with water help to maintain fluid levels and replace some of the lost potassium, as well as supplying energy and nutrients. Vegetable soups and stewed fruits are easy to digest and help to replace lost potassium and, in the case of soup, sodium.

Bananas are well tolerated and rich in potassium. **White rice, white pasta**, and rice pudding are low in insoluble fiber and supply energy without overstimulating colon movement.
Yogurt helps to replenish beneficial bacteria lost through diarrhea. It also supplies protein, carbohydrate, and calcium.

✖ FOODS TO AVOID
Coffee, tea, and sodas containing caffeine should not be consumed for at least 48 hours after diarrhea, since they have a diuretic effect.
Any foods to which a person is intolerant should be removed from the diet.
Candies and drinks containing sorbitol and manitol speed up the action of the digestive tract and are best avoided by those with diarrhea.

◷ OTHER MEASURES
❑ Drink plenty of water and other fluids.
❑ Zinc supplements may help chronic diarrhea.
❑ Avoid taking more than 6g of vitamin C daily.

See Also Infections, page 212

FLATULENCE

KEY FOODS

GINGER
page 114

SEEDS
pages 103–105

HERBS
page 108

YOGURT
page 128

EXCESSIVE GAS, OR FLATULENCE, can be caused by bacteria acting on undigested proteins and carbohydrates in the colon. More than 250 gases are expelled from the body in the form of flatus, or gas. Nitrogen, oxygen, hydrogen, carbon dioxide, and methane make up 99 percent of these gases.

✪ SYMPTOMS Flatulence causes bloating and abdominal discomfort, and this is often only relieved by the expulsion of gas.

✚ CONVENTIONAL TREATMENT In the absence of any other symptoms, general advice on diet and lifestyle is usually given.

✔ BENEFICIAL FOODS
Rosemary, sage, thyme, and fennel help the digestion and may be eaten with brussels sprouts, cabbage, and legumes, which can cause flatulence.
Cinnamon has antispasmodic and antimicrobial properties. It is thought to help reduce flatulence.
Caraway seeds and fennel seeds are used by herbalists for their powerful calming effects on the digestive system.

Chamomile tea may help to reduce inflammation in the digestive tract and relieve flatulence.
Yogurt eaten daily can help to maintain levels of beneficial bacteria essential to digestion.
Peppermint made into a tea relaxes the colon, helping to relieve the discomfort of gas.

✖ FOODS TO AVOID
Legumes contain carbohydrates called stacchyose and raffinose, which cause bacteria in the colon to produce gas. Jerusalem artichokes contain inulin, which has a similar effect.
Rutabaga, brussels sprouts, cabbage, and corn are known for creating excess gas.
Sorbitol, a sweetener used in diet drinks, is difficult to digest and causes gas in many people.

◷ OTHER MEASURES
❑ Exercise helps to prevent the gas in the colon from becoming trapped and causing discomfort.
❑ Massaging the stomach can help to release trapped gas so that it can be expelled.

See Also Bloating, page 179

LIVER DISEASE

KEY FOODS

ARTICHOKES
page 48

GARLIC
page 66

APPLES &
PEARS
pages 74–75

LEGUMES
pages 58–60

MEATS
page 122

FISH
pages 118–121

POULTRY
page 124

DAIRY
PRODUCTS
pages 126–128

NUTS &
SEEDS
pages 100–105

WHOLE GRAINS
pages 92–99

THE LIVER IS THE SECOND-LARGEST ORGAN of the body. It filters more than a 4 cups of blood per minute, removing bacteria, toxins, antigens, and antibodies from the circulation. It is by this route that many other substances in the blood, including histamine, hormones, drugs, and pesticides, are excreted. The liver is responsible for producing bile, which is stored in the gallbladder, and helps the digestion of fats and absorption of fat soluble substances, including vitamins. Many vitamins and minerals are stored in the liver, as is glucose in the form of glycogen, which helps to maintain blood sugar levels.

All of these functions and many others are affected by liver disease, which may be acute or chronic. Acute liver disease is caused by viruses or toxins, including alcohol. The liver has a remarkable capacity to regenerate itself, but the effects of persistent and long-term alcohol abuse can lead to chronic alcoholic hepatitis and cirrhosis. Cirrhosis is an inflammation of the liver. This leads to the formation of scar tissue, which affects liver function. Chronic liver diseases can also be caused by drugs, viral infections, and autoimmune disease.

✪ SYMPTOMS Signs of chronic liver disease can include jaundice, fever, loss of body hair, distension of the abdomen, and fatty deposits around the eyelids.

✚ CONVENTIONAL TREATMENT Since the liver's role in metabolism and nutrition is so diverse, a number of nutritional imbalances can occur due to poor functioning. Hospital treatment is required to identify the underlying cause of liver disease and to assess the nutritional status of the patient. Nutritional therapy varies depending on the symptoms. In addition to nutritional therapy, treatment may include various drugs, diuretics, and fluid restrictions.

✔ BENEFICIAL FOODS
For those who do not have a serious liver disease but wish to improve their liver function, the following dietary steps can be taken.
Artichokes are believed to help reduce levels of fats and cholesterol by stimulating liver function. This could reduce fatty buildups in the liver and improve its ability to detoxify, as well as its capacity for repair.
Garlic has antibiotic, antiviral, and antibacterial effects that may help to protect the liver. Garlic also appears to lower cholesterol levels and contains sulfurous compounds that may detoxify

harmful metals such as mercury, which would otherwise be dealt with by the liver.
Apples and pears contain pectin, a soluble fiber that helps to lower cholesterol levels and takes some strain off the liver.
Oats and legumes contain soluble fiber and have a similar effect to pectin.
Meat, fish, poultry, eggs, and dairy products are rich sources of high value protein required for the growth, repair, and maintenance of body tissues. A diet lacking in protein affects the liver by drawing on its protein stores.
Legumes, nuts, seeds, and cereals are good sources of protein for those who avoid animal products.
Green leafy vegetables and whole-grain foods are good sources of the B vitamin folate, which can become depleted when the liver is under strain.
Nuts, seeds, avocados, and vegetable oils supply vitamin E. Citrus fruits, berries, green leafy vegetables, and peppers contain vitamin C, and wholegrains, fish, and Brazil nuts supply selenium. All have antioxidant properties that help to protect the liver from free radicals.
Dandelion leaves ease liver congestion and are said to reduce toxicity. They can be added to salads, or drunk as dandelion tea or coffee.
Turmeric stimulates the flow of bile and can be a useful addition to meals in treating liver disease.

✖ FOODS TO AVOID
Fried foods, pastries, meat products, dairy products, oils, cakes, cookies, and chocolate are rich in animal fat, which can overload the liver.
Alcohol, in large amounts, can lead to fatty deposits in the liver, which interfere with its functions. It is thought that the liver can safely process the equivalent of two glasses of wine per day. More than this is not recommended.
Ready-made meals, bacon, smoked foods, pastries, and meat products supply large amounts of sodium. A low-sodium diet may reduce water retention associated with liver problems.
Vegetables and fruits should be washed or peeled before use to remove traces of pesticides.

◎ OTHER MEASURES
❑ Liver functioning may be greatly assisted by taking daily supplements of milk thistle.
❑ Psyllium husks are rich in soluble fiber and mucilaginous compounds that help to absorb toxins and eliminate them from the digestive tract, which reduces the toxin load on the liver.

See Also Alcohol, page 19

KEY FOODS

LEAN MEATS
page 122

POULTRY
page 124

WHOLE GRAINS
pages 92–99

YOGURT
page 128

FRUITS
pages 72–91

VEGETABLES
pages 42–71

CELERY
page 50

OBESITY

OBESITY IS ONE OF THE MOST COMMON nutritional disorders in the West, and the number of people who are considered to be obese is increasing steadily. Today, obesity is a serious public health problem. Obese people have a higher risk of developing disorders such as high blood pressure, heart disease, diabetes, gallstones, and arthritis than people who are not overweight or obese. The degree to which a person is overweight or obese is measured through the use of the Body Mass Index (BMI), which is a person's weight in kilograms divided by their height in meters squared. Health risks are thought to increase dramatically once a person's BMI exceeds 30. Occasionally attributed to various uncontrollable factors, such as hormone imbalance or genes, obesity in most people is due to the fact that they are consuming more calories than they use up.

⊗ SYMPTOMS
In addition to carrying excessive amounts of body fat, symptoms such as shortness of breath, aching legs, swollen ankles, low self-esteem, and depression are common.

⊕ CONVENTIONAL TREATMENT
Drugs that interfere with fat absorption may be prescribed. More drastic measures include wiring the jaw, stomach stapling, and liposuction. Other treatments, such as counseling, can be successful. Very low-calorie diets may be appropriate in some cases. Joining a weight-loss group may be helpful to some people, and increasing exercise is recommended. Long-term changes in eating habits are also required.

⊘ BENEFICIAL FOODS
Foods that are low in fat and release energy into the bloodstream slowly and steadily are the most useful for obese people trying to lose weight.
Lean beef, pork, lamb, chicken, turkey, and white fish are all good sources of protein that do not supply large amounts of fat. These foods can be alternated with those containing vegetable protein, such as peas, beans, lentils, and tofu.
Protein-rich foods should be included in each meal, since they appear to help trigger the parts of the brain that tell us when we are full.
Pasta, basmati rice, rye bread, and cooked cereals are useful carbohydrates for those wishing to lose weight. These foods are digested slowly and lead to a gradual rise in blood sugar levels, which leaves the body feeling full longer.
Yogurts and fruits make good snacks since they cause only small rises in blood sugar, helping to keep the biochemistry of the blood balanced.

CASE HISTORY
John Philips, aged 54, gradually gained weight after he gave up playing football in his twenties. By the age of 30, his weight had risen to over 194lbs (88kg), and by his 50th birthday, he weighed 238lbs (108kg). His doctor advised a low-fat diet, supplying 1,500 calories a day. John gave up eating high-calorie breakfasts and had cereal with skim milk and fruit instead. As a mid-morning snack he ate a banana, and for lunch he had sandwiches with lean meat or chicken, and an apple. For his evening meals he ate lean protein foods with plenty of vegetables. Over two years, he lost 55lbs (25kg).

Pears contain soluble fiber, and are low in calories. They release sugars slowly, making the body feel full for longer.
Vegetables such as salad greens, brassicas, and sprouting vegetables are very low in calories and have a low-calorie density, which means that they can be consumed in large volumes without providing the body with large amounts of energy.
Celery, in particular, contains very few calories and virtually no fat, making it a useful addition to a weight-watcher's diet.
Whole-grain breads, cereals, rice, pasta, fruits and vegetables contain fiber, which leaves the body feeling full for longer.

⊗ FOODS TO AVOID
Fried foods, sausages, burgers, and other processed meat products are rich in fat, and have twice the calories of carbohydrate- and protein-rich foods.
Butter, margarines, oils, and lard are high in fat and should be consumed in moderation. Olive oil contains as much fat as any other oil.
Cookies, cakes, pies, and chocolates are high in fat and should be avoided whenever possible.
Sugary foods cause a rapid increase in the amount of sugar in the bloodstream, which results in the release of the hormone insulin. Insulin removes excess sugar from the blood, which may then be stored as fat.

⊘ OTHER MEASURES
Counseling or behavioral therapy, alongside nutritional advice, will improve the chances of successful weight loss for those who are obese.
❏ Slimming clubs can provide useful support.
❏ Increased exercise is essential.

See Also Heart Disease, page 152

EATING PLAN FOR OBESITY

The key to treating obesity is to take a long-term approach and to accept that, over time, losses of 1lb a week can lead to significant weight reduction.

An easy way to reduce calorie intake is to reduce the total amount of fat in the diet and to fill up on fruits, vegetables, and complex carbohydrates.

BREAKFASTS	LIGHT MEALS	MAIN MEALS	SNACKS
A bacon sandwich made with 2 slices of bread, 2 slices of lean bacon broiled, and a sliced tomato	Smoked turkey sandwich made with 2 slices of wholewheat bread spread with a teaspoon of low-fat salad dressing, plus 1 1/2 oz (50g) smoked turkey, a sliced tomato, and watercress	4oz (100g) roast chicken served with two small roast potatoes and plenty of fresh, steamed vegetables	Low-fat yogurt ◆ Fruit scone ◆ Slice of malt loaf ◆ Apple ◆ Pear ◆ Orange ◆ Plums
◆ 1/2 cup (40g) bowl of branflakes with a chopped peach, plus 1 cup (200ml) skim milk and a glass of grapefruit juice	◆ Hot egg and ham muffin, made with a wholewheat muffin, with a slice of ham on each side; one half topped with a poached egg, the other with slices of tomato	◆ 5oz (150g) cod baked with leeks, mushrooms, and half a can of condensed mushroom soup; served with 1 cup (100g) mashed potatoes and 3/4 cup (100g) peas	
◆ Large fresh fruit salad with low-fat yogurt			

BLOATING

ABDOMINAL BLOATING is often caused by a change in the diet, liver disease, or a disease of the stomach or small intestine. With this disorder, carbohydrates and proteins may only be partially digested when they reach the colon, where they create gas. Bloating is a symptom of irritable bowel syndrome, and is also associated with premenstrual syndrome. It can also be caused by water retention.

SYMPTOMS
A swelling occurs around the abdomen, which is frequently uncomfortable. Bloating may be accompanied by flatulence.

CONVENTIONAL TREATMENT
If food intolerances are identified in the diet, specialist dietary advice is required. For bloating caused by water retention, diuretic drugs may be prescribed.

BENEFICIAL FOODS
Fruits, vegetables, and oats are rich in soluble fiber, which is easier for the digestive system to handle than foods with added processed bran. **Soy milks, yogurts, and cheeses** with added calcium are useful for people who have bloating due to an intolerance to the lactose in milk.

FOODS TO AVOID
Rutabagas, cabbage, legumes, and coarse bran that is added to food can cause bloating. **Carbonated drinks** introduce air into the digestive tract, which contributes to bloating. **Foods containing milk** should be avoided by those with a lactose intolerance, except for yogurt, which may be tolerated in small amounts. **Meat products** and ready-made meals are high in salt. Cutting down on these foods may reduce bloating associated with water retention.

OTHER MEASURES
❑ Food should be eaten slowly and chewed well.
❑ Drink from a glass rather than from a bottle to reduce the amount of extra air swallowed.
❑ If bloating is caused by a food intolerance, consult a nutritionist.
❑ Exercise can help to relieve the discomfort of bloating caused by premenstrual syndrome.
❑ A supplement of vitamin B_6 taken prior to and during a menstrual period may be beneficial.

See Also Irritable Bowel Syndrome, page 173; Premenstrual Syndrome, page 222

KEY FOODS

VEGETABLES
pages 42–71

RICE & OATS
pages 94–95

GINGER
page 114

EGGS
page 129

DAIRY PRODUCTS
pages 126–128

FRUITS
pages 72–91

FENNEL
page 108

NAUSEA

THE SENSATION OF FEELING sick, or nauseous, may be caused by food poisoning, overindulgence in food or alcohol, motion sickness, morning sickness, or as a side effect of certain drugs. Nausea can also be the result of gallbladder and kidney disease, or a poorly functioning liver. If the liver is unable to detoxify substances such as the various hormones produced during pregnancy, these toxins circulate in the blood, eventually reaching the brain, where they stimulate nausea and vomiting. High temperatures in children, migraines, ear infections, and anxiety can also cause nausea.

SYMPTOMS Nausea creates a feeling of queasiness, often associated with paleness, sweating, and an overproduction of saliva. The person is likely to feel generally unwell, faint, with a loss of appetite, and may vomit.

CONVENTIONAL TREATMENT Before any treatment can be given, it is necessary to diagnose the underlying cause and treat it accordingly. Antinausea drugs known as antiemetics may be given, but these drugs are inappropriate for nausea during pregnancy.

BENEFICIAL FOODS

Vegetable soups without added spices are usually acceptable, as are steamed vegetables.
Rice, cooked cereals, oats, oatcakes, dry toast, bread, and crackers are high in carbohydrates and can often be eaten without causing nausea.
Ginger helps to quell feelings of sickness, especially motion sickness. Two teaspoons of sliced ginger should be placed in a cup of boiling water. Steep, covered, for five to ten minutes, then strain and drink hot. Ginger cookies, ginger ale, or ginger tea may also help to relieve nausea.
Boiled eggs or baked beans with dry toast are often tolerated.
Low-fat, milky drinks and milk puddings, lean cold meats, and yogurts are high-protein foods without strong aromas or flavors.
Fruit salads and cottage cheese are low in fat, plain, and well tolerated by those with nausea.
Fennel can help to relieve nausea if made into an infusion. Place two teaspoons of fresh fennel in a cup and pour in boiling water. Steep, covered, for five to ten minutes. Strain, and drink hot.

FOODS TO AVOID

Greasy, fatty, and fried foods worsen symptoms.
Spicy and strong-smelling foods such as cooked cabbage can cause nausea in susceptible people.

OTHER MEASURES

❑ Minimize odors when preparing hot foods.
❑ Remove foods that are associated with nausea.

See Also Food Safety, page 242

EATING PLAN FOR NAUSEA

People experiencing nausea need to avoid being in the vicinity of cooking smells, especially those of fried and spicy foods. Eating plain foods that require little preparation is advisable, as is selecting dishes that have no negative thought associations. Try adding fresh, grated ginger to main meals.

BREAKFASTS	LIGHT MEALS	MAIN MEALS	SNACKS
Cooked cereal with fruit compote	*Chicken and cucumber sandwich without butter*	*Pea risotto*	*Ginger cookies*
◆	*Pear*	*Sorbet*	◆
Unbuttered wholewheat toast with fruit spread	◆	◆	*Oatcakes*
◆	*Baked beans on plain wholewheat toast*	*Cold roast pork with rice and green salad*	◆
Low-fat, plain yogurt with chopped banana and apple	*Peach*	◆	*Crackers*
◆	◆	*Tuna salad with plain, hot ciabatta bread*	◆
Muesli with skim milk	*Slices of cold turkey with tomato salad*	◆	*Dry toast*
	Banana	*Cold, lean roast meat or poultry without skin, with boiled potatoes and salad*	◆
			Low-fat yogurt

ANOREXIA NERVOSA

THE CONDITION KNOWN as anorexia nervosa is an eating disorder characterized by an intense fear of gaining weight, a disturbance in the way the affected person perceives his or her weight, size, and shape, and a body weight that is 15 percent less than that expected. Anorexia nervosa is a psychiatric disorder and must be taken seriously, since it can result in death.

✪ SYMPTOMS
In women, in addition to loss of weight, weakness, and lack of menstruation, a downy covering of hair can often be seen on the body and face. Many people with anorexia nervosa display an obsessional interest in food, yet eat very little. In prolonged anorexia, estrogen levels and bone mass fall, bone-marrow activity decreases, and there is a reduction in red and white blood-cell counts. Liver abnormalities and muscular atrophy can occur. Infertility in women is also common.

✚ CONVENTIONAL TREATMENT
In the past, treatment included force-feeding, tube-feeding, and drugs to stimulate appetite. Today, treatment is based more on combined psychiatric and dietary advice. A key target is to correct a person's abnormal attitudes toward food and to reduce their fear of dietary change. People who have developed anorexia nervosa learn or relearn normal eating behavior, and are taught how to deal with feelings of panic during meals, and with underlying emotional and psychiatric problems that may resurface as weight is gained. They are also taught how to cope with the triggers that previously sent them spiraling out of control and into starvation mode.

✔ BENEFICIAL FOODS
Many people with anorexia nervosa have a good knowledge of the calorie content of foods but do not know how to plan a healthy diet. Foods are often classified as "good" or "bad" by an anorexic, according to their calorie content and irrespective of their nutritional value. People with anorexia need to begin to consume a normal range of foods again, working toward a regular eating pattern and a diet that provides proteins, fruits, vegetables, starchy foods such as potatoes and bread, as well as essential oils and some fat.
Meats, oily fish, shellfish, and whole-grain foods supply the mineral zinc, which is often very low in those who have anorexia nervosa. A deficiency of zinc in the diet leads to a loss of taste. Foods that are rich in zinc, such as shellfish, may help to restore this.

CASE HISTORY
Alexandra Baker was 15 years old when she started a diet for her summer vacation. Her weight loss rapidly became an obsession, and over a year her weight fell from 145 to 72lbs (66 to 32.75kg). Diagnosed with anorexia, Alexandra was force-fed in a psychiatric unit, without success. Her recovery came later through a long-term stay at a specialist eating disorder center, where she received therapy and nutritional education. She was made to take responsibility for planning her weekly menu, and was gradually reintroduced to a varied diet that included potatoes, bread, chicken, and fish. Her perception of food and her body image slowly changed, and she now maintains a healthy weight.

Citrus fruits, berries, peppers, and green vegetables are good sources of vitamin C, which is needed for the repair of tissues and cells that may have been damaged during a period of self-imposed starvation as a result of the disease. **Avocados, vegetable oils, nuts, and seeds** are rich in vitamin E, which is needed for the repair of body tissues.

✖ FOODS TO AVOID
A person with anorexia nervosa requires a wide variety of foods, some of which need to be high in calories. It is unwise to allow a recovering anorexic to eat only low-calorie foods such as fruits and vegetables. These foods should form part of an overall, balanced diet that also supplies proteins, fats, and carbohydrates.

❂ OTHER MEASURES
❑ Long-term help is often required for a person with this condition as he or she learns gradually how to eat in social situations. People who are recovering from anorexia nervosa also need a great deal of emotional support from their families and friends to enable them to maintain their body weight at a reasonable level.
❑ Teenagers should be discouraged from focusing on diets, weight, and body shape. From an early age, children need to eat regular main meals and to consume a wide variety of foods.
❑ Processed foods and high-energy, low-nutrient snacks should be limited during childhood, in order to avoid the excess weight gain that can trigger the dieting process later on in life.

See Also Stress & Anxiety, page 231; Women & Nutrition, page 140

RESPIRATORY SYSTEM

EVERY CELL IN THE BODY needs oxygen in order to function. The gas is obtained via the respiratory and circulatory systems, which are also responsible for removing carbon dioxide, a waste product of body processes. Oxygen is diffused into arteries through the lung walls for transportation through the body, and carbon dioxide is diffused from the veins into the lungs for exhalation.

DIET & RESPIRATION

Despite years of research, it seems that little can be done to prevent infections of the respiratory tract that cause the common cold. Of the many cold "cures" and recommendations available, a high vitamin C intake is one of the few to show positive effects. Evidence indicates that asthma responds to nutritional manipulation, and there is also some evidence that regular consumption of certain vegetables and fruits may reduce the risk of lung cancer.

A BREATH OF FRESH AIR

The health of the respiratory tract depends on being able to inhale germ-free, unpolluted air. Regular intake of a variety of nutrients, such as vitamin A, helps to keep the respiratory tract linings healthy, while omega-3 and omega-6 essential fatty acids are believed to maintain the functioning of cells throughout the system.

HOW THE LUNGS WORK

Each lung consists of an intricate network of fine, branching tubes enveloped by an equally delicate network of blood vessels. Air moves in and out of the lungs as a result of pressure changes produced automatically by movement of the diaphragm.

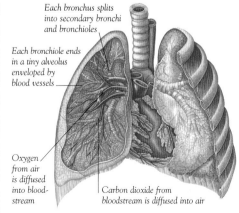

Each bronchus splits into secondary bronchi and bronchioles

Each bronchiole ends in a tiny alveolus enveloped by blood vessels

Oxygen from air is diffused into blood-stream

Carbon dioxide from bloodstream is diffused into air

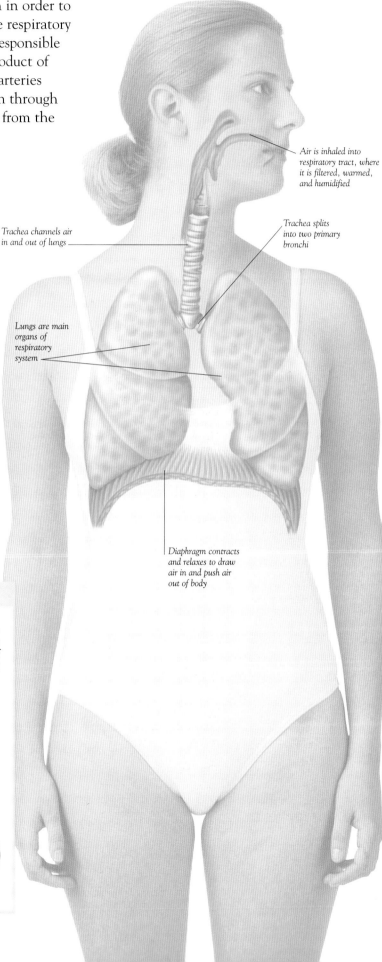

Air is inhaled into respiratory tract, where it is filtered, warmed, and humidified

Trachea splits into two primary bronchi

Trachea channels air in and out of lungs

Lungs are main organs of respiratory system

Diaphragm contracts and relaxes to draw air in and push air out of body

TOP HEALING FOODS

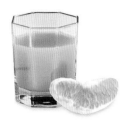

ORANGE JUICE PAGE 88

Benefits A daily glass may bolster antioxidants in the respiratory-tract linings and may protect against atmospheric pollutants.
Useful for Those with asthma or colds, smokers.
Nutrients Vitamin C.

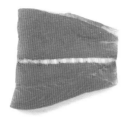

SALMON PAGE 118

Benefits Contains fatty acids that reduce inflammation and improve resistance to viral invasion of cells in respiratory linings.
Useful for Those with chronic bronchitis or asthma, smokers.
Nutrients Omega-3 fatty acids.

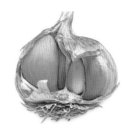

GARLIC PAGE 66

Benefits Has antiviral and antibacterial properties, and good intakes may help to reduce the risk of respiratory infections.
Useful for Colds, flu.
Nutrients The phytonutrient allicin, iron, zinc.

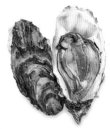

SHELLFISH PAGE 120

Benefits May help to reduce the risk of infections by boosting the immune system.
Useful for Colds, flu, and recurrent infections of the respiratory tract.
Nutrients Zinc, protein.

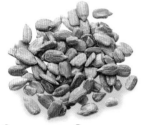

SUNFLOWER SEEDS PAGE 104

Benefits May boost antioxidant levels in alveolar fluid and reduce free-radical activity from inhaling cigarette smoke. Regular intakes may help prevent lung cancer.
Useful for Smokers.
Nutrients Vitamin E.

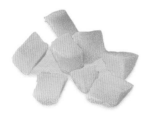

MANGOES PAGE 91

Benefits May protect those with vitamin A deficiency from recurrent respiratory infections.
Useful for Children, the elderly, and active and passive smokers.
Nutrients Beta carotene, which the body converts into vitamin A.

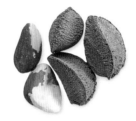

BRAZIL NUTS PAGE 100

Benefits Aid the formation of an enzyme thought to promote antioxidant action in the lungs.
Useful for Asthma sufferers, smokers, those exposed to polluted air.
Nutrients Selenium, protein.

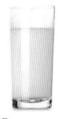

DAIRY PRODUCTS PAGE 126

Benefits Contain all nine essential amino acids needed for growth and maintenance of the body and to fight infections.
Useful for Colds, flu, and other respiratory-tract infections.
Nutrients Protein.

OTHER BENEFICIAL FOODS

HERRINGS PAGE 119

Benefits May protect the lungs against pollution and reduce respiratory-tract inflammation.
Useful for Smokers and people exposed to air pollution.
Nutrients Fatty acids, calcium.

AVOCADOS PAGE 51

Benefits Boost antioxidants in the linings of the respiratory tract.
Useful for Fighting the effects of air pollution and preventing cancerous changes in cells.
Nutrients Vitamin E.

PEPPERS PAGE 68

Benefits Boost antioxidant levels in the airways and may protect against air pollutants.
Useful for Smokers and people exposed to air pollution.
Nutrients Vitamin C.

FORTIFIED CEREALS PAGE 92

Benefits Contain substances, such as folic acid, essential for a strong immune system.
Useful for Colds, flu.
Nutrients Folate, vitamin B_6, protein.

FOODS TO AVOID

EGGS

Eggs are quite common triggers of asthma attacks, particularly in young children, but also in some adults. If eggs produce this effect, they could be excluded from the diet and the number of attacks monitored in order to establish whether or not they have been reduced.

MONOSODIUM GLUTAMATE

It is possible that this flavor enhancer, often referred to simply as MSG, may trigger asthma. MSG is a common ingredient in many popular dishes in Chinese cooking. However, thus far, no conclusive evidence of a clear link between MSG and asthma has been produced.

ORANGE SODAS

Orange sodas and orange-colored foods that contain the food coloring tartrazine, such as carbonated drinks and certain confectionery items, should be avoided by those susceptible to asthma. Tartrazine has been reported to cause attacks in some sensitive people.

SALICYLATES

There is evidence that a naturally occurring group of chemicals called salicylates, resembling aspirin, may provoke asthma attacks, particularly in children. People who have allergic reactions to aspirin may also be sensitive to foods that contain salicylates. Many processed, canned, and packaged foods contain salicylates, as do such varied foods as honey, licorice, green beans, yeast products, peppermint sweets, almonds, and peanuts.

FOOD PRESERVATIVES

There is evidence that sulfite preservatives can trigger asthma attacks. Sulfite preservatives are found in various food products, such as shrimp, dried fruit, and processed potatoes, and they are also used to make some wines and beers. People susceptible to asthma attacks should avoid consuming these foods and ready-made meals containing preservatives.

COLDS & INFLUENZA

KEY FOODS

BERRIES
pages 82–85

CITRUS FRUITS
pages 86–88

WHOLE GRAINS
pages 92–99

LEGUMES
pages 58–60

GARLIC
page 66

OILY FISH
page 118

POULTRY
page 124

BRASSICAS
pages 44–45

MEATS
page 122

DAIRY PRODUCTS
pages 126–128

THERE ARE MORE THAN 200 known viruses that can affect the upper respiratory tract and cause the common cold. In most cases, colds are mild and usually last for about a week, as the cold virus burns itself out on its own. Influenza, or "flu," as it is commonly known, is the name given to a more severe and highly infectious viral infection that affects the upper respiratory tract. The name "influenza" is derived from the old belief that the illness was due to divine influence.

⊗ SYMPTOMS Cold symptoms usually appear two or three days after a cold virus enters the body. Common symptoms include a sore throat, a runny or stuffy nose, coughing, sneezing, and aching limbs. Restlessness, watery eyes, and sleep problems may also occur. When symptoms last for longer than a week and include severe headaches, weakness, a loss of appetite, and thirst, the infection is more likely to be due to an influenza virus. Feverishness is also common.

✚ CONVENTIONAL TREATMENT For viral infections of the upper respiratory tract, it is only possible to treat the symptoms, not the cause of the illness. For the common cold, plenty of rest, large amounts of fluids, and gargling with warm saltwater may help alleviate symptoms. Pain relievers can ease headaches and lower the temperature. Antibiotics are appropriate only if a bacterial infection follows the viral infection. With influenza, it is essential that bed rest is taken and that fluid intake is maintained. The very young, pregnant women, the elderly, and those with other problems such as diabetes or kidney disease may need further medical advice. Immunization is sometimes recommended for alderly "at risk" groups to help prevent infection.

✔ BENEFICIAL FOODS
The immune system must receive the nutrients essential for its optimum functioning in order to give the body the best chance of warding off cold and influenza viruses.
Oranges, grapefruits, black currants, strawberries, sweet potatoes, potatoes, peppers, and green leafy vegetables, such as cabbage and broccoli, are some of the most significant natural suppliers of vitamin C. Regular large intakes of vitamin C appear to help reduce the incidence, severity, and duration of the common cold.
Whole grains and legumes are good suppliers of the B vitamin pantothenic acid. A deficiency of pantothenic acid may result in frequent upper respiratory infections.

Garlic and onions contain allicin, which is believed to boost the immune system and reduce the risk of infections.
Mackerel, salmon, and sardines are oily fish rich in omega-3 fatty acids. Flaxseeds, pumpkin seeds, and hemp oil are other good sources. Sunflower, pumpkin, and sesame seeds are rich sources of omega-6 fatty acids. These fatty acids may help the cells in the respiratory tract to fight off cold infections.
Liver, canned red salmon, mackerel, herring, butter, fortified margarine, and eggs supply vitamin A. Carrots, sweet potatoes, mangoes, apricots, and dark green vegetables provide beta carotene, which is converted into vitamin A. Repeated respiratory infections have been recorded in children with depleted vitamin A stores. A mixed diet containing these foods provides adequate intakes for a growing child.
Fish, poultry, lean meats, dairy foods, and combinations of legumes, nuts, seeds, and whole-grain foods provide protein. Poor intakes increase the risk of susceptibility to infections.
Meats, milk, cereals, and legumes supply vitamins B_6 and pantothenic acid, which are needed for a healthy immune system.
Fortified breakfast cereals, breads, and yeast extracts provide folic acid, important for a robust immune system. Beets, black-eyed peas, kale, and brussels sprouts are particularly good sources of folate, the natural form of folic acid.
Shellfish such as oysters, lean red meats, and whole-grain cereals contain zinc, a mineral needed for a strong immune system.

✖ FOODS TO AVOID
Prepackaged, manufactured foods low in vitamins and minerals should be replaced with fresh fruits, vegetables, meats, fish, cereals, nuts, and seeds.

⊘ OTHER MEASURES
❏ Vitamin C supplementation has been studied in depth in relation to the common cold. It appears that while supplements of between 500–1,000mg a day cannot prevent infections, they may help to lessen the severity and possibly the duration of a cold. In some circumstances, symptoms have been reduced by 19 percent on taking 1,000mg over an extended period. Vitamin C may work by increasing levels of interferon in the body, which fights infections.
❏ Supplements of certain micronutrients, including 20mg of zinc, 100mcg of selenium, 120mg of vitamin C, 15mg of vitamin E, and 6mg of beta carotene, have been shown in trials

COLDS & INFLUENZA

to decrease the incidence of respiratory infections in elderly people in long-term care.

❏ Zinc salts, taken in lozenge form, have been shown to improve symptoms of the common cold in several clinical trials. In spite of these positive results and possible theories for zinc's beneficial effect, ranging from it preventing the cold virus attaching to the nose lining, to improving the action of the immune system, and acting as an anti-inflammatory, there are an equal number of research programs that suggest that zinc lozenges have no effect on symptoms. It should be left to the individual doctor to decide whether or not it is worth prescribing zinc lozenges for a patient. It should also be noted that taking high levels of 150mg of zinc a day can actually increase a person's susceptibility to infection. **Seek medical advice before taking these steps**.

❏ Goldenrod infusion or goldenrod tincture is used by herbalists as an anti-inflammatory for the mucous membranes and for watery mucus.

❏ Elder infusion or tincture is a beneficial antiphlegm herbal remedy.

❏ Echinacea has long been recognized as a home remedy for colds and influenza. Echinacea drops (ten drops, two or three times a day) are recommended for their antiviral properties. Three 200mg capsules of echinacea can also be taken up to three times a day when cold or influenza symptoms first become apparent.

❏ Garlic tablets or capsules containing extracts of garlic may help to prevent colds, due to the antiviral effects of the phytonutrient allicin.

❏ Wash hands frequently to prevent cold viruses from spreading, and avoid close contact with and exposure to those with colds and influenza.

❏ Use a tissue when coughing or sneezing.

❏ A steam inhalation can help nasal stuffiness. Pour hot water into a bowl, place a towel over the head and over the bowl, and inhale deeply through the nose for ten minutes. This can be repeated three times a day. Menthol or eucalyptus oil can be added to the water or to a hot bath to ease breathing.

❏ Plenty of fluids are necessary. During severe bouts of influenza, it may be necessary to take nutritious fluids such as meal-replacement drinks, which contain the correct balance of nutrients.

❏ Rest and sleep as much as possible. The immune system needs plenty of rest in order to repair itself. Ignoring the symptoms of a viral infection and trying to work through them can lengthen the time that they linger.

See Also Minerals, page 30; Vitamins, page 26

EATING PLAN FOR COLDS & INFLUENZA

It is often difficult to taste foods if you have a severe cold or influenza. It is essential to drink plenty of fluids, such as soups and juices, even if you do not wish to eat solid foods. The body can quickly become dehydrated without adequate fluids, which makes the symptoms worse.

BREAKFASTS	LIGHT MEALS	MAIN MEALS	SNACKS
Whole-grain breakfast cereal fortified with folic acid, plus grated apple and skim milk	Salmon and alfalfa sprout pita bread	Chicken satay with wholewheat pitas, plus a carrot and orange salad	Breakfast cereal with skim milk
◆	Large fruit salad	Baked pears with ginger	◆
Strawberry smoothie made with strawberries, banana, yogurt, and skim milk	◆	◆	Fresh vegetable soups
◆	Baked sweet potato with feta cheese and cucumber salad	Trout and caramelized onions with new potato salad and fresh greens	◆
Wholewheat muffin with poached egg and broiled tomatoes	◆	Cinnamon baked bananas	Smoothies made from blended orange juice, bananas, and mangoes
Freshly squeezed orange juice	Mushroom omelette with wholewheat roll	◆	◆
	Apricot and mango fruit salad	Wholewheat spaghetti served with seafood sauce	Oranges, tangerines, strawberries, and raspberries
		◆	
		Fresh fruit	

BRONCHITIS

KEY FOODS

ROOT
VEGETABLES
pages 54–57

GREEN
VEGETABLES
pages 44–50

AVOCADOS
page 51

WHOLE GRAINS
pages 92–99

OILY FISH
page 118

DAIRY
PRODUCTS
pages 126–128

EGGS
page 129

AN INFLAMMATION OF the air passages, or bronchi, that lead to the lungs is commonly known as bronchitis. This condition may be acute and temporary, or chronic, which has long-term effects on health. Acute bronchitis often follows a respiratory tract infection, such as a cold. Chronic bronchitis results from frequent irritation of the lungs, often caused by environmental pollution or by smoking.

SYMPTOMS
There may be excessive secretion of mucus from the mucus-producing glands in the bronchi, a productive cough, wheezy breathing, and breathlessness. In simple chronic bronchitis, the mucus-producing glands tend to be permanently enlarged. The cough continues for at least three months and symptoms occur for at least two years. In obstructive chronic bronchitis, the bronchial tubes become so swollen that they are narrowed. Breathlessness may be severe and is associated with a persistent, productive cough.

CONVENTIONAL TREATMENT
Cough medicine may be given to soothe the coughing, and antibiotic drugs to treat any secondary bacterial infections. Inhaled drugs that open the airways may relieve the symptoms of chronic bronchitis. Long-term medical treatment is often necessary for this condition.

BENEFICIAL FOODS
Population studies that look at the food intakes of people and the kinds of disease that they develop reveal that those who consume the most vegetables appear to have the lowest risk of chronic bronchitis. High intakes were defined as more than seven servings of vegetables a week.
Carrots, sweet potatoes, apricots, mangoes, and green vegetables are good sources of beta carotene. Population research studies show that the occurrence of chronic bronchitis is low in people who have high intakes of beta carotene. This supports the idea that higher intakes of vegetables may protect against this illness.
Avocados, green leafy vegetables, and whole-grain cereals are among the best sources of vitamin E, which may help to protect against bronchitis.
Mackerel, canned red salmon, anchovies, whole milk, cheese, and egg yolks supply vitamin A. Beta carotene can be converted into vitamin A in the body if levels are low. Research using vitamin A supplements suggests that smokers who are otherwise healthy may have a deficiency

of vitamin A in the respiratory tract. It may therefore be wise for people who smoke to eat plenty of foods that are rich in vitamin A, as well as beta carotene, on a regular basis.
Herrings, kippers, mackerel, pilchards, salmon, sardines, trout, fresh tuna, and crab supply omega-3 fatty acids. These fatty acids interfere with the body's inflammatory responses and help to relieve inflammatory conditions. Research shows that the omega-3 fatty acids found in oily fish may protect against chronic bronchitis and deterioration of lung function in cigarette smokers. This protection may come from the fatty acids' interference with the inflammatory damage usually caused by smoking.

FOODS TO AVOID
Poorly balanced diets lacking in protein foods, vegetables, and fruits are to be avoided. Replace monotonous food intakes that involve little variety with a wide range of fresh produce. Frozen vegetables and fruits are an acceptable alternative to fresh vegetables.

OTHER MEASURES
Chronic bronchitis may be more likely to occur in adults who were underweight at birth, who were underweight at one year old, and who contracted a respiratory tract infection during the first two years of their life. A well-balanced diet during pregnancy, including adequate calories from a mix of proteins, carbohydrates, and fats, plus a wide range of fruits and vegetables, may help to reduce the risk of chronic bronchitis in children later in life.
❑ Vitamin C supplements of 500mg a day, taken daily, may be beneficial to people who are affected by bronchitis.
❑ Eucalyptus and sweet thyme oil may be added to a bowl of steaming water and the steam inhaled. Placing a towel over the bowl and head intensifies the treatment.
❑ Elecampane root is used by herbalists as a tonic for relieving coughs and congestion, and weakness following episodes of bronchitis. The tincture may also be used for chronic bronchitis, and a syrup can be made for treating coughs.
❑ Thyme infusions, tinctures, and syrups for bronchitis appear to help loosen phlegm.
❑ White horehound tincture helps to relax the airways and eases congestion.
❑ Smokers are advised to give up the habit, and those with bronchitis should avoid smoky areas.

See Also Colds & Influenza, page 184

ASTHMA

KEY FOODS

CITRUS
FRUITS
pages 86–88

BERRIES
pages 82–85

BRASSICAS
pages 44–47

SWEET
POTATOES
page 55

BRAZIL NUTS
page 100

OILY FISH
page 118

WHOLE GRAINS
pages 92–99

MILK
page 126

IN THE WEST, ASTHMA affects about five percent of people at some time in their lives. It occurs when the smooth muscle in the bronchioles suddenly contracts, usually due to a foreign substance in the air. Most asthmatic attacks in people under the age of 30 are brought on by an allergic reaction, particularly to pollen, and possibly to certain foods. Over the age of 30, asthma is often caused by irritants, such as air pollution, colds, or bronchitis. Allergens, for example pollen, appear to trigger the release of histamine and bradykinin, which cause swelling, secretion of mucus, and spasm in the bronchiole walls. The effect is to restrict the airways, making exhalation difficult.

✪ SYMPTOMS Wheezing, shortness of breath, tightness in the chest, and a dry cough are the main symptoms. An attack can cause sweating, rapid heartbeat, and gasping for breath. Severe asthma attacks can be fatal.

✚ CONVENTIONAL TREATMENT Drugs known as bronchodilators taken through an inhaler can keep mild asthma under control. Steroid inhalers may be necessary for more severe cases to reduce swelling and inflammation of the bronchioles. After an acute and severe attack, steroidal drugs may be given for a short period. Inhalers that deliver drugs capable of blocking allergic reactions are also available, and these are useful for childhood asthma.

✔ BENEFICIAL FOODS
Diets rich in fresh fruits and vegetables may increase the antioxidant defenses of the lungs against inhaled irritants and allergens and reduce susceptibility to harmful inhaled substances.
Oranges, grapefruits, strawberries, raspberries, peppers, brassicas and other green leafy vegetables, sweet potatoes, and parsley are some of the richest natural sources of vitamin C. High intakes of these foods may help to protect against asthma caused by environmental pollution. Population studies show that asthmatic individuals tend to have lower than normal concentrations of vitamin C circulating in the bloodstream. Vitamin C is the major antioxidant substance in the surface liquid of the lung and it could protect against oxidants breathed in via polluted air, particularly cigarette smoke. It may also help to block the release of histamine in hypersensitive people. Increasing intakes of vitamin C may help to reduce the risk of asthmatic attacks in both adults and children.

Brazil nuts and oily fish are particularly good sources of selenium, which has been found to be low in some people with asthma. It is needed for the action of an enzyme called glutathione peroxidase, which is thought to be involved in the antioxidant function of the lungs.
Fruits, vegetables, cereals, and milk provide magnesium, which is needed for relaxation of the smooth muscle in the bronchioles. A low intake has been reported in people with asthma.
Herrings, mackerel, salmon, and other oily fish supply good amounts of omega-3 fatty acids. Research into the diets of children has shown that regular consumption of oily fish is associated with a reduced risk of asthma in childhood. It seems that the fatty acids in fish oil reduce inflammatory substances involved in the asthmatic reaction in the lungs.

✖ FOODS TO AVOID
Studies have shown that allergic reactions to food trigger asthma in about six out of 10,000 people. Food-induced asthma occurs within minutes to an hour of eating, leading to deep, repetitive coughing, shortness of breath, and wheezing. Acute attacks must be treated immediately, as they may lead to anaphylactic shock, and even death. Tests can be performed to establish an allergic reaction. If an allergy or food sensitivity is found, a well-balanced diet that excludes the offending foods must be followed.
Milk and eggs have been associated with asthma in children. In adults, common allergens are peanuts, shellfish, and soy and dairy products.
Processed potatoes, dried fruits, wine, and beer contain sulfites, which can trigger attacks.
Tartrazine (the food coloring), aspirin, and natural substances in foods called salicylates, have caused asthmatic symptoms in some people.
Monosodium glutamate (MSG) added to food as a flavor enhancer, has been said to cause asthma, but as yet the relationship is not established.

⊘ OTHER MEASURES
❑ Avoid cigarette smoke and wood-burning fires.
❑ Avoid sudden changes in temperature.
❑ Try to keep the home environment free of dust.
❑ Relaxation therapies, such as yoga, massage, and aromatherapy, can improve symptoms.
❑ A few drops of peppermint oil added to a bowl of hot water may be inhaled to ease breathing.
❑ An infusion of the herb elecampane may help.

See Also Food Allergies, page 210

URINARY SYSTEM

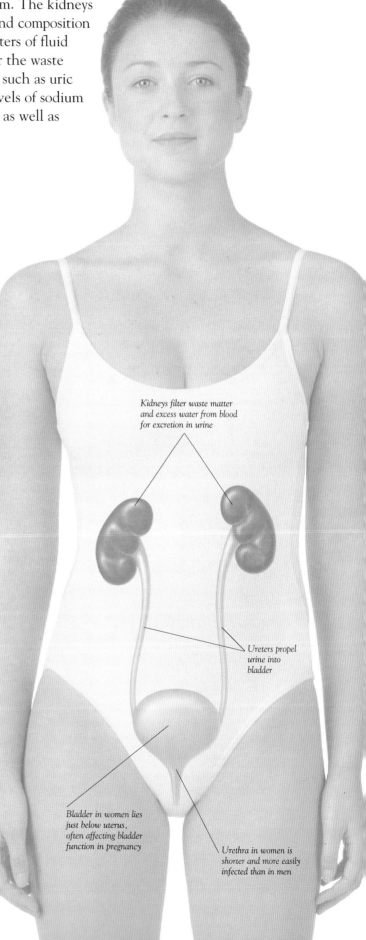

FLUID LEVELS AND THE FILTERING of waste products in the body are controlled by the urinary system. The kidneys are responsible for regulating the volume and composition of fluids in the body, often filtering several liters of fluid from the bloodstream every day. They filter the waste products generated by metabolic processes, such as uric acid, from the blood, and determine the levels of sodium and potassium in the body. Waste products as well as excess water are excreted as urine.

DIET & THE URINARY TRACT

Research indicates that specific diets controlling intakes of protein and sodium may help to prolong function in diseased kidneys. Specific dietary advice must be sought from a dietitian by those with kidney failure. Purine-rich foods such as organ meats have been linked to gout and kidney stones, while foods rich in folic acid may help to reduce the risk of stone formation.

KEEPING HEALTHY

Drinking up to two liters of water a day helps to avoid dehydration and avert the formation of stones. A glass of cranberry juice daily may help to relieve infections of the urinary-tract tubes. Reducing salt intake can help to maintain efficient kidney function.

Kidneys filter waste matter and excess water from blood for excretion in urine

Ureters propel urine into bladder

Bladder in women lies just below uterus, often affecting bladder function in pregnancy

Urethra in women is shorter and more easily infected than in men

MALE URINARY SYSTEM

The urinary tract consists of the kidneys, ureters, bladder, and urethra. In men, the urethra is five times as long as in women, while in women the bladder is lower than in men.

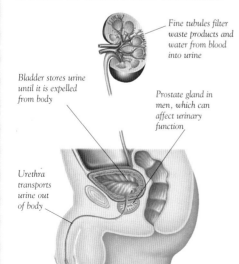

Fine tubules filter waste products and water from blood into urine

Bladder stores urine until it is expelled from body

Prostate gland in men, which can affect urinary function

Urethra transports urine out of body

TOP HEALING FOODS

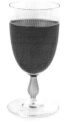

CRANBERRY JUICE   PAGE 85

Benefits Can help treat and prevent urinary infections by stopping *E-coli* bacteria from attaching themselves to the walls of the urinary tract.
Useful for Those with cystitis.
Nutrients Phytonutrients.

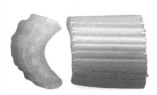

CELERY   PAGE 50

Benefits Used by herbalists, in the East and West, to cleanse the system of uric acid.
Useful for Those who are prone to gout and urinary infections.
Nutrients Phytonutrients with diuretic properties, apiin.

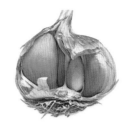

GARLIC   PAGE 66

Benefits Has natural antibiotic properties that help to fight against bacterial infections.
Useful for People who have recurrent urinary infections.
Nutrients Phytonutrients such as allicin.

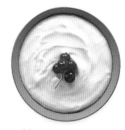

LIVE YOGURT   PAGE 128

Benefits Contains bacteria that are beneficial to the colon.
Useful for Those who, following antibiotic treatment for urinary infections, need to re-establish beneficial organisms in the gut.
Nutrients Calcium, magnesium.

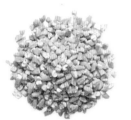

OATS   PAGE 95

Benefits This carbohydrate-rich food is an excellent source of energy that is low in sodium.
Useful for Those with kidney disease who need to follow a diet that is low in sodium.
Nutrients Zinc, carbohydrates.

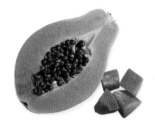

PAPAYAS   PAGE 89

Benefits Supply nutrients that are capable of boosting the immune system's effectiveness.
Useful for Helping to fight off and aid recovery from infections.
Nutrients Vitamin C, beta carotene.

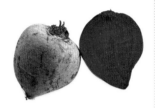

BEETS   PAGE 57

Benefits Contain substances that may help to inhibit the action of the enzyme that is involved in the production of uric acid.
Useful for Those who are susceptible to attacks of gout.
Nutrients Folate, vitamin C.

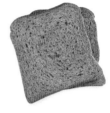

WHOLEWHEAT BREAD   P 98

Benefits Can help to provide valuable minerals that may be at lower than recommended levels in people affected by gout.
Useful for Those affected by recurrent attacks of gout.
Nutrients Zinc, carbohydrates.

OTHER BENEFICIAL FOODS

BROWN RICE   PAGE 92

Benefits A good source of energy that is low in sodium.
Useful for People with kidney disorders on low-sodium diets.
Nutrients Carbohydrate, B vitamins, potassium.

POULTRY   PAGE 124

Benefits Cooked without the addition of salt, it is a source of lean, low-sodium protein.
Useful for Easing kidney strain by reducing sodium in the diet.
Nutrients Protein.

OILY FISH   PAGE 118

Benefits May be helpful in reducing inflammation.
Useful for Those affected by infections of the urinary tract.
Nutrients Omega-3 fatty acids, protein, calcium.

DANDELION COFFEE   PAGE 108

Benefits Can help to cleanse the system by acting as a diuretic.
Useful for Those susceptible to infections and those who wish to cleanse the system of toxins.
Nutrients Caffeic acid.

FOODS TO AVOID

ORGAN MEATS

Liver, kidneys, hearts, and other organ meats contain substances known as purines. When purines are broken down in the body during digestion, they produce uric acid. A failure to flush uric acid out of the body can lead to the formation of urate crystals. These crystals can be deposited in the joints, causing great pain. Reduced purine levels are sometimes recommended for people who still experience attacks of gout in spite of being prescribed drug treatment.

SPICY FOODS

Peppery and spicy foods and condiments are best avoided by people with infections of the urinary tract, since these foods may cause irritation to the bladder and the walls of the urinary tract.

SALTY SNACKS

Potato chips, salted nuts, tortilla chips, and similar snack foods, as well as many ready-made meals, should be eaten in strict moderation, to reduce sodium in the diet and therefore possible excessive kidney strain.

COFFEE, TEA & SODAS

Drinks such as coffee, tea, and sodas contain significant amounts of caffeine, which is capable of stimulating the bladder wall and increasing the urge to urinate. Consequently, to avoid excessive caffeine intakes, the number of drinks containing caffeine that are drunk daily should be strictly limited. Many products that are sold as remedies for the common cold also contain caffeine. Consumption of these products should be similarly restricted.

OXALATE

Most kidney stones contain a substance called oxalate, and the tendency to form stones is often due to faulty oxalate metabolism. Oxalate occurs naturally in a range of foods, including wheat bran, nuts, tea, chocolate, spinach, beets, and rhubarb. Those prone to stones, which may be hereditary, should avoid oxalate-rich foods.

CYSTITIS

KEY FOODS

CRANBERRIES
page 85

CELERY
page 50

GARLIC
page 66

DANDELION
LEAVES
page 108

A COMMON AILMENT, cystitis is an inflammation of the bladder, usually caused by a bacterial infection. About one in three women have cystitis at some stage in life, and the condition is most prevalent in women between the ages 25 and 54. This is because the urethra, which transports urine from the bladder, is shorter in women than in men, making it easier for bacteria such as *Escherichia coli* to work their way up the urinary tract and into the bladder.

⊕ SYMPTOMS The main symptom of this ailment is a frequent urge to pass urine with only small amounts of urine passed, coupled with a painful, burning sensation. The urine is likely to smell strong and it may contain blood. There may also be back or abdominal pain, and fever.

⊕ CONVENTIONAL TREATMENT A urine sample is taken for analysis and antibiotic drugs are prescribed. Pain can be relieved by aspirin or acetaminophen. Over-the-counter remedies are also available.

⊘ BENEFICIAL FOODS
Cranberry juice contains phytonutrients that seem to prevent the bacterium *E. coli* from attaching itself to the urinary tract, allowing it to be flushed out of the bladder and into the urine. This action may reduce or prevent the symptoms of cystitis. A daily $1\frac{1}{2}$ cup (300ml)

glass of cranberry juice is estimated to be sufficient to prevent *E. coli* attachment. Blueberries contain similar phytonutrients and appear to be effective in fighting this bacterium. **Celery** cleanses uric acid from the system. An infusion taken three times a day may help. **Garlic** has natural antibiotic properties and is worth eating regularly to help fight infections. **Dandelion leaf tea** and dandelion extract are diuretics that can help to cleanse the system.

✖ FOODS TO AVOID
Coffee, tea, cola, and cold remedies contain caffeine, which makes bladder irritation worse. **Citrus fruits, spicy foods,** tomatoes, alcohol, and chocolate may make symptoms worse.

⊘ OTHER MEASURES
❑ Initially, drink $1\frac{1}{2}$ cups (300ml) of water every 20 minutes or so in order to flush out the system.
❑ Bicarbonate of soda dissolved in $1\frac{1}{2}$ cups (300ml) of water twice daily reduces urine acidity. The taste can be disguised with fruit juice.
❑ Supplements of vitamins C and A help to protect against urinary tract infections.
❑ Bearberry is a known antiseptic. The herb can be made into an infusion by simmering $\frac{1}{4}$ cup (15g) with 2 cups (500ml) of water.

See Also Women & Nutrition, page 140

EATING PLAN FOR CYSTITIS

It is important for people with cystitis to drink fluids throughout the day, including plenty of water with each meal. Drink cranberry juice whenever possible during the day, and select fruits and vegetables rich in vitamin C to boost the immune system and fight infections.

BREAKFASTS	LIGHT MEALS	MAIN MEALS	SNACKS
Bowl of whole-grain cereal with chopped banana	Freshly baked ciabatta roll with crumbled feta cheese and sliced tomatoes	Stir-fried vegetables with tofu and cashews	Carrot, cucumber, and celery crudités
Glass of cranberry juice	Glass of apple, ginger, and celery juice	Blueberry crumble	Wholewheat muffin with a banana
Fresh, bran muffin	Bagels with smoked salmon and low-fat cream cheese	Roast monkfish with freshly steamed zucchini, and lemon and garlic couscous	Wholewheat and fruit or plain scone
Glass of cranberry juice	Fruit salad including green apples	Vegetable lasagne with green salad	Glass of cranberry juice
Large bowl of fruit salad including berries	Turkey and cranberry wholewheat bread sandwich with watercress	Fresh, homemade berry sorbet	Serving of yogurt
Large serving of yogurt	Fresh apricots and plums		Apple and pear
Glass of cranberry juice			

PROSTATE DISORDERS

THE PROSTATE GLAND in men secretes prostatic fluid into the semen, supplying nutrients to keep sperm in good condition and hormonelike substances to aid their movement in the female genital tract. An inflammation or infection of the prostate gland is known as prostatitis. It may be caused by a sudden bacterial infection that is carried to the prostate via the bloodstream or the urethra. Prostatitis can occur from about the age of 25. Benign prostatic hyperplasia (BPH) is a swelling of the gland that can occur from about the age of 45. It is also possible for cancer to develop in this gland.

SYMPTOMS

Acute prostatitis can cause flu-like symptoms, with pain in the back, around the thighs, and between the scrotum and anus. It is often difficult to pass water and painful to ejaculate. The symptoms of chronic prostatitis are similar to those of acute prostatitis, and there may be a watery discharge from the penis and blood in the semen. The symptoms of BPH include difficulty in urinating and incontinence. Cancer of the prostate gland leads to fatigue, blood in the urine and sperm, painful bones, and a loss of appetite and weight.

CONVENTIONAL TREATMENT

Acute prostatitis is treated with antibiotics for about a month. Chronic prostatitis is treated for a longer period. Anti-inflammatory drugs can also be taken. BPH is treated with drugs called 5-alpha-reductase inhibitors, which prevent the male hormone testosterone from being converted into the substance that triggers prostatic swelling. Alpha-blocker drugs, which relax the urethra, may also be prescribed. Treatment for prostate cancer depends on how far it has progressed.

BENEFICIAL FOODS

Research has shown that men living in the US are 26 times more likely to develop prostate problems than men living in China and Japan. It appears that traditional diets in the East may offer some protection against prostate disease.

Soybeans, tofu, and other soy products are rich in isoflavones and lignans, plant estrogens that are thought to reduce the effect of the male hormones responsible for benign prostate swellings. Tests show that Japanese men generally have 50 times more plant estrogens in their blood than men living in the West.

Vegetables, such as brassicas, root vegetables, squashes, and salad leaves, contain antioxidant vitamins, minerals, and phytonutrients, which may offer protection against this disease.

Cabbage contains indoles, phytonutrients that appear to decrease the activity of enzymes that are associated with prostate problems.

Beans and other legumes contain small quantities of isoflavones. Research has shown a significant relationship between intakes of baked beans and peas and a reduced risk of prostate cancer.

Alfalfa seeds and alfalfa sprouts contain isoflavones called daidzein and genistein. These latch onto receptors in the prostate gland and may help to reduce the risk of prostate cancer.

Tomatoes appear to offer moderate protection against prostate cancer, possibly due to the lycopene that they contain. In one study, tomato sauce, tomatoes, and pizza were significantly associated with a lower risk of prostate cancer.

Mackerel, salmon, sardines, and other oily fish rich in omega-3 fatty acids may help to reduce inflammation in the prostate. These fatty acids are converted into prostaglandins, which have anti-inflammatory properties.

Flax and hemp seeds contain omega-3 fatty acids and may be worth including in the diet on a regular basis. They can be ground and sprinkled on breakfast cereals and yogurt.

FOODS TO AVOID

There appears to be some association with high meat consumption and prostate cancer, so it is best to alternate servings of lean meat with fish, poultry, and legumes, especially soybeans.

Fatty foods, such as mayonnaise, pies, pastries, cakes, cookies, butter, lard, and oil, contain large amounts of fat. High-fat diets seem to increase the activity of the enzyme 5-alpha-reductase, which may ultimately lead to prostatic swelling.

OTHER MEASURES

❑ Saw palmetto (*Sereno repens*) berries contain substances that appear to inhibit the activity of 5-alpha-reductase, which in turn seems to reduce the swelling of the prostate gland in people with BPH. Saw palmetto can be taken in the form of a dietary supplement.

❑ Rye pollen extract has been shown to help prostatitis and BPH, probably through its fatty acid, protein, and hormone extracts.

❑ Vitamin E supplements have been shown in trials to lead to a significant decrease in the risk of prostate cancer.

See Also Cancer, page 214; Men & Nutrition, page 142; Plant Nutrients, page 34

KIDNEY DISORDERS

KEY FOODS

WHOLE GRAINS
pages 92–99

POTATOES
page 54

MEATS
page 122

POULTRY
page 124

FISH
pages 118–121

VEGETABLES
pages 42–71

HERBS &
SPICES
pages 108–114

FRUITS
pages 72–91

LEMON JUICE
page 87

THE KIDNEYS MAINTAIN many aspects of the body's internal chemistry. They filter the blood and remove surplus water and minerals, and waste products such as uric acid. They also produce important substances, including hormones that regulate the release of red blood cells from the bone marrow. By varying the amount of urine produced daily, the kidneys can respond to variable fluid intakes and demands created by exercise and climate. In this way, they maintain the body's fluid balance.

Kidney failure can be acute and sudden, or chronic and long term, and may involve the formation of kidney stones. Acute kidney failure can result from another disorder, such as heart failure, prostate enlargement, or postoperative bladder problems. Chronic kidney failure can be caused by glomerula disorders, vascular problems, diabetes, kidney infections, kidney tumors, and cystic disease. An inflammation of the glomerular filters in the kidney causes high blood pressure, a lack of urine, blood in the urine produced, and water retention. Inflammation of the glomerulus can progress to nephrotic syndrome, which causes bloating and loss of protein in the urine.

✪ **SYMPTOMS** The symptoms of acute kidney failure include those causing the underlying disease, plus a period of low urine production followed by excessive urine production. If water retention and raised potassium levels accompany the underlying disorder, acute kidney failure can be life-threatening. The symptoms of chronic kidney failure depend on the underlying cause. They include anemia, bone pain, and itching. If kidney stones are present, there is an excruciating pain when a stone moves from the kidneys down the urinary tract. This pain is relieved once the kidney stone is passed out of the body or removed by a surgeon.

✚ **CONVENTIONAL TREATMENT** Kidney stones can usually be surgically removed or dispersed using ultrasound. Dietary advice and drugs may be given to help prevent further stones. If the person is overweight, weight loss is advisable. Glomerular inflammation may need treatment with drugs such as steroids and other immunosuppressants, which work by reducing inflammation. Treatment includes fluid restriction, a low-sodium diet, and sometimes diuretic drugs. In severe cases, dialysis or a kidney transplant may be necessary. Nephrotic syndrome is often also treated with controlled protein intake. Fluid replacement is essential, and kidney

CASE HISTORY

Jerry Pringle, aged 52, was unaware that he had kidney stones until one moved from his kidneys along his urinary tract. The pain was so excruciating that he thought he was having a heart attack. His doctor diagnosed kidney stones. He was treated medically for these but also followed dietary advice to reduce the chances of the kidney stones recurring. He gave up tea, coffee, and chocolate, and started to eat oatmeal for breakfast. Instead of eating meat pies and sausages for lunch he chose lean roast meats with vegetables, and snacks of potato chips and salted nuts were replaced with fruits. Jerry has not experienced kidney problems since.

dialysis may be necessary. Treatment is monitored by regular blood tests to see how much protein, energy, and sodium is needed. Individuals' needs vary greatly, and plans must be worked out by a doctor and dietician.

Treatment for acute kidney failure often takes place in an intensive care unit and includes fluid replacement and dialysis. The aim of treatment for chronic kidney failure is to prevent further deterioration and to prevent or treat any complications. Treatment includes control of blood pressure, and dietary restriction of protein, potassium, and phosphate. Sodium and calcium intakes also need to be carefully controlled. Various drugs can be helpful, including ACE inhibitors, and diuretics to control fluid balance. In severe cases, kidney failure may require kidney dialysis or transplant.

✔ **BENEFICIAL FOODS**
Anyone with a kidney disorder must seek specialist advice from their doctor and dietician. Puffed wheat, oatmeal, oats, rice, pasta, and potatoes are good sources of carbohydrate for those who need to restrict sodium intake.
Lean meat, poultry, game, and fresh fish provide dietary sources of protein that are relatively low in sodium for those required to restrict sodium intake.
Fresh and frozen vegetables, fresh, canned, or stewed fruits, fruit juices, and unsalted nuts are often suitable for those with kidney disorders.
Herbs and spices make useful alternatives to salt when following a reduced sodium eating plan.
Fresh vegetables, unsalted nuts, and fresh fruits, such as grapes, are good sources of potassium for those needing to increase intakes of this mineral.
Wholemeal pita bread, brown pasta, brown rice, and whole-grain cereals are beneficial for kidney stones that are caused by high levels of calcium.

EATING PLAN FOR KIDNEY STONES

Drinking plenty of fluids may help to reduce the risk of kidney stone formation, so try to consume water with and between meals. Adding a little lemon juice to foods and drinks may reduce the risk further. Avoid eating foods rich in oxalates, such as spinach, peanuts, chocolate, and rhubarb.

BREAKFASTS	LIGHT MEALS	MAIN MEALS	SNACKS
Fresh fruit salad with yogurt	Turkey and cranberry ciabatta sandwich with watercress	Roast chicken with potatoes and vegetables, excluding spinach	Oatcakes
Large glass of water	Apple and pear	Baked apple with custard	Wholewheat fruit scone
◆	Large glass of water	◆	Wholewheat roll
Broiled tomatoes and mushrooms with baked beans	◆	Seafood spaghetti with large salad	Wholewheat crispbreads
◆	Baked potato with red kidney bean, pepper, and corn filling, plus salad	Ice cream or sorbet with wafer	Banana
Wholewheat toast with unsalted butter and marmalade	Peach or plums	◆	Apricots
Large glass of orange juice	Large glass of water	Stir-fry with tofu and aromatic steamed rice	Plums
	◆	Large serving of melon with raspberries	
	Large bowl of vegetable soup with wholewheat roll		
	Fruit salad with fromage frais		
	Large glass of water		

The phytic acid in these foods helps to bind calcium in the intestine and reduces absorption. **Cereals, potatoes,** and other vegetables provide magnesium. High intakes of this mineral may help to prevent the formation of kidney stones. **Water and other fluids** should be consumed regularly every day by those prone to kidney stones. A good flow of urine helps to wash out the gravel particles that may be building up. At least two quarts of water needs to be drunk daily. **Lemon juice** contains citrate, which may help to prevent calcium-based kidney stones. Two quarts of lemonade (consisting of about $1/2$ cup of reconstituted lemon juice mixed with 2 quarts of water), drunk throughout the day, has been found to increase urinary citrate levels more than twofold in volunteers over a six-day period.

✖ FOODS TO AVOID

Bacon, ham, sausages, canned meats, meat pastes, meat pies, and burgers must be avoided by those restricting their sodium intakes. Stock cubes and yeast extracts are also high in sodium. **Canned fish,** large amounts of dairy products, vegetables canned in saltwater, instant potatoes, dried fruits, salted nuts, and peanut butter are best avoided by those on low-sodium diets. **Liver, kidneys, anchovies,** and sardines are particularly rich in proteins called purines. About 25 percent of people with uric acid kidney stones have a condition known as "hyperuricosuria,"

which in most cases is due to excessive intakes of dietary purines. Although drugs can prevent the formation of uric acid stones from purines, it is sometimes still advisable to avoid purine-rich foods.

Rhubarb, spinach, beets, peanuts, chocolate, and tea contain oxalates which, together with calcium, form about 70 percent of kidney stones in people living in the West. These foods need to be eaten in moderation by those people who experience kidney stones regularly.
Seek medical advice before taking these steps.

⊘ OTHER MEASURES

❑ Supplements of vitamin B_6 may be useful for those with calcium oxalate kidney stones. A lack of B_6 can lead to increased amounts of oxalic acid in the urine, which causes stone formation.
❑ Fenugreek seeds are given as a decoction by herbalists and are recommended in Chinese medicine as a way of strengthening the kidneys.
❑ Cinnamon, taken as a decoction, infusion, or in the form of capsules, is thought to be warming and tonifying for weak kidneys.
❑ Citrate supplements can be useful for those with calcium-based kidney stones.
Seek medical advice before taking these steps.

See Also Diabetes, page 218; Prostate Disorders, page 191; Urinary System, page 188

MUSCLES, BONES & JOINTS

BONES ARE LIVING, dynamic tissue composed of protein and mineral salts, such as calcium, magnesium, and phosphorus. There are more than 200 bones in the human skeleton, which has five essential functions: to support, protect, allow movement, store minerals, and facilitate the production of red blood cells in the bone marrow. Joints are the points connecting individual bones. There are several types of joint, each permitting a specific range of skeletal movement. Any movement is effected by one or more of over 600 skeletal muscles.

THE IMPORTANCE OF DIET

It has been shown that bone density and strength in maturity depend critically on a person's diet during the first two decades of life. Poor nutrition can increase the risk of developing osteoporosis in later life, and other nutritional deficiencies may weaken bone tissue and increase the risk of fractures. Dietary intake may relieve diseases of the joints, such as rheumatoid arthritis. Research into sports nutrition has revealed the importance of eating a diet rich in carbohydrates for the skeletal muscles.

MAINTAINING HEALTH

Regular weight-bearing activities, such as walking and running, exercise the skeletal muscles and help to maintain bone density. A balanced intake of proteins, minerals, vitamins, fats, and carbohydrates helps to maintain healthy bones muscles and bones.

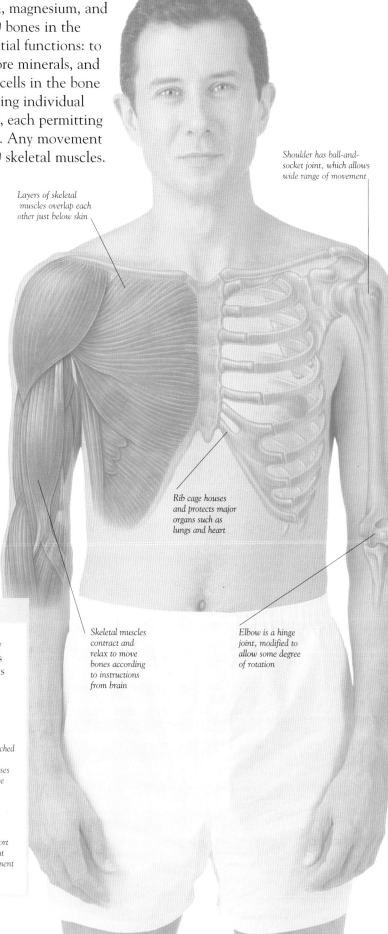

Shoulder has ball-and-socket joint, which allows wide range of movement

Layers of skeletal muscles overlap each other just below skin

Rib cage houses and protects major organs such as lungs and heart

Skeletal muscles contract and relax to move bones according to instructions from brain

Elbow is a hinge joint, modified to allow some degree of rotation

STRUCTURE OF A JOINT

Joints may be fixed, such as the skull, slightly moveable, such as the spine, or mobile, such as the knee, which is a hinge joint. Mobile joints also include ball-and-socket joints.

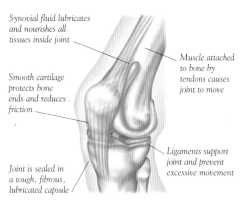

Synovial fluid lubricates and nourishes all tissues inside joint

Smooth cartilage protects bone ends and reduces friction

Joint is sealed in a tough, fibrous, lubricated capsule

Muscle attached to bone by tendons causes joint to move

Ligaments support joint and prevent excessive movement

TOP HEALING FOODS

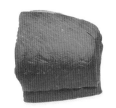

OILY FISH   PAGE 118

Benefits Contains essential fats that may reduce inflammation caused by rheumatoid arthritis.
Useful for Rheumatoid arthritis, bone building and maintenance.
Nutrients Omega-3 fatty acids, vitamin D, protein.

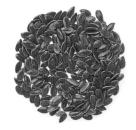

FLAX SEEDS   PAGE 105

Benefits Both the seeds and flax-seed oil are an alternative source of essential fats found in oily fish.
Useful for Vegetarians who do not eat fish, and people with inflammatory joint problems.
Nutrients Essential fats, protein.

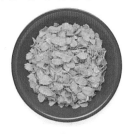

BREAKFAST CEREALS PAGE 93

Benefits If fortified with folic acid, help to replenish levels of this important nutrient.
Useful for People taking regular aspirin-based painkillers, which can reduce folic acid levels.
Nutrients Folic acid, B vitamins.

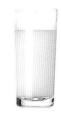

SEMI-SKIM MILK   PAGE 126

Benefits Rich in bone-building minerals to help establish and maintain bone strength.
Useful for Growing children, adults, and elderly people for whom osteoporosis is a risk.
Nutrients Calcium, phosphorus.

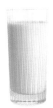

SOY MILK   PAGE 60

Benefits If fortified with calcium, may help prevent menopausal bone deterioration in women.
Useful for Vegetarians, people with cow's milk intolerance, and menopausal women.
Nutrients Calcium, protein.

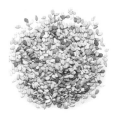

SESAME SEEDS   PAGE 103

Benefits The seeds and foods made from them, such as tahini, are rich sources of mineral salts needed for healthy bones.
Useful for Non-dairy eaters.
Nutrients Calcium, protein, zinc, iron.

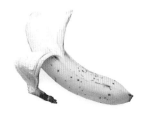

BANANAS   PAGE 90

Benefits May help with muscle cramps and restore energy levels depleted by exercise.
Useful for Those who exercise regularly or whose low potassium levels cause them to have cramps.
Nutrients Potassium, magnesium.

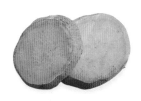

SWEET POTATOES   PAGE 55

Benefits Rich in antioxidant nutrients that may reduce muscle and bone inflammation.
Useful for Those with rheumatoid arthritis and those who get regular exercise.
Nutrients Vitamins C and E.

OTHER BENEFICIAL FOODS

CANNED SARDINES PAGE 119

Benefits Eaten with bones, they provide calcium and vitamin D, needed to aid calcium absorption.
Useful for Useful for building and maintaining strong bones.
Nutrients Calcium, vitamin D.

BLUEBERRIES   PAGE 83

Benefits Supply antioxidants that may help to strengthen blood vessel walls.
Useful for Those who suffer cramps due to poor circulation.
Nutrients Vitamin C.

SOY YOGURT   PAGE 60

Benefits Source of plant estrogens, which may help to slow down loss of bone calcium during menopause.
Useful for Menopausal women.
Nutrients Plant estrogens.

RYE BREAD   PAGE 99

Benefits Good source of magnesium, needed to maintain the nerve impulses to muscles and to balance calcium levels.
Useful for Pregnant women.
Nutrients Magnesium, iron.

FOODS TO AVOID

SOFT DRINKS

These are rich in phosphorus, excessive intakes of which can lead to calcium loss. This may reduce the ability of a child's or teenager's absorption of calcium by the bones and so build up bone density. Regular, large intakes may also contribute to an increased loss of calcium from the bones in adulthood.

WHOLEWHEAT PITA

Unleavened breads, such as pita made from wholewheat flour, contain phytates. These substances can combine with calcium and magnesium, and this has the effect of reducing the amounts of these minerals available for the body to absorb. Yeasts present in leavened breads largely break down any phytates.

RHUBARB

This fruit contains oxalates, which reduce the availability of calcium to the body by combining with it in the digestive system. Beets and spinach are other dietary sources of oxalates, and they may also have the effect of reducing calcium supplies.

FRIED FOODS

Since fried foods are rich in fat, their regular consumption is likely to contribute to weight gain. Excess weight increases wear and tear on bones and joints, and it can also lead to osteoarthritis.

MEAT PRODUCTS

Sausages, burgers, and other meat products are rich in fat and, if eaten regularly, may increase body weight and the wear on bones. Such foods should be eaten in strict moderation and, ideally, in reduced-fat forms.

BRAN

Bran, often sprinkled over breakfast cereals and on soups by people trying to increase their fiber intake, is rich in phytates. These impair the body's capacity to absorb calcium, which is essential for building and maintaining good bone structure. The type of fiber that does not impede absorption is found in vegetables and most fruits.

GOUT

WHEN LEVELS OF URIC ACID in the blood increase excessively, urate crystals form in the joints. Uric acid is a by-product of substances in food called "purines." The body usually eliminates uric acid in the urine, but in some people, the kidneys cannot flush out the uric acid quickly enough, which can lead to attacks of gout.

SYMPTOMS Gout usually affects one joint, often in the big toe, which becomes red, swollen and extremely painful for a few days at a time.

CONVENTIONAL TREATMENT Drugs may be given to inhibit the production of uric acid and to increase its excretion. People with gout are advised to reach a normal body weight and to eat foods that are low in purines.

BENEFICIAL FOODS
Whole-grain cereals and wholewheat breads supply zinc, which may be decreased during gout attacks. **Breakfast cereals and breads** fortified with folic acid may help to reduce uric acid production. **Breads, pasta, milk**, low-fat milk products, eggs, lettuce, and tomatoes are low in purines.

Fruits and vegetables supply vitamin C, which may help the kidneys to excrete uric acid.

FOODS TO AVOID
Meats, including liver, are rich in purines, as are asparagus, spinach, cauliflower, and mushrooms. Beans, peas, lentils, herrings, mackerel, sardines, crabs, and shrimp supply significant amounts. **Alcohol** increases the production of uric acid from purines in foods. Beer also contains purines. **Dried fruits** should be eaten in moderation since fructose (fruit sugar) increases urate production.

OTHER MEASURES
❏ Drinking at least two quarts of water a day will help to flush urate crystals out via the kidneys.
❏ Fish oil and evening primrose oil supplements can help to reduce inflammation caused by gout.
❏ Losing weight is important if it is above normal, since uric acid levels increase as weight creeps up. Drastic diets should, however, be avoided, since they may cause urate levels to rise.

See Also Kidney Disorders, page 192

MUSCLE CRAMPS

SUSTAINED CONTRACTIONS of the muscles, or cramps, may be caused by low blood sugar levels, losses of sodium or calcium, dehydration, or food poisoning. Stomach cramps are associated with premenstrual syndrome and poor circulation.

SYMPTOMS Cramps cause the muscles to become painful. Premenstrual cramps are characterized by pains in the lower abdomen.

CONVENTIONAL TREATMENT The underlying cause of the cramps must be diagnosed and treated first. Painkillers may be prescribed.

BENEFICIAL FOODS
Low-fat dairy products, tofu, sardines, sesame seeds, and nuts supply calcium, which is needed if cramps are associated with a loss of calcium. **Green vegetables, breads**, pasta, and potatoes are good sources of magnesium, needed by muscle fibers. A lack of this nutrient can lead to cramps. **Bananas, apricots, figs,** raisins, black currants, potatoes, onions, and tomatoes are beneficial if cramps are due to low potassium levels. **Mackerel, salmon, sardines,** and kippers supply

omega-3 fatty acids, which may help to relieve cramps caused by poor circulation.
Berries, which contain flavonoids, may help those with cramps due to poor circulation.
Legumes, oats, pasta, and rye bread are sources of carbohydrates, which are helpful for cramps that are associated with dips in blood sugar levels.

FOODS TO AVOID
Sugary foods such as cakes are best avoided if cramps are caused by dips in blood sugar levels.
Spinach and beets should be limited if cramps are caused by calcium imbalances.
Oxylates in rhubarb block calcium absorption, as do phytates in unleavened breads such as pita. Pregnant women may limit intake of these foods.

OTHER MEASURES
❏ Keeping well hydrated helps to prevent cramps brought on due to a lack of fluids.
❏ Eating snacks throughout the day may help to control cramps caused by low blood sugar levels.

See Also Premenstrual Syndrome, page 222

RHEUMATOID ARTHRITIS

THIS INFLAMMATORY DISEASE is one of the more common forms of arthritis. Inflammation often occurs in the membranes of the joints, which become swollen. The disease varies greatly in its severity, from very mild forms to severe attacks that permanently damage joints, cartilage, and bone. The precise cause of this condition is still unknown and is a subject of much debate, although it seems to be associated with an overactivity of the immune system. It may also be caused by a microscopic organism, or "microbe."

✪ SYMPTOMS The fingers, knuckles, and wrists are usually the first joints affected, followed by the knees and feet. Later, other joints may be affected, including the elbows, shoulders, hips, ankles, and even the jaw. The joints become uncomfortably swollen and stiff and may be difficult to move. Rheumatoid arthritis may also be accompanied by influenza-like symptoms.

✚ CONVENTIONAL TREATMENT The treatment for rheumatoid arthritis involves anti-inflammatory drugs, which dampen down inflammation to prevent it from affecting the cartilage and bone. It is important that an individual with rheumatoid arthritis does not alter or stop their prescribed medication unless they are advised to do so by their specialist.

✔ BENEFICIAL FOODS
The following foods contain nutrients that may be beneficial for rheumatoid arthritis because they help to reduce inflammation or deal with other problems that may arise.
Salmon, sardines, mackerel, tuna, kippers, and other oily fish supply the omega-3 fatty acids. These fatty acids are broken down by the body into prostaglandins, which have anti-inflammatory effects, and may help to reduce symptoms of rheumatoid arthritis.
Flax and hemp seeds supply omega-3 fatty acids. Vegetarians can take these fatty acids in the form of flaxseeds or flax oil supplements.
Lean red meats, such as beef, supply omega-3 fatty acids. Meat must be extra lean to ensure that saturated fat content is reduced.
Berries, oranges, orange juice, grapefruits, grapes, papayas, peppers, dark green vegetables, and sweet potatoes are rich sources of vitamin C, which is important for healing. These foods should be eaten regularly by those with rheumatoid arthritis who bruise easily.
Skim milk and low-fat milk products, sesame seeds, tahini, tofu, fortified soy milks, sunflower seeds, dark green vegetables, and nuts supply calcium. This mineral is important for those with rheumatoid arthritis, as they have a higher than normal risk of osteoporosis.
Carrots, sweet potatoes, green leafy vegetables, apricots, papayas, and mangoes are good sources of beta carotene, and avocados, green leafy vegetables, and whole-grain cereals supply vitamin E. Beta carotene and vitamin E are antioxidants that may help to reduce the damaging effects of inflammation.

✖ FOODS TO AVOID
Butter, fatty meats, and meat products, cookies, and pastries should be eaten in strict moderation since these foods are rich in saturated fats.
Corn and wheat may provoke symptoms of rheumatoid arthritis. Bacon and other pork products, whole milk, oats, and rye may also worsen symptoms. Some specialists have found that people benefit from avoiding these foods.
Carry out elimination diets only under the supervision of a qualified dietician.

⊘ OTHER MEASURES
❑ Supplements of fish oils and evening primrose oil combined have been proven to be useful in helping those with rheumatoid arthritis.
❑ Losing weight if carrying excess weight is essential in order to reduce unnecessary strain on the joints. Reducing the amount of fat consumed can help with weight reduction and may also allow the fatty acids obtained from oily fish, nuts, and seeds to be fully effective.

See Also Immune System, page 208; Muscles, Bones & Joints, page 194

CASE HISTORY

Joan Jackson was diagnosed with mild rheumatoid arthritis in her hands at the age of 40, and was prescribed nonsteroidal anti-inflammatory drugs to control the pain and swelling. With the help of a dietician, Joan's consultant then arranged for her to follow an exclusion diet avoiding wheat and dairy products. Joan was prescribed a daily supplement of fish oil and evening primrose oil and was advised to include more oily fish in her diet. After taking the supplements for 12 weeks and after increasing her weekly consumption of oily fish, Joan began to notice a significant reduction in pain and was able to reduce her intake of anti-inflammatory drugs from then on.

OSTEOARTHRITIS

KEY FOODS

OILY FISH
page 118

SEEDS
pages 103–105

WHOLE GRAINS
pages 92–99

LEAN RED
MEATS
page 122

CITRUS
FRUITS
pages 86–88

THIS IS THE MOST common form of arthritis, in which the smooth layers of cartilage that cover and cushion the ends of the bones gradually break down. The space between the joint and bone narrows, making the surrounding ligaments looser and the joint less stable. Osteoarthritis affects elderly people in particular, but can also occur in younger people, often after an injury.

☻ SYMPTOMS As small lumps of bone called osteophytes grow outward from a joint, the joints become enlarged and deformed. Pain, swelling, and stiffness of the joints are common. As the disease progresses, the cartilage may become eroded, causing great discomfort.

✚ CONVENTIONAL TREATMENT
Painkilling drugs, such as aspirin, and nonsteroidal anti-inflammatory drugs may be prescribed.

✔ BENEFICIAL FOODS
Oily fish and flax and hemp seeds may be useful for inflammation resulting from osteoarthritis.
Breakfast cereals and breads fortified with folic acid, and legumes, spinach, cabbage, asparagus, and cauliflower, which provide folate, are useful for those taking aspirin and other painkilling drugs, which can create a deficiency of this B vitamin.
Lean red meats, fish, and fortified breakfast cereals supply plentiful amounts of iron, which may be depleted in those taking long-term doses of nonsteroidal anti-inflammatory drugs.
Citrus fruits, berries, and vegetables can help to replace vitamin C lost through long-term use of aspirin, and all fruits and vegetables can replace potassium lost as a result of taking aspirin.

✘ FOODS TO AVOID
Pies, pastries, fried foods, butter, margarine, oils, cream, whole-milk dairy products, cakes, cookies, and chocolate should be restricted by those who are overweight. Weight loss can improve symptoms of osteoarthritis, especially in the hips and knees.

⊘ OTHER MEASURES
❏ Fish oil and evening primrose oil supplements may be useful for those with inflammation.

See Also Muscles, Bones & Joints, page 194

OSTEOPOROSIS

KEY FOODS

LOW-FAT
DAIRY
PRODUCTS
pages 126–128

OILY FISH
page 118

LEGUMES
pages 58–60

NUTS &
SEEDS
pages 100–105

AS PEOPLE GROW OLDER, the density of the bones decreases and their fragility increases, making them prone to fracturing. This is osteoporosis. Causes include a lack of calcium during the first two decades of life, hormonal disorders, and use of corticosteroid drugs. Women are commonly affected by osteoporosis after menopause, because their ovaries no longer produce estrogen, which helps to maintain bone mass. Osteoporosis is not only potentially debilitating, but also life-threatening, with 20 percent of people dying within six months of sustaining a hip fracture.

☻ SYMPTOMS There may be no symptoms, but obvious signs are a loss of height and a hump on the back. Bones in the hips, spine, and wrists are commonly affected. The teeth may become loose and, as the spine crumbles, the loss of height can cause internal organs to become compacted, often resulting in digestive problems.

✚ CONVENTIONAL TREATMENT The single most effective treatment in preventing osteoporosis in older women is to replace lost estrogen during the years after menopause. It is essential that anyone who is at risk of osteoporosis seeks and follows medical advice. This may include calcium supplementation with etidronate, a drug that helps calcium lock onto the bones. Another drug, alendronate, may help to improve established osteoporosis when used in conjunction with calcium supplements. The hormone calcitonin can be given by injection to improve the levels of calcium in the body.

✔ BENEFICIAL FOODS
Low-fat milk and dairy products provide an source of calcium that is relatively easy for the body to absorb. An intake of at least 700mg of calcium is recommended per day; $2^1/_2$ cups of skim milk supplies this amount.
Oily fish, such as herrings, kippers, mackerel, sardines, and tuna, supply vitamin D, which enables the body to absorb calcium from the intestines. Eggs, butter, and fortified margarine also supply vitamin D. Research suggests that the omega-3 fatty acids in oily fish may help to reduce the amount of calcium excreted in the urine and stools. These fatty acids also appear to increase the amount of calcium absorbed directly

OSTEOPOROSIS

KEY FOODS

EGGS
page 129

SPROUTING
VEGETABLES
page 69

GREEN
VEGETABLES
pages 44–51

BERRIES
pages 82–85

PINEAPPLES
page 78

from the intestines, as well as encouraging it to be deposited on the bones. Flax and hemp seeds and lean meats also provide omega-3 fatty acids.

Canned sardines, shelled shrimp, figs, baked beans, tofu, almonds, spinach, sesame seeds, tahini, and white bread are very useful sources of calcium. So too are some bottled mineral waters.

Soy milk enriched with calcium is a good source of calcium for vegetarians and vegans who wish to avoid eating dairy products.

Soybeans, tofu, and alfalfa sprouts provide plant estrogens that mimic the effects of human estrogen, and may help to preserve bone density in women during and after menopause.

Lentils, sardines, peanuts, hazelnuts, and walnuts are rich suppliers of magnesium, and lean meats, most fish, milk, peas, green vegetables, potatoes, black currants, and pineapples are also good sources. Magnesium intakes should be roughly half those of calcium. This means that intakes need to be approximately 300–400mg a day.

✖ FOODS TO AVOID

Colas and other carbonated drinks contain phosphoric acid. This, along with phosphates in products such as ham, turkey, processed meats, some sausages, and pâté, may contribute to calcium losses and thereby osteoporosis. Check food labels for phosphoric acid.

Alcohol may lead to loss of minerals from the bones and should be moderated.

Unleavened breads, such as soda, pita, and naan bread, contain phytates, especially if they are made with wholewheat flour. Phytates bind with calcium and magnesium, which reduces the amounts of these minerals that are available to the body. Phytates are largely broken down by yeast when the bread is leavened.

Bran sprinkled over foods such as breakfast cereals and soups to increase the fiber intake in the diet is not advisable, since bran contains mineral-blocking phytates.

Rhubarb, beets, and spinach contain substances called oxalates, which bind with calcium and reduce its availability in the body. The calcium in spinach is so strongly bound with the oxalates that only three to five percent can be absorbed. Oxalates also bind manganese, which is needed for the maintenance of strong bones. It may be appropriate for vegans, who rely on vegetable sources of calcium rather than dairy products, and who may not always have adequate intakes of calcium, to ensure that spinach is eaten in moderation and, preferably, separated from calcium-rich foods.

Tannin in tea can block calcium absorption. Tea should not be drunk with meals or directly after meals that are rich in calcium.

Caffeine, found in coffee, tea, cola, and cold remedies, may increase the amount of calcium lost through the stools and urine.

Soups, meat products, canned meats and fish, and ready-made meals are sources of large amounts of sodium. This may affect calcium absorption by decreasing vitamin D synthesis in the body. Reducing the amount of sodium that is consumed at mealtimes is advisable, especially for postmenopausal women.

Meat pies, sausages, and other animal products containing saturated fats should be restricted in order to allow the essential fats to perform optimally in the body.

⊘ OTHER MEASURES

❑ For very strong bones, and to avoid the risk of developing osteoporosis in later life, it is essential to eat foods rich in calcium regularly throughout the first two decades of life. Bone mass is accumulated during the early years, peaking in the late teens and early twenties. It is important to encourage children to consume a diet that is rich in calcium from an early age.

❑ Fish oil supplements containing essential fatty acids appear to show an ability to increase calcium absorption from the intestines, and to reduce calcium losses through urine and stools.

❑ Regular exercise, such as walking, is important because it helps to strengthen the bones.

❑ Smokers are advised to give up the habit, since smoking encourages loss of bone density.

See Also Minerals, page 30; Vitamins, page 26; Women & Nutrition, page 140

EYES, EARS, NOSE, MOUTH & THROAT

BECAUSE DIET HAS COME TO PLAY an increasingly influential role in the knowledge of how to maintain healthy body systems, it has become clear that the foods and drinks that people regularly consume are able to affect the health of their visual, olfactory, and auditory systems as well as their throats and mouths. While it has been acknowledged for some time that good dental health is partly dependent upon the timing and quantity of sugary foods consumed, less obvious links are now coming to light between dietary intake and the prevention of diseases of the eyes, ears, nose, and throat.

THE INFLUENCE OF DIET

Links have recently been established between diets that are rich in certain antioxidant substances and a reduced risk of eye problems such as cataracts and glaucoma. Research trials using children have shown that giving them drinks and chewing gum containing a natural sweetener called xylitol may render them less prone to middle ear infections. This measure has the added advantage of leading to a reduction in the use of antibiotics.

KEEPING A CLEAR HEAD

Maintaining the health of the eyes, ears, nose, throat, and mouth requires a generally balanced diet that is rich in fruits and vegetables and limits intake of sugary and fatty products. A diet that excludes foods known to cause allergic reactions may prevent the irritation of mucous membranes lining some of these parts of the body.

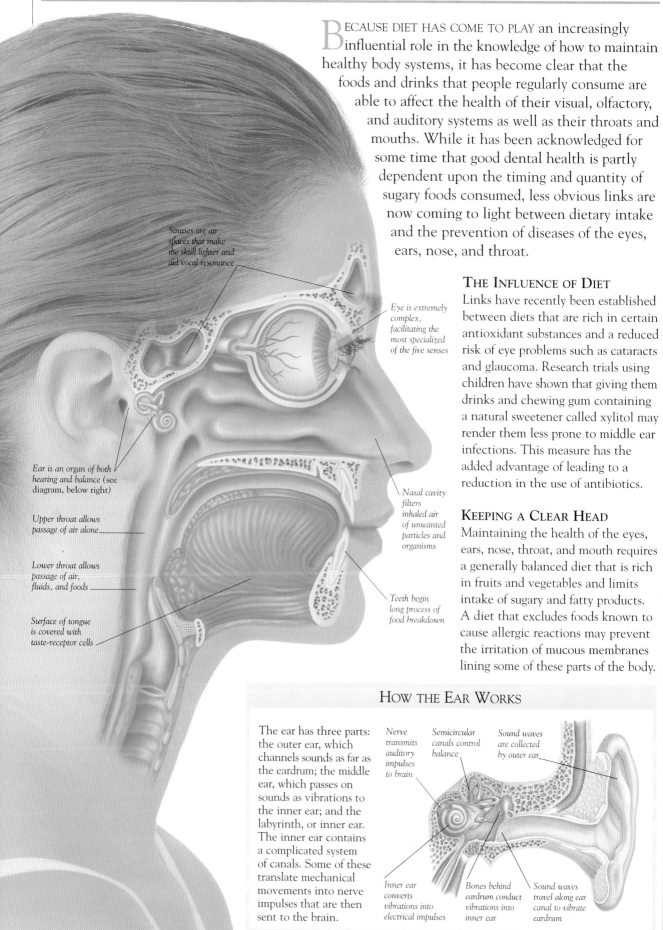

Sinuses are air spaces that make the skull lighter and aid vocal resonance

Eye is extremely complex, facilitating the most specialized of the five senses

Ear is an organ of both hearing and balance (see diagram, below right)

Upper throat allows passage of air alone

Lower throat allows passage of air, fluids, and foods

Surface of tongue is covered with taste-receptor cells

Nasal cavity filters inhaled air of unwanted particles and organisms

Teeth begin long process of food breakdown

HOW THE EAR WORKS

The ear has three parts: the outer ear, which channels sounds as far as the eardrum; the middle ear, which passes on sounds as vibrations to the inner ear; and the labyrinth, or inner ear. The inner ear contains a complicated system of canals. Some of these translate mechanical movements into nerve impulses that are then sent to the brain.

Nerve transmits auditory impulses to brain

Semicircular canals control balance

Sound waves are collected by outer ear

Inner ear converts vibrations into electrical impulses

Bones behind eardrum conduct vibrations into inner ear

Sound waves travel along ear canal to vibrate eardrum

TOP HEALING FOODS

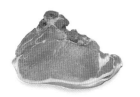

PORK   PAGE 122

Benefits Contains vitamin B and may therefore help to maintain the health of the optic nerve, which is essential for good vision.
Useful for People who are susceptible to glaucoma.
Nutrients Vitamin B_1.

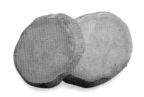

SWEET POTATOES   PAGE 55

Benefits May reduce the risk of elevated pressure in the eye, protect against pollution, and minimize free-radical damage.
Useful for Those with glaucoma and those prone to cataracts.
Nutrients Beta carotene.

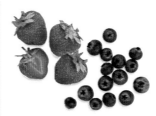

BERRIES   PAGE 82

Benefits May reduce the risk of elevated pressure in the eye, boost the immune system, and minimize free-radical damage.
Useful for Glaucoma, cataracts, and ear and throat infections.
Nutrients Vitamin C.

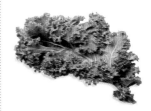

KALE   PAGE 44

Benefits Contains large amounts of beta carotene which is needed by the eyes to allow them to adjust to darkness.
Useful for Night vision.
Nutrients Beta carotene, which the body converts into vitamin A.

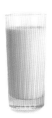

SOY MILK   PAGE 60

Benefits Being lactose-free, soy milk can replace dairy products that may trigger sinusitis.
Useful for Those who have an allergic reaction to lactose.
Nutrients Protein and, if fortified, calcium.

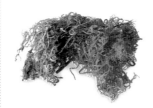

SEAWEEDS   PAGE 70

Benefits Contain iodine, which helps to maintain good hearing.
Useful for Improving the hearing of those people who experience hearing loss as a result of low iodine intakes.
Nutrients Iodine.

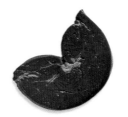

LIVER   PAGE 123

Benefits The vitamin A in liver maintains good health in the part of the inner ear where sound is converted into nerve impulses.
Useful for Those with a hearing defect linked to lack of vitamin A.
Nutrients Vitamin A.

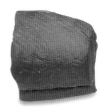

OILY FISH   PAGE 118

Benefits Contains essential fats, which can reduce inflammation and may help to guard against malformations of the ear bones.
Useful for Sinusitis, infections.
Nutrients Omega-3 fatty acids, protein, vitamin D.

OTHER BENEFICIAL FOODS

RED MEATS   PAGE 122

Benefits May help in the restoration of the sensorineural type of hearing loss.
Useful for People with low iron intakes and low iron stores.
Nutrients Iron, selenium.

CHEESE   PAGE 127

Benefits After a meal, helps to restore the mouth's alkaline pH, reducing the risk of tooth decay.
Useful for People susceptible to tooth decay and erosion.
Nutrients Calcium, phosphorus.

BREAST MILK   PAGE 134

Benefits Breastfeeding can protect against middle-ear infections in young children.
Useful for Protection from ear infections and antibiotic overuse.
Nutrients Calcium, fatty acids.

SUGAR-FREE GUM   PAGE 207

Benefits Sugar-free gum protects teeth against decay. Sweetened with xylitol, gum may reduce the risk of middle-ear infections.
Useful for Ear infections.
Nutrients Natural sugar xylitol.

FOODS TO AVOID

COFFEE, TEA & SODAS

Drinking excessive amounts of coffee, tea, and carbonated beverages containing caffeine, may lead to increases in pressure in the eyes. These drinks should be avoided by those affected by, or likely to develop, glaucoma.

DAIRY PRODUCTS

Milk and milk products should be avoided by people with allergic sinusitis, which involves a reaction to the milk sugar lactose. Other dairy foods and foodstuffs that contain dairy derivatives

should also be avoided. People with general lactose intolerance should also avoid eating these foods, since the galactose in milk may build up and damage the eyes.

SUGAR

Sugary foods and drinks should be avoided between meals in order to help reduce the risk of tooth decay. Sugar is a source of food for the bacteria that occur naturally in the mouth. In the course of processing such food, the bacteria produce acids, and it is this that causes cavities.

CARBONATED DRINKS

Carbonated drinks contain phosphoric acid, which is capable of corroding teeth. These drinks should only be taken infrequently, and then preferably with meals, to limit the potential damage.

CITRUS FRUIT JUICES

Grapefruit and orange juices both contain citric acid, which is potentially highly corrosive. If taken between meals, these juices can cause corrosion of tooth enamel. Drink at meal times, with food, to reduce the damage.

ARGININE

Studies have revealed that the amino acid arginine is used by the *Herpes* virus to help it replicate. People who are susceptible to cold sores or genital herpes are advised to restrict arginine-rich food in their diet to help prevent the virus from spreading. Such foods include cereal grains, chocolate, seeds, nuts, gelatin, and raisins.

CATARACTS

KEY FOODS

GREEN
VEGETABLES
pages 44–51

ROOT
VEGETABLES
page 54

CITRUS
FRUITS
pages 86–88

BERRIES
pages 82–85

A CLOUDY AREA in the lens of the eye is known as a cataract. This condition develops when the protein fibers in the lens, which are normally transparent, gradually coagulate, creating an opaque film. Most cataracts occur in the elderly.

✪ SYMPTOMS Cataracts are usually painless, causing blurred vision, which gradually worsens. Left untreated, cataracts can lead to blindness.

✚ CONVENTIONAL TREATMENT The damaged lens may be replaced with an artificial one, but not every case requires this treatment.

✔ BENEFICIAL FOODS
Cabbage and other green leafy vegetables, and also carrots, apricots, and other yellow and orange fruits and vegetables supply carotenes. High intakes of carotenes have been associated with a lower risk of cataracts. Carotenes probably help to protect the eyes by deactivating harmful free radicals. Spinach, in particular, may help to lower the risk of developing cataracts.
Oranges, grapefruits, berries, green leafy vegetables, and potatoes supply vitamin C. This vitamin appears to protect against free radicals that can damage the eyes. Good intakes may reduce the risk and slow the development of cataracts. People who eat more than four servings of vegetables and fruits a day appear to be less at risk of developing the condition.

✘ FOODS TO AVOID
Dairy products should be avoided by those with a lactose intolerance because the milk sugar galactose may build up and worsen cataracts.
Prepackaged foods are low in important nutrients, and are best avoided by those with cataracts.

⊘ OTHER MEASURES
❑ Vitamin C may help to reverse cataracts when supplements of at least 350mg are taken daily.
❑ Bilberry extracts and bioflavonoid supplements may be beneficial for those with cataracts.
❑ Smoking should be stopped, because it lowers vitamin C levels in the blood, robbing the body of its antioxidant protection.

See Also Food Supplements, page 36

GLAUCOMA

KEY FOODS

CITRUS
FRUITS
page 86–88

WHOLE GRAINS
pages 92–99

MEATS
page 122

NUTS
pages 100–102

THIS IS A DISEASE in which the pressure inside the eye rises above normal, causing part of the optic nerve to become compressed. Glaucoma blocks drainage systems in the eye and is thought to prevent nutrients from reaching the nerves.

✪ SYMPTOMS Often there are no symptoms. However, in some cases the eyes may be painful and bloodshot, especially in the morning. The vision is blurred and the eyes are unable to adjust to the dark. Glaucoma can lead to blindness.

✚ CONVENTIONAL TREATMENT Eye drops, pills, or liquids may be given to reduce the high pressure in the eye. If these are unsuccessful, surgery is possible. This involves making a small opening in the iris to allow the eye to drain.

✔ BENEFICIAL FOODS
Pork, wholewheat bread, brown rice, pasta, whole-grain breakfast cereals, liver, nuts, and legumes are all good sources of vitamin B$_1$. A lack of this vitamin may be associated with glaucoma.
Liver and eggs supply vitamin A, and yellow and orange fruits and vegetables, such as apricots and carrots, provide beta carotene, which is converted into vitamin A in the body. A deficiency of this vitamin can cause increased pressure in the eyes.
Citrus fruits and berries are some of the richest sources of vitamin C. High intakes may help to reduce the risk of glaucoma. People with daily intakes of 1,200mg of vitamin C have been shown to have significantly lower pressure in the eyes than people with intakes of 75mg a day.

✘ FOODS TO AVOID
Protein-rich foods such as meats, fish, poultry, and eggs are not advisable in excessive amounts.
Caffeine may lead to an increase in eye pressure. Coffee, tea, cola, cold remedies, chocolate, and cocoa are best avoided by those with glaucoma.

⊘ OTHER MEASURES
❑ Rutin, a flavonoid found in many citrus fruits and red wine, is available as a supplement. Taking 20mg of rutin three times daily can result in at least a 15 percent reduction in eye pressure.

See Also Alcohol, page 19; Plant Nutrients, page 34

EAR DISORDERS

DISORDERS OF THE EAR include otitis media, an infection of the middle ear that can lead to a burst eardrum, and Ménière's disease, a condition resulting from a buildup of fluid in the inner ear. Diet may have a role to play in these disorders.

✪ SYMPTOMS The symptoms depend on the specific ailment. Otitis media is the most common cause of earache. There may be loss of hearing and a raised temperature. Ménière's disease usually causes intermittent, progressive vertigo, deafness, and tinnitus (ringing or buzzing in the ears).

✚ CONVENTIONAL TREATMENT For earache, analgesic drugs may be given; the underlying cause is also treated.

✔ BENEFICIAL FOODS
Oily fish, shellfish, eggs, milk, yogurt, meats, and seaweed supply iodine. A mild to moderate iodine deficiency has been associated with hearing loss. In China, hearing improved among children who lived in iodine-deficient areas, following the introduction of iodized salt.
Liver, whole milk, eggs, and oily fish such as mackerel, red salmon, and anchovies supply vitamin A. The cochlea, a spiral canal in the inner ear, usually has a high concentration of vitamin A, and depends on it in order to function properly. Lack of vitamin A may be associated with disorders of the inner ear.
Carrots, squashes, peppers, green leafy vegetables, and orange and yellow fruits such as mangoes and apricots provide beta carotene, which is converted into vitamin A in the body.
Oily fish, eggs, fortified breakfast cereals, butter, and margarine supply vitamin D. Very low levels of vitamin D have been found in people who have otosclerosis, a condition of the inner ear that can cause deafness.
Red meats, fish, dark green vegetables, and fortified breakfast cereals provide iron. An iron deficiency may be associated with hearing loss. Low iron intakes are a problem for those on a vegetarian diet, especially women.
Whole-grain cereals, red meats, and seafoods contain zinc. Concentrations of zinc are usually high in the sensory areas of the inner ear. Tinnitus may be associated with low zinc levels.

✪ FOODS TO AVOID
Sugar, honey, molasses, syrup, and foods containing sugar are thought to cause inner ear disorders by triggering an overproduction of insulin, followed quickly by low blood sugar

CASE STUDY

Abigail Edelman, aged 11, had experienced middle-ear infections since the age of three. The antibiotics prescribed were sometimes effective, but did not always work, which left Abigail in great pain. Abigail's mother decided to give her daughter chewing gum containing xylitol regularly, and within a year the infections had virtually ceased. As a result, Abigail was able to reduce her intake of antibiotics dramatically, and no longer needed to take days off school. Now, Abigail's mother also encourages her other children to chew gum containing xylitol, to prevent the risk of ear infections.

levels. This, in turn, causes an adrenaline release and constriction of blood vessels. In tests on people with Ménière's disease, many were shown to have high insulin levels. Once they were following a low-carbohydrate, high-protein diet, nearly all them were able to control their vertigo and for several of them their hearing improved.
Potatoes, breads, bagels, croissants, and English muffins all cause relatively rapid rises in blood sugar levels. It may be advisable for people with ear disorders such as Ménière's syndrome to eat these foods in moderation, and to concentrate their carbohydrate intakes on slowly absorbed foods such as oatmeal, rice, rye bread, and pasta.
Raspberries, cherries, dried dates, prunes and liquorice contain aspirinlike substances called salicylates. Some people with tinnitus may be sensitive to salicylates.

⊘ OTHER MEASURES
❏ Zinc sulfate supplements may improve the symptoms of tinnitus in some people.
❏ Breast-feeding infants for the first four months of life can protect them against otitis media until at least one year old. The longer the period of time that a child is breast-fed, the lower the chance of developing middle-ear infections.
❏ Some sugar-free chewing gums contain a substance known as xylitol, which can reduce the risk of otitis media. Xylitol inhibits the growth of the bacteria pneumococci and appears to reduce its ability to stick to the eustachian tube, which links the back of the throat to the inner ear.
❏ Xylitol syrup can help to reduce the risk of middle-ear infections and is suitable for infants and children under five years of age, for whom chewing gum is not recommended.

See Also Infections, page 212

KEY FOODS

OILY FISH
page 118

SHELLFISH
page 120

RED MEATS
page 122

WHOLE GRAINS
pages 92–99

NUTS & SEEDS
pages 100–105

BERRIES
pages 82–85

CITRUS FRUITS
pages 86–88

VEGETABLES
pages 42–71

SOY PRODUCTS
page 60

SINUSITIS

THE SINUSES ARE SMALL, air-filled cavities in the skull, lined with delicate membranes that link up with membranes inside the nose. When these membranes become inflamed the condition known as sinusitis occurs. Sudden, temporary sinusitis is known as acute sinusitis. This is frequently caused by colds or by bacterial and viral infections of the nose, throat, and upper respiratory tract. Long-term, or chronic, irritation of the synovial membranes may be caused by cigarette smoke and exposure to pollution, pollen, and certain smells. Chronic sinusitis tends to make breathing difficult and it can lead to the development of polyps in the nose. Allergic reactions to certain foods can also cause sinus problems (*see page 210*).

✪ SYMPTOMS There may be a blocked nose, headache, earache, toothache, facial pain, and an impaired sense of smell. In some cases, sinusitis may also cause fever.

✚ CONVENTIONAL TREATMENT Medical advice should be sought. Asthma, bronchitis, laryngitis, and pneumonia can be precipitated by the infection that caused the sinusitis. Antibiotics and decongestants may be prescribed for sinus infections and nasal polyps can be removed surgically.

✔ BENEFICIAL FOODS
Eating plenty of foods that boost the immune system is important for those with sinusitis. If the problem is caused by an allergic reaction to certain foods, these must be removed from the diet. Tests should be carried out by an allergy specialist, and a diet needs to be devised with a dietician to ensure that all the essential nutrients are present in the foods and drinks allowed.
Seafood, red meats, wholewheat breads, wholegrain breakfast cereals, nuts, and seeds supply zinc. This mineral is essential for the immune system to function properly. A diet that is rich in zinc may help the body to fight off infections that can lead to sinusitis.
Strawberries, black currants, and papayas, oranges, grapefruits, and other citrus fruits, sweet potatoes, potatoes, peas, peppers, and green leafy vegetables provide good amounts of vitamin C. This vitamin appears to help the cells of the immune system to mature and improves the performance of antibodies. It also seems to have antiviral and antibacterial properties, and can help to dampen down inflammation, as well as boost immunity.

Carrots, sweet potatoes, spinach, kale, and brussels sprouts all contain beta carotene, which is converted into vitamin A in the body. A lack of vitamin A can lead to changes in the cells lining the respiratory tract, which may make infections more likely. Natural, or "preformed," vitamin A is found in foods such as liver, whole milk and cheese, egg yolks, and butter, as well as in some oily fish, including anchovies, mackerel, and red salmon.
Soybeans, tofu, sesame seeds, sunflower seeds, peanuts, and some soy milks contain calcium. These non-dairy foods are important for those whose sinusitis is triggered by a milk allergy.
Mackerel, sardines, salmon, kippers, pilchards, nuts, and seeds contain omega-3 fatty acids, which may help to dampen down inflammation associated with sinusitis.

✪ FOODS TO AVOID
Food allergies can be the cause of sinusitis. If a food allergy is suspected, a doctor should perform an allergy test to detect problem foods.
Milk and dairy products, such as yogurt, cheese, and fromage frais, may cause allergic sinusitis. If this is so, such foods should be removed from the diet. A completely milk-free diet requires the exclusion of all types of milk, including fresh, condensed, dried, evaporated, and skim milk, and also butter, cream, margarine, ice cream, and milk shakes. Food labels must be checked, since some breakfast cereals, desserts, cakes, cookies, and meat products contain milk. Instant mashed potatoes, toffee, butterscotch, milk chocolate, malted drinks, soups, sauces, gravies, and some sweeteners also contain milk derivatives.

✪ OTHER MEASURES
❏ Hot drinks encourage mucus to flow, which relieves congestion and pressure in the sinuses.
❏ Ground ivy infusion helps to dry out mucus.
❏ Goldenseal tincture relieves mucus. Taking 1ml three times a day can ease symptoms.
❏ A supplement of 1,000mg of vitamin C a day may help to strengthen the immune system.
❏ Drinking 15 drops of echinacea in warm water three times a day helps to strengthen the immune system.
❏ Smoky and polluted environments are best avoided by people with sinusitis, because fumes can worsen this condition.

See Also Food Allergies, page 210; Food Supplements, page 36; Vitamins, page 26

EATING PLAN FOR SINUSITIS

For individuals who are prone to sinusitis, it is important to eat plenty of foods that are rich in zinc and vitamin C in order to maintain a healthy immune system. Vegetables such as garlic and onions can be added to the savory dishes shown below, since they are thought to have antibacterial effects.

BREAKFASTS

Peach-filled crêpes made with wholewheat flour

Glass of freshly squeezed orange juice

◆

Apple and dates added to a high fiber cereal, with soya milk

Glass of ruby red grapefruit juice

◆

Poached egg and mushrooms on wholewheat toast

Ready-made or freshly prepared fruit salad

LIGHT MEALS

Grilled mackerel with a carrot and cilantro salad and hot French bread

Slice of melon

◆

Wholewheat bread roll filled with peanut butter and fresh watercress

Ready-made or freshly prepared fruit salad

◆

Whole-grain pita bread filled with egg salad (made with low-fat salad dressing) and mustard and cress

Large apple and banana

MAIN MEALS

Baked salmon fishcakes with stir-fried beansprouts and noodles

Summer pudding with fat-free soya yogurt

◆

Grilled chicken with spinach and brown rice

Poached peaches

◆

Steamed mussels with garlic and wine sauce and hot wholewheat bread

Spiced winter fruit salad with honey-roasted sunflower seeds

SNACKS

Whole-grain breakfast cereal with low-fat milk or soy milk

◆

Orange or grapefruit juice with two wholewheat cookies

◆

Whole-grain crispbreads with lean ham and sliced tomatoes

◆

Mixture of sesame seeds, pumpkin seeds, and sunflower seeds, with cup of herbal tea

---

COLD SORES

KEY FOODS

FRUITS
pages 72–91

GREEN VEGETABLES
pages 44–51

ONIONS
page 67

RED MEATS
page 122

A COLD SORE IS CAUSED by the *Herpes simplex* virus, which sits in the facial nerves. It may be triggered by stress, colds, influenza, menstruation, and fatigue. The virus migrates to the end of the nerve, usually around the lip margins. It then enters the cells and sets up an infection that develops into a cold sore.

✪ SYMPTOMS
The first sign is a tingling sensation. Within 24 hours this usually turns into one or several blisters. The infection can lead to influenza-like symptoms. After several days the cold sore dries up and the skin eventually heals.

✚ CONVENTIONAL TREATMENT
Certain painkillers can be taken to reduce pain. Antiviral drugs, such as acyclovir, may be applied in a cream form. Severe or recurrent herpes infections may be treated orally with acyclovir.

⊘ BENEFICIAL FOODS
Oranges, grapefruits, berries, peppers, green leafy vegetables, sweet potatoes, and potatoes are good sources of vitamin C. High intakes of this vitamin may help to prevent cold sores.

Onions, apples, grapes, and tea are rich in bioflavonoids, which may help to prevent the development of blisters after the tingling phase.
Meats, milk, fish, chicken, and eggs contain the amino acid lysine, which blocks the action of the virus-promoting amino acid arginine.

✖ FOODS TO AVOID
Chocolate, peanuts and other nuts, raisins, and seeds contain arginine, which is needed by the herpes virus if it is to multiply.

⊘ OTHER MEASURES
❑ Supplements of 200mg each of vitamin C and bioflavonoids taken three to four times a day may prevent full-blown outbreaks of herpes.
❑ Zinc lozenges taken during periods of stress help to stimulate the immune system.
❑ *Melissa officinalis* lip salve is a useful preventive measure against cold sores.
❑ Drinking 15 drops of echinacea in warm water three times a day boosts the immune system.

See Also Infections, page 212

GUM DISEASE

KEY FOODS

FRUITS
pages 72–91

GREEN VEGETABLES
pages 44–51

GARLIC & ONIONS
pages 66–67

TEA
page 110

WHOLE GRAINS
pages 92–99

OILY FISH
page 118

CARROTS
page 56

DAIRY PRODUCTS
pages 126–128

RED MEATS
page 122

THE MOST COMMON gum disorder is inflammation of the gums, known as gingivitis, which is often the result of an infection. Gingivitis is thought to be caused by the buildup of dental plaque (a sticky mixture of food particles, saliva, and bacteria). It may also result from hormonal changes associated with pregnancy. If gingivitis is left untreated, it can progress to periodontitis, a disease that affects the gums, teeth, and bone.

SYMPTOMS Gingivitis causes the gums to swell, creating pockets next to the teeth that accumulate plaque. The gums become shiny, red, and tender. If allowed to progress to periodontitis the gums become inflamed, painful, and often bleed. The disease causes bad breath, erosion of the jawbone, and abscesses.

CONVENTIONAL TREATMENT It is essential to seek the advice of a dentist if gum disease is suspected. Regular, thorough brushing and flossing are recommended, and the use of electric toothbrushes can be helpful. The gums should be brushed using a soft toothbrush. Plaque-finding tablets can help to identify areas of plaque that have been missed when brushing. Advanced periodontitis may require surgery to reshape the gum and bone.

BENEFICIAL FOODS
Oranges, grapefruits, green leafy vegetables, berries, peppers, and potatoes are good sources of vitamin C, important for strengthening the gums. Deficiency of vitamin C in the diet is associated with increased swelling and redness of gingivitis.
Onions, apples, and tea are very good suppliers of bioflavonoids, which promote gum healing.
Garlic contains antibacterial substances that help to fight infections in the mouth.
Fortified breakfast cereals, breads, and yeast extracts supply folic acid, the B vitamin needed for tissue health. People with low levels of folic acid may be able to reduce gum inflammation by increasing intakes of these foods, along with those that naturally contain folate, such as beets, kale, asparagus, spinach, and legumes.
Sardines and pilchards, canned whole with their bones, are excellent sources of vitamin D and calcium. A lack of vitamin D impairs calcium absorption, which may aggravate periodontitis.
Sweet potatoes, carrots, mangoes, apricots, and green leafy vegetables supply beta carotene, which boosts vitamin A levels. A lack of this vitamin is associated with a risk of periodontal disease. Pregnant women, who are prone to

periodontal disease due to hormonal changes, should eat foods rich in beta carotene to ensure that their vitamin A reserves are full. Supplements of vitamin A are not advised because it is possible to overdose and damage the developing fetus.
Milk, yogurt, cheese, fortified soy milk, tofu, sesame seeds, and tahini supply calcium. Good intakes of this mineral help to ensure strong jawbones. A lack of calcium in the diet may contribute to gum disease.
Red meats, seafood, and whole-grain cereals provide zinc. A deficiency of this mineral may make the gum tissues prone to damage.

FOODS TO AVOID
Sugar, sweet drinks, cookies, cakes, honey, molasses, and corn syrup increase plaque and should be eaten in strict moderation.
Carbonated drinks, canned meats, and processed foods contain phosphorus in the form of additives, such as sodium phosphate, potassium phosphate, phosphoric acid, and polyphosphate. Some phosphorus is vital for healthy bone, but too much can damage the calcium-to-phosphorus ratio, leading to calcium loss. This may weaken the jawbone, which can worsen gum disease.

OTHER MEASURES
❑ Chewing gum sweetened with xylitol helps to clean the teeth after eating and between meals. Xylitol is a natural sweetener that reduces the activity of bacteria in the mouth and helps to prevent the buildup of plaque.
❑ Folic acid mouthwashes may help to reduce inflammation and infection of the gums. Folic acid supplements may be helpful for those with low levels of folate in their diet.
❑ Vitamin C supplements of 60–70mg a day are beneficial for treating gingivitis. Easily obtainable from fruits and vegetables, this amount helps to decrease bleeding associated with gingivitis.
❑ Vitamin E capsules can be bitten in half and the oil applied directly to the affected area.
❑ Supplements of coenzyme Q10 can help to reduce the depth of pockets around the teeth and help to stop deterioration of the gums.
❑ Goldenseal is a herbal remedy with natural antibacterial properties. Brushing the teeth with goldenseal powder daily may help gum disease.
❑ Smokers are advised to give up the habit, because smoking is associated with an increased risk of periodontal disease.

See Also Minerals, page 30; Vitamins, page 26

TOOTH DECAY

KEY FOODS

DAIRY
PRODUCTS
pages 126–128

ALSO KNOWN AS DENTAL CARIES, tooth decay occurs when areas of the hard enamel covering on the teeth become damaged by acids in the mouth. This initially occurs in the subsurface of the tooth, but if it is not stopped, a cavity forms and this can progress through the enamel and into the soft dentine below.

✪ SYMPTOMS There may be a mild toothache when eating sweet, hot, or cold foods. In more severe cases, there is a sharp, stabbing pain if the dentine below the surface is affected.

✚ CONVENTIONAL TREATMENT Decayed teeth can be filled by a dentist. Today there is much emphasis on the prevention of tooth decay through oral hygiene and the topical application or oral ingestion of the mineral fluoride.

✔ BENEFICIAL FOODS
The kinds of food and drink consumed and the timing of meals can play an important role in helping to prevent tooth decay.
Milk and cheese are alkaline, so they can help to restore the pH balance in the mouth if consumed at the end of a meal. The protein called casein in cheese helps to prevent tooth enamel from being dissolved by acids from food, drinks, and bacteria. Milk and cheese are also good sources of calcium and phosphorus, needed for strong teeth.

✖ FOODS TO AVOID
Candies, sugar, honey, molasses, syrup, and sugary foods and drinks should be reduced. **Dried fruits** should be avoided between meals if it is not possible to clean the teeth afterward.

❂ OTHER MEASURES
❑ Cleaning the teeth or chewing gum containing xylitol after meals may reduce the risk of decay. Sugar-free gum containing xylitol stimulates the production of saliva, which helps to stop acid attacking the teeth. Xylitol reduces the quantity of acid-producing bacteria and plaque.
❑ Fluoridated toothpaste helps to prevent tooth decay and fluoridated mouthwashes may help to reverse early signs of tooth demineralization.

See Also Minerals, page 30; Vitamins, page 26

TOOTH EROSION

KEY FOODS

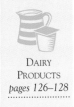

DAIRY
PRODUCTS
pages 126–128

TEA
page 110

SHALLOW AREAS OF EROSION on the teeth are caused by repeated exposure to acid, which washes over the teeth. The acid can be a result of heartburn, or of eating acidic foods and drinks.

✪ SYMPTOMS Erosion leads to sensitive, painful teeth, which often have chips on the cutting edges and may be darker in color than other teeth due to the absence of enamel.

✚ CONVENTIONAL TREATMENT If the erosion is severe and painful, dentine is exposed and the tooth is at risk of fracturing. Advice should be sought from a dentist. Veneers of resin, porcelain, gold, or nickel chrome are usually placed over the teeth to stabilize the problem. Dietary advice is given and the cause and effect of acid reflux are treated, if appropriate.

✔ BENEFICIAL FOODS
Milk, tea, coffee, and water are alkaline, and should be drunk in place of fruit juices and carbonated drinks, which are acidic. Milk and other dairy products are also rich in calcium, which is important for strong teeth.

✖ FOODS TO AVOID
Oranges, grapefruits, and lemons contain citric acid and should be eaten only with meals unless it is possible to chew sugar-free gum or consume an acid-lowering food, such as cheese, afterward. Grapefruit and orange juice contain citric acid and apple juice contains malic acid. Both these substances are highly erosive, so acidic fruit juices should be avoided between meals.
Colas and other carbonated drinks contain phosphoric acid, which erodes the teeth. They should be kept to a minimum between meals.

❂ OTHER MEASURES
❑ Chewing gum, sugar-free candies, toothpastes, and mouthwashes containing xylitol help to improve saliva flow and reduce the pH of the mouth after eating acidic foods and drinks.
❑ The teeth should not be brushed immediately after eating acidic foods, since this causes erosion.
❑ A straw should be used when drinking colas and other acidic drinks to minimize erosion.

See Also Heartburn, page 170; Minerals, page 30

IMMUNE SYSTEM

THE IMMUNE SYSTEM is comprised of a number of defenses that are able to combat the effects of bacteria, viruses, and irritants that invade the body. These defenses include the skin, mucous membranes in the nose and throat, and acid in the digestive system. The immune system also has at its disposal many millions of individual immune cells that circulate in body fluids as part of the lymphatic system.

DIET & DISEASE

It is becoming increasingly clear that the foods and drinks people consume on a regular basis can profoundly affect their ability to fight disease. Research indicates that a diet poor in vitamin C, beta carotene, and zinc diminishes the immune system's ability to overcome invasions from hostile organisms and other damaging substances. It also appears likely that specific nutrients may be able to reduce the risk of cancers forming.

HELPING IMMUNITY

The avoidance of smoking is crucial to maintaining a healthy immune system. A lifestyle that is as stress-free as possible, combined with plenty of physical exercise and a diet rich in plant nutrients, is thought to give the system the best chance of working to its highest level of efficiency.

HOW A LYMPH NODE WORKS

Lymph is a clear, watery liquid that circulates around the body in the lymphatic system. In lymph nodes (glands) this liquid is filtered of disease-causing organisms by white blood cells called lymphocytes and macrophages.

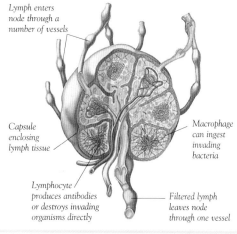

Lymph enters node through a number of vessels

Capsule enclosing lymph tissue

Macrophage can ingest invading bacteria

Lymphocyte produces antibodies or destroys invading organisms directly

Filtered lymph leaves node through one vessel

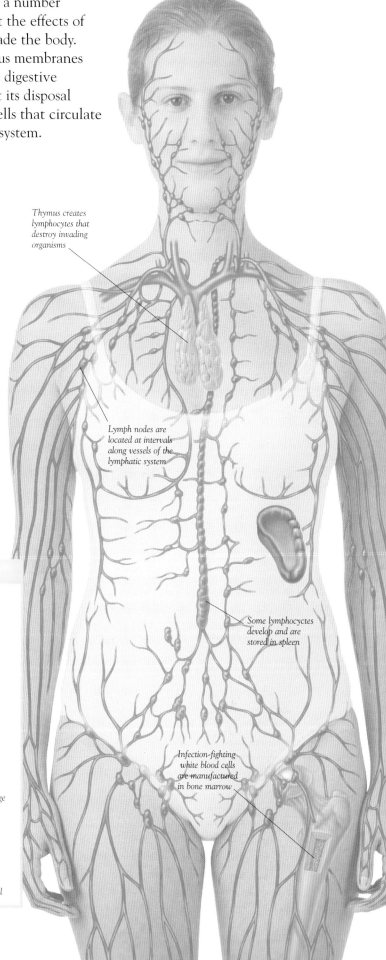

Thymus creates lymphocytes that destroy invading organisms

Lymph nodes are located at intervals along vessels of the lymphatic system

Some lymphocytes develop and are stored in spleen

Infection-fighting white blood cells are manufactured in bone marrow

TOP HEALING FOODS

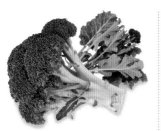 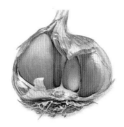 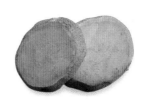 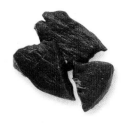

BROCCOLI   PAGE 46
Benefits May help to block carcinogens before they are able to harm cells in the body and trigger the growth of tumors.
Useful for Helping to reduce the risk of lung and colon cancers.
Nutrients Vitamins C and E.

GARLIC   PAGE 66
Benefits Thought to help reduce the risk of contracting viral, bacterial, and fungal infections.
Useful for Bolstering the immune system of children and adults, especially in winter.
Nutrients Phytonutrient allicin.

SWEET POTATOES   PAGE 55
Benefits Supply beta carotene, which the body converts to vitamin A that protects against respiratory infections.
Useful for Those with lowered vitamin A levels, such as vegans.
Nutrients Beta carotene.

RED MEATS   PAGE 122
Benefits Lean red meats supply minerals that lymph tissue needs in order to function correctly.
Useful for Those needing good sources of protein and minerals following a series of infections.
Nutrients Iron, zinc, protein.

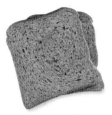 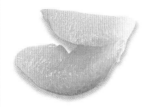 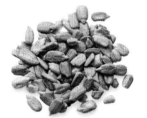 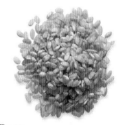

WHOLE-GRAIN BREAD P 98
Benefits Rich in insoluble fiber, which can bind with carcinogens and remove them in the stools.
Useful for Reducing the risk of colonic cancer and for improving bowel movements.
Nutrients Carbohydrates, iron.

ORANGES   PAGE 88
Benefits Good restorers of antioxidants, levels of which seem to fall at times of infection.
Useful for Alleviating symptoms of colds and helping to prevent tissue damage during infections.
Nutrients Vitamin C.

SUNFLOWER SEEDS PAGE 104
Benefits Contain essential fats that enhance the antibacterial strength of mucous membrane.
Useful for Boosting the immune system's effectiveness.
Nutrients Essential omega-6 fatty acids, vitamin E, protein.

RICE   PAGE 94
Benefits Rice contains no gluten, a protein found in wheat and other cereals that causes food intolerance in some people.
Useful for People who are affected by celiac disease.
Nutrients Carbohydrates.

OTHER BENEFICIAL FOODS

SOYBEANS   PAGE 60
Benefits Increases levels of plant estrogens in the body.
Useful for Potentially, the prevention of breast cancer.
Nutrients The phytonutrients daidzein and genistein.

TURKEY   PAGE 124
Benefits Good source of low-fat protein. Has low allergenicity.
Useful for Helping the body to fight breast cancer.
Nutrients Protein, plus some iron in the dark meat.

ONIONS   PAGE 67
Benefits Onions and scallions may help to fight off viral, bacterial, and fungal infections.
Useful for Helping to fight off infections prevalent in winter.
Nutrients Phytonutrient allicin.

CARROTS   PAGE 56
Benefits Fights *Listeria*, bacteria that cause food poisoning.
Useful for People who are at greatest risk from *Listeria*, such as pregnant women.
Nutrients Beta carotene.

FOODS TO AVOID

CHARRED MEATS
Meats that have been cooked to the point of being charred contain substances that are believed to trigger cancers in the body. This is also the case with charred fish. Avoid eating foods that have been either over-barbecued or over-broiled, and also avoid eating juices from meats that have been overcooked.

PROCESSED MEATS
There are many different kinds of processed meats. These should be eaten in moderation since many of them contain mineral salts called nitrites, which may trigger cancerous cell growth, especially in the stomach.

ALCOHOL
There is evidence that alcohol, when consumed regularly and in large amounts, increases the risk of cancer not only of the liver, but also in the upper respiratory tract. The World Cancer Research Fund has recommended that intakes are limited to no more than two alcoholic drinks a day for men and one for women.

ORANGE SODA
A common additive found in orange soda and a number of other brightly colored orange foods, such as jellies, soups, and cookies, is tartrazine, an artificial food coloring. Research has identified this substance as one that may stimulate an allergic reaction in some people. Children and adults who appear to produce allergic reactions to this artificial coloring are strongly advised to check food labels in order to avoid consuming products containing this food additive.

FOOD SUPPLEMENTS
It is thought by some nutritionists that supplementing the diet with certain nutrients, such as vitamin C, beta carotene, and the mineral selenium, may help to reduce the risk of certain cancers and generally boost the body's resistance to infections. There is, however, no conclusive evidence available to confirm this view.

FOOD ALLERGIES

KEY FOODS

POULTRY
page 124

CARROTS
page 56

BRASSICAS
pages 44–47

VEGETABLE
OILS
page 106

RICE
page 94

FRUITS
pages 72–91

A TRUE FOOD ALLERGY is a reaction to a small amount of a specific food or foods. It involves the immune system and, in most cases, the antibody IgE. Antibodies are usually formed in the body to fight bacterial, viral, and parasitic infections. They bind on to the invading agent and make it harmless. When IgE antibodies come into contact with an allergen, the body releases histamine into the bloodstream, making blood vessels dilate, or muscles in the lung, stomach, or bladder contract. When someone is allergic to a food, the response may occur within minutes of eating it. In some cases an allergic reaction, such as a peanut allergy, can be life-threatening.

☻ SYMPTOMS
An allergy can cause itching, vomiting, swelling in the mouth and throat, and breathing difficulties. Allergic reactions are usually immediate and may worsen asthma, rhinitis, and eczema. If a reaction is very severe, it can result in anaphylactic shock.

✚ CONVENTIONAL TREATMENT
A full diagnosis must be made before treatment is given. An allergy test may be carried out, although these have varying degrees of accuracy. The radioallergosorbent test, or RAST, involves testing a sample of blood. Skin-prick tests are available for a few foods, including milk, eggs, peanuts, and soybeans. Removing a particular food from the diet, then reintroducing it under the supervision of a doctor is another type of test (*see* Exclusion diets, *page 245*). The only treatment for a true food allergy is avoidance of the offending food. Antihistamine drugs may relieve symptoms, but they can mask warning signs of a severe reaction and are not advisable.

✔ BENEFICIAL FOODS
Exclusion diets (*see page 245*) aim to remove potential allergens then reintroduce them and observe the response. It is important to seek advice from a doctor and dietician before embarking on an exclusion diet. In such diets, plain chicken, turkey, rabbit, carrots, cauliflower, broccoli, rice, sweet potatoes, tapioca, sago, buckwheat, peaches, pears, and sunflower and olive oils are considered to be foods that are unlikely to cause reactions.
Soy milk, and soy milk products, such as drinks, yogurt, cheese, and spreads, are useful alternatives for those avoiding dairy products. Clarified butter and vegetable margarines can be used instead of dairy butter.
Gluten-free flour, made from corn, rice, split peas, soy, or carob, is suitable for those with

wheat allergies. Rye bread, rye flour, oatcakes, and oats may also be suitable. Buckwheat flour can often be used in place of wheatflour if wheat causes an allergic reaction.
Egg-free mayonnaise is suitable for those avoiding eggs. Gelatin may be used in desserts that need the setting qualities of eggs. One teaspoonful of gelatin is equivalent to one egg.

✖ FOODS TO AVOID
It is estimated that food allergy occurs in about six percent of children and just over one percent of adults in the West. Foods should not be eliminated from the diet until a diagnosis has been made and a balanced diet has been planned with a dietician. The following foods may be the cause of IgE allergic reactions in certain people.
Cow's milk protein may cause allergic reactions in children. All fresh, dried, evaporated, and low-fat milks must be avoided, plus all dairy products, many baby cereals and instant desserts, some confectionery, some soups, and even certain salad dressings. Check food labels. A dietician can supply a full list of foods and drinks to avoid.
Hen's eggs are more likely to cause allergic reactions in children than in adults. An egg-free diet involves avoiding whole eggs, dried eggs, egg yolk, albumin, and lecithin, as well as some types of pasta, cookies and cakes, baked products, meringues, and mayonnaise.
Shrimp and other seafood, such as crustaceans, shellfish, and cod, may cause allergies.
Peanuts and other nuts can cause severe allergic reactions in children and adults and may result in anaphylactic shock and even death. Whole peanuts, peanuts in sweets, chocolates, peanut butter, cookies, cheesecake bases, peanut oil, and other manufactured products must be avoided. Checking food labels is essential.
Soybeans and foods containing their derivatives, such as soy lecithin, may spark allergic reactions. Avoiding soy products can be difficult because soy flour is added to many foods. Vegetable protein, tofu, and soy milk, cheese, and yogurt also need to be eliminated.
Wheat can cause allergic reactions. It is in wheat flour, pasta, breakfast cereals, cakes, and cookies. Some people may react to oats, rye, corn, and barley.
Additives may cause allergies. Azo dyes cause the most problems, including tartrazine (E102), sunset yellow (E110), and amaranth (E123).

See Also Asthma, page 187; Eczema, page 165

NONALLERGIC FOOD INTOLERANCES

UNLIKE TRUE FOOD-ALLERGY REACTIONS, which involve the immune system, nonallergic intolerances to food have pharmacological, psychological, metabolic, and toxic causes. The causes of these reactions are different, although the symptoms are often similar, and can create confusion for the doctor and the person with the problem. Food intolerances can develop over time and often involve foods that are eaten regularly in the diet.

✪ SYMPTOMS Pharmacological intolerances to certain substances may provoke flushing, a drop in blood pressure, and skin rashes. For example, tyramine in cheese and red wine can provoke migraine, and monosodium glutamate causes flushing, headaches, and stomach pains in some people. A metabolic cause, such as an intolerance to the milk sugar lactose, can manifest itself as stomach cramps and chronic diarrhea. Toxic reactions to chemicals such as food additives can cause diarrhea and vomiting. There may be a link between certain foods and Crohn's disease, irritable bowel syndrome, canker sores, bloating, and even rheumatoid arthritis.

✚ CONVENTIONAL TREATMENT A doctor can refer a person with a food intolerance to a dietician, who will conduct a controlled elimination diet, then plan a nutritionally adequate maintenance diet for the individual.

✔ BENEFICIAL FOODS
It is important to eat a balanced diet that provides all the nutrients required in the correct proportions according to your age and gender. A dietician will help to plan such a diet, taking into account the foods that need to be excluded.
Soy milk, soy milk infant formulas, and soy milk products such as yogurt and cheese, make good alternatives for those with cow's milk intolerance. Choose dairy products that are fortified with calcium whenever possible.
Turkey, lamb, rabbit, and beef are good sources of protein, and these foods are unlikely to cause any intolerances.
Carrots, cauliflower, and broccoli are vegetables that are unlikely to cause food intolerances.
Rice, potatoes, sweet potatoes, tapioca, sago, and buckwheat are well tolerated and they provide the body with starchy forms of energy giving carbohydrates.
Pears, peaches, and most other fruits, with the exception of citrus fruits, which may be too acidic, are usually well tolerated.

✖ FOODS TO AVOID
Nonallergic food intolerances are unique to the individual and must be investigated by a doctor. It is important to organize a nutritionally adequate maintenance diet with a dietician in order to ensure that no nutrients are compromised as a result of leaving out certain foods or groups of foods from the diet.
Milk needs to avoided by those who are lactose intolerant due to a lack of the enzyme lactase. This is known as a "metabolic intolerance."
Fruits, fruit juices, and fruit derivatives must be avoided by those who lack the enzyme fructose and who are fructose intolerant.
Cheese, spinach, tomato, sausages, anchovies, sardines, canned foods, wine, and beer contain histamine, which may lead to pharmacologically induced, nonallergic adverse reactions in susceptible people. These can involve the skin, blood vessels, and bronchioles, causing urticaria (hives), difficulty in swallowing, swelling, wheezing, and migraines.
Cheese, beer, wine, yeast, marinated herring, avocados, and raspberries contain tyramine, which can have similar effects to histamine. Phenylethylamine present in chocolate may have a similar effect.
Coffee, tea, cola drinks, some cold remedies and painkillers, and dark chocolate contain caffeine, which has pharmacological effects on the nervous system. In large quantities caffeine can cause tremors, sweating, rapid breathing, palpitations, and insomnia.
Green potatoes contain solanine and chaconine. These alkaloids can cause a toxic-induced intolerance leading to drowsiness, stomachache, diarrhea, and even paralysis.
Honey produced by bees that have been feeding on rhododendrons can cause toxic-induced intolerance, resulting in tingling and numbness in the extremities minutes after eating. Eat honey only from reliable sources.

◉ OTHER MEASURES
It may be possible to help a person to overcome an aversion that has psychological roots with a course of therapy. If the food is nutritionally important to the diet, it may be possible to disguise it. For example, milk may be associated with a bad experience and cause a psychological reaction, but when taken in a white sauce, custard, or yogurt, it may be quite acceptable.

See Also Nausea, page 180

KEY FOODS

MEATS
page 122

POULTRY
page 124

FISH
pages 118–121

DAIRY PRODUCTS
pages 126–128

LEGUMES
pages 58–60

NUTS & SEEDS
pages 100–105

EGGS
page 129

AVOCADOS
page 51

WHOLEGRAINS
pages 92–99

GARLIC
page 66

INFECTIONS

AN INFECTION IS CAUSED by bacteria, parasites, viruses, or fungi entering the body and damaging cells, which sparks a reaction by the immune system. Infections raise the body's metabolic rate, increasing the rate of tissue breakdown and the need for a wide range of nutrients. How this affects an individual's nutritional status depends on how long the infection lasts, how severe the infection is, how nutritious the person's diet is prior to the infection, and what foods are eaten during the infection. If any nutrient is lacking in significant quantities, the immune system may be impaired and the healing process slows down.

✪ SYMPTOMS

These vary according to the type of microorganism that has taken hold and on how widespread the infection is. An infection tends to reduce the appetite and affects the absorption of nutrients from the digestive tract. A rise in temperature may occur, and there may be fatigue, headaches, and other types of pain.

✚ CONVENTIONAL TREATMENT

Drugs such as antibiotics may be given to treat the cause. Acetaminophen may be given to ease pain, aspirin to lower temperature.

✔ BENEFICIAL FOODS

Pork, beef, lamb, poultry, fish, milk and dairy products, nuts, seeds, and legumes are good sources of protein. Infections can cause an average loss of 0.6g of protein per 2lbs (1kg) per day, which is about equal to an adult's daily protein needs. Protein losses are higher when there is diarrhea and higher still with severe infections. Protein foods should be eaten daily.
Eggs, liver, and whole-milk dairy products, such as cheese, supply vitamin A. Mangoes, apricots, carrots, sweet potatoes, and green leafy vegetables, such as broccoli, provide beta carotene, which is converted into vitamin A in the body. People with deficiencies of vitamin A have an increased susceptibility to infectious organisms.
Orange and grapefruit juices, citrus fruits, berries, papayas, peppers, and dark green vegetables supply vitamin C, which decreases in infected individuals. Vitamin C is required in increased amounts during infections to stop tissue damage.
Milk, meats, and cereal foods provide vitamins B₆ and B₂, needed for the maintenance of glutathione, an important antioxidant. Levels of vitamin B₂ are adversely affected by infections and care should be taken to maintain intakes.
Avocados, nuts, seeds, wheat germ, vegetable oils, eggs, and green leafy vegetables all supply vitamin E. This vitamin is needed to limit tissue damage and to improve resistance to infections.
Shellfish, red meats, and whole-grain cereals supply zinc, which is diminished during infections. Zinc deficiency also affects immunity.
Wholewheat breads and whole-grain cereals are rich in copper, a mineral that is depleted in the body as a result of infectious diseases.
Pumpkin, sunflower, and sesame seeds provide omega-6 fatty acids, which appear to improve the body's defensive barriers against bacteria such as *Staphylococci*.
Garlic has antimicrobial and antifungal properties, and may help to reduce the risk of infections if consumed on a regular basis.

✖ FOODS TO AVOID

It is best to avoid foods that supply few essential nutrients. This is important when trying to boost the immune system to help it to resist disease, and during and after infections, when it is crucial to maintain good vitamin and mineral intakes.
Meat products can supply large amounts of fat but relatively small proportions of protein for their volume and weight, so these foods should be eaten in moderation.
Tea, coffee, artificial fruit-flavored drinks, and carbonated drinks should be replaced with drinks that can supply nourishment, such as milk or soy-based drinks, or fruit juices.
Candies, potato chips, and chocolate should be replaced by more nourishing snacks, such as chunks of cheese, and nuts and seeds, which provide the body with important minerals and, in the case of nuts and seeds, essential fats.

◑ OTHER MEASURES

❑ Supplements containing zinc, selenium, and vitamins C, E, and beta carotene appear to be beneficial for respiratory and urinary infections.
❑ Echinacea helps to strengthen the body's resistance to infections. Powdered echinacea root and tincture preparations are available.
❑ Excessive iron intakes appear to make people more susceptible to infection, so large supplements of this mineral are best avoided.
❑ Breast milk is thought to protect infants against gastroenteritis and diarrhea and may reduce the risk of respiratory tract infections. In addition, prolonged breastfeeding appears to protect children from otitis media (*see page 203*).

See Also Colds & Influenza, page 184; Ear Disorders, page 203; Immune System, page 208

HIV & AIDS

KEY FOODS

FISH
pages 118–121

MEATS
page 122

POULTRY
page 124

DAIRY
PRODUCTS
pages 126–128

NUTS &
SEEDS
pages 100–105

WHOLE GRAINS
pages 92–99

FRUITS
pages 72–91

VEGETABLES
pages 44–71

INFECTION WITH the human immunodeficiency virus (HIV) is responsible for the condition known as acquired immunodeficiency syndrome (AIDS). The HIV virus can be transmitted through sexual intercourse, via infected blood, or from an infected mother to her child during pregnancy or via breast milk. About 21 million people worldwide are infected with the HIV virus and 90 percent of them live in developing countries. It is not yet known if every HIV-positive person will develop AIDS. When AIDS does develop, the immune system is profoundly affected, making a person very susceptible to life-threatening infections.

SYMPTOMS After initial infection, there may be an illness similar to mononucleosis lasting for a few weeks, after which the person may have no further symptoms for ten years or more. At some time after the initial infection, HIV may cause fever, diarrhea, and weight loss. Other possible symptoms include recurrent infections, cancers, and disorders of the nervous system, such as dementia. A diagnosis of AIDS depends on the presence of certain conditions, such as malignant, blue-red skin tumors known as Kaposi's sarcoma. Some people can remain physically well with full-blown AIDS for a considerable time.

CONVENTIONAL TREATMENT As yet, there is no cure or vaccine against HIV, but the symptoms of the HIV disease respond to drugs and radiation therapy. Antinausea, antidiarrheal, and appetite-stimulant drugs are often used. Other drugs are given according to particular problems, and include those for fungal, bacterial, parasitic, and herpes infections. Cancer treatments such as chemotherapy may be used.

BENEFICIAL FOODS
Nutritional support depends on the development stage of the HIV infection. A well-balanced diet that boosts the immune system at the onset of an infection may help to reduce problems at a later stage. Good nutrition is essential for those with full-blown AIDS, who require specialist help.
Seek advice from a doctor and a dietician before taking any dietary steps.
Fish, meats, poultry, and milk, cheese and other dairy products, nuts, seeds, legumes, and soy supply protein, which is needed to help prevent weight loss. During infections it is important to keep up protein intakes.
Breads, potatoes, pasta, rice, oats, rye, bulgur wheat, and other cereals help to boost calorie

intake and provide B vitamins and minerals.
Fruits and vegetables should be consumed in as much variety as possible to ensure good intakes of vitamins, minerals, and phytonutrients, which help to maintain immune functions.
Oily fish, nuts, and seeds should be included in the diet to provide essential fatty acids that may help to protect the body against some infections.
Yogurt, milk shakes, soups, and other foods and drinks with a smooth, thick consistency may be easy to swallow for those who are experiencing swallowing difficulties or whose mouths are sore as a result of yeast infection or Kaposi's sarcoma.
Frequent drinks, especially sips of carbonated drinks, and candies to suck on may help those with dry mouths as a result of yeast infection.
Strong-smelling foods and well-seasoned dishes may be helpful for people whose taste perceptions have changed as a result of a yeast infection.
Drinks and snacks that are high in nutrients are useful in situations where the metabolic rate has increased due to infections.
Isotonic drinks are helpful for those with night sweats since they replace body fluids and salts.

FOODS TO AVOID
A healthy, balanced diet can be planned by a dietician in order to ensure that food is rich in as wide a range of nutrients as possible. Foods of low nutritional value should be replaced with high-nutrient foods. For people with AIDS, specific advice is required for particular problems. The following are examples of foods that may worsen particular symptoms.
Rich cakes, fatty fried foods, sauces, pastries, and spicy foods can worsen nausea and vomiting.
Salty, acidic, and spicy foods should be avoided by people with sore mouths.
Hot foods are best avoided by people who have experienced taste changes.

OTHER MEASURES
❑ Supplements containing the recommended daily intake of each nutrient are advised.
❑ Artificial saliva sprays can be helpful for a dry mouth, and lips can be moistened with lip balm.
❑ High-energy supplements may be needed by those with swallowing difficulties.
❑ Small, frequent meals and antinausea medication may lessen nausea and vomiting.

See Also Candidiasis, page 224; Digestive System, page 168; Respiratory System, page 182

KEY FOODS

FRUITS
pages 72–91

VEGETABLES
pages 42–71

**ONIONS &
GARLIC**
pages 66–67

CARROTS
page 56

TOMATOES
page 65

**CITRUS
FRUITS**
pages 86–88

WHOLE GRAINS
pages 92–99

SOYBEANS
page 60

BERRIES
pages 82–85

CANCER

MALIGNANT TUMORS, or growths, in any part of the body are referred to as cancer. Evidence suggests that both genetic and environmental factors play important roles in the development of this disease. Malignant tumors can be triggered by smoking, exposure to pollutants or viruses, ultraviolet light, or as a result of inappropriate eating or drinking habits. There may also be a family predisposition to the disease.

Some forms of cancer are more likely to be caused by overnutrition, such as too much fat in the diet, while others may arise through a lack of certain nutrients. The study of diets gives an insight into the kind of dietary factors that may affect certain cancers. Economically developed countries tend to have relatively high rates of cancers of the colon and rectum, and hormone-related cancers such as breast and prostate cancers. Developing countries tend to have higher rates of mouth, stomach, liver, and cervical cancers. By making dietary changes, it may be possible to lower the risk of developing certain cancers.

As well as observing the patterns of diet and cancer in different populations, research is being carried out to see if the rates of certain cancers decline if diets are changed. It can take years for the results of such work to emerge. Studying the action of certain food substances on cancer cells in a laboratory setting makes it possible to learn how diet may help to prevent cancer.

⊕ SYMPTOMS These depend on the type of cancer and its stage of development and position. Pain is not necessarily an obvious symptom, since malignant cells can cause a painless swelling, for example in the breast. A tumor in the brain may cause headaches, vomiting, or disturbed vision. A tumor in the colon can cause blood in the stools, and cancer of the bladder may cause blood in the urine. Cancer of the liver may create a distended feeling, and cancer of the lung may cause blood in the sputum and shortness of breath. Skin cancers tend to reveal themselves as itchy moles that gradually increase in size. One of the first signs of cancer may be an unexplained loss of weight, which may be due to a loss of appetite or taste, or an increased metabolic rate.

⊕ CONVENTIONAL TREATMENT This depends on the type, position, and stage of cancer, and whether or not it is possible to cure it, or to treat the symptoms and accept that a cure is not feasible. A combination of treatments is often given, including radiation

and chemotherapy. Malignant tumors may be treated with surgery and radiotherapy. Surgery involves physically removing the malignancy. For some types of cancer, such as cancer of the larynx, radiation is preferable to surgery. It involves exposing the tumor cells to ionizing radiation, which damages the genetic material in the tumor and can halt its reproduction and growth. Certain types of cancer, such as leukemia, are highly sensitive to chemotherapy. This involves the administration of oral, intramuscular, and intravenous drugs. These drugs are designed to arrest or eradicate the cancerous cells while doing minimum damage to healthy tissues. Tumors in organs that depend on hormones, such as the breast and prostate gland, may also be treated with "endocrine therapy." This involves drugs that inhibit the action of the hormones.

If active treatment is not appropriate, terminal care is a priority. Pain relief and the relief of other symptoms is crucial, in association with appropriate help for the individual, their family, and friends, to help deal with the emotional difficulties that lie ahead.

✅ BENEFICIAL FOODS

People with cancer need to eat as well as possible in order to avoid weight loss. It is essential to consult a specialist for advice regarding food, drink, and the best way to meet nutritional needs. Eating the following foods on a regular basis may help to prevent cancer from developing.
Fruits and vegetables contain a wide variety of vitamins, minerals, and phytonutrients, which are believed to play a role in cancer prevention. It is recommended that 14oz (400g), or five servings, of fruits and vegetables are consumed each day and that the sources are as varied as possible.
Green vegetables appear to be particularly protective against cancers of the mouth, pharynx, esophagus, and lung. Brassicas such as broccoli and cabbage contain indoles, plant chemicals that appear to block harmful carcinogens before they have a chance to damage cells. These foods also contain isothiocyanates (ITCs), which seem to suppress tumor growth in laboratory experiments.
Onions, garlic, leeks, chives, and green vegetables are thought to help reduce the risk of stomach cancer, especially when eaten raw. Laboratory studies suggest that the sulfurous substances in these foods interfere with cancer-causing enzymes and stop the formation of harmful nitrosamines. Onions and garlic also contain plant chemicals called saponins, which appear to help inhibit the substances that encourage tumor growth.

CANCER

Carrots, tomatoes, and citrus fruits may protect against cancer of the colon. These foods contain phenolic acids which, in tests, prevent carcinogens from triggering excessive cell growth.

Carrots, sweet potatoes, apricots, and green leafy vegetables are rich in carotenoids, which may protect against cancers of the esophagus, lung, colon, rectum, stomach, breast, and cervix.

Citrus fruits, berries, peppers, sweet potatoes, and green leafy vegetables are high in vitamin C, which probably helps to protect against cancer of the stomach, and possibly cancers of the mouth, pharynx, esophagus, lung, pancreas, and cervix.

Whole-grain cereals, such as wholewheat bread, brown rice, and brown pasta, may lower the risk of cancers of the colon and rectum. These foods bulk up the stools and increase the speed with which they pass through the colon. It is thought that the cancer-causing substances are carried out of the body and have less time to attach to the colon and rectum walls, where they could trigger cancers. There is also evidence that diets rich in insoluble fiber may reduce the risk of breast cancer. The fiber may increase the movement of the stools, carrying estrogens out of the body via the colon, and lowering the levels of estrogen. Whole grains also contain lignans, which are phytonutrients that, in tests, block cancerous changes.

Soybeans are rich in the isoflavones genistein and daidzein. These are plant estrogens that are consumed regularly in countries where breast cancer rates are quite low. It is thought that soybeans and, to a lesser extent, soy derivatives such as tofu may offer some protection against breast cancer by blocking the action of the body's own estrogen. Excess human estrogen is thought to increase the chances of breast cancer.

Onions, tea, apples, grapes, and citrus fruits such as oranges and grapefruits are rich in flavonoids. These phytonutrients are antioxidants which, in laboratory tests, suppress malignant changes in cells and block cancer-causing substances.

Strawberries, raspberries, grapes, and apples contain ellagic acid. In tests, ellagic acid seems to neutralize some of the harmful free radicals present in cigarette smoke.

✗ FOODS TO AVOID

Burned or charred meats and fish should be avoided. Overcooking these foods produces compounds called heterocyclic aromatic amines, some of which may be carcinogenic.

Red meats such as beef, pork, and lamb, and meat products may increase the risk of cancer of the colon, rectum, pancreas, breast, prostate, and kidneys, if eaten regularly in substantial amounts. The World Cancer Research Fund recommends consuming no more than 3oz of red meat a day.

Processed meats that have been treated with nitrites contain substances called N-nitrosamines, which may be carcinogenic. No risk to humans has yet been firmly established, but they should be eaten in moderation.

Smoked meats, fish, cheese, and other smoked foods contain polycyclic aromatic hydrocarbons produced through the burning of wood. Evidence is inconclusive, but laboratory tests suggest that these substances may trigger cancerous changes, so they should be eaten in moderation.

Salty foods eaten in large quantities may increase the risk of stomach cancer. These foods include obviously salted products such as potato chips and salted peanuts, and manufactured ones containing hidden sodium. A maximum of 6g of table salt per day is advised for adults and half this amount for children.

Fatty cuts of meat, and pies, pastries, cakes, cookies, butter, lard, margarine, and oils need to be limited. High intakes of these foods increase the risk of obesity. This in turn probably increases the risk of postmenopausal breast cancer, cancer of the endometrium, and cancer of the colon.

Alcohol, consumed regularly in large amounts, has been convincingly linked to cancers of the mouth, pharynx, larynx, esophagus, and liver. Alcohol probably also increases the risk of cancers of the colon, rectum, and breast. The World Cancer Research Fund advises that alcohol should be limited to no more than two drinks a day for men and one for women.

Foods that are beyond their "best before" date, appear to be moldy, or have not been stored properly, may be contaminated.

⊘ OTHER MEASURES

❑ All perishable foods should be stored under chilled conditions, preferably in a refrigerator.
❑ Maintaining a normal body weight throughout life is important for reducing the risk of breast and prostate cancer. So, too, is maintaining a good level of regular physical activity.
❑ Supplements of vitamin C, selenium, and carotenoids may prove to be helpful in preventing certain types of cancer.

See Also Men's & Women's Health, page 220; Plant Nutrients, page 34; Vitamins, page 26

ENDOCRINE SYSTEM

THE ENDOCRINE SYSTEM, like the nervous system, is one of the major systems controlling the body. Several important glands produce hormones that act as chemical messengers. They are released into the blood and transported around the body until they reach their target cells. The endocrine system affects growth and development, body defenses, reproduction, the maintenance of a variety of blood constituents, and the regulation of cell metabolism and energy balance.

DIET & HORMONAL BALANCE

The effectiveness of dietary manipulation in the treatment of malfunctions of the pancreas and thyroid gland demonstrates the importance of specific dietary requirements in the maintenance of hormonal balance in the body. Plant chemicals found in soybeans, for example, are believed to modulate the effects of human estrogen.

HELPING HORMONES TO WORK

The health of the endocrine system may be improved by regular exercise, plenty of sleep, and the avoidance of stress. The diet should contain adequate amounts of calcium for hormone secretion, vitamin C for the production of adrenal hormones, iodine for thyroid hormones, and zinc and chromium for insulin regulation.

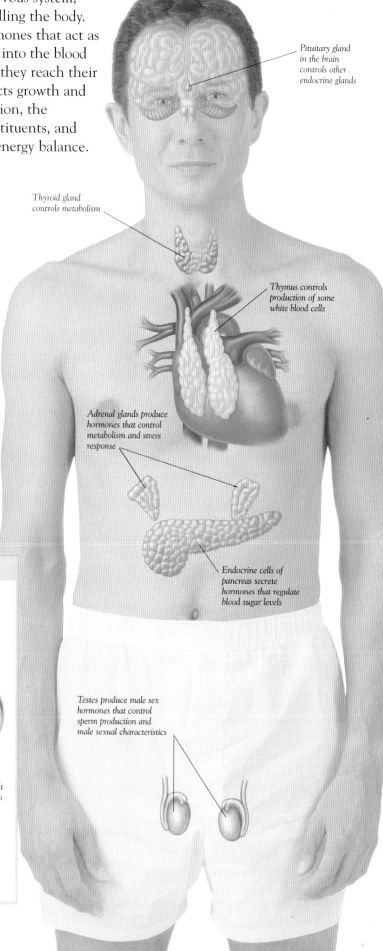

Pituitary gland in the brain controls other endocrine glands

Thyroid gland controls metabolism

Thymus controls production of some white blood cells

Adrenal glands produce hormones that control metabolism and stress response

Endocrine cells of pancreas secrete hormones that regulate blood sugar levels

Testes produce male sex hormones that control sperm production and male sexual characteristics

FEMALE SEX HORMONES

In the female, sex hormones produced in the ovaries stimulate the production of eggs and the progress of the menstrual cycle, as well determine secondary sexual characteristics, such as the development of breasts.

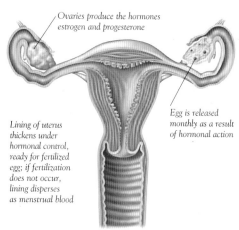

Ovaries produce the hormones estrogen and progesterone

Egg is released monthly as a result of hormonal action

Lining of uterus thickens under hormonal control, ready for fertilized egg; if fertilization does not occur, lining disperses as menstrual blood

TOP HEALING FOODS

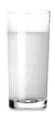

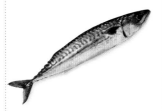

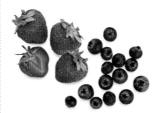

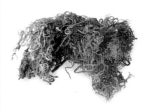

MILK
PAGE 126

Benefits A source of calcium that is easily digestible.
Useful for Maintaining body systems involved in hormone release from the endocrine glands.
Nutrients Calcium, protein, B vitamins.

MACKEREL
PAGE 118

Benefits Helps in the production of certain prostaglandins, which are hormonelike substances that can reduce inflammation.
Useful for People with psoriasis and rheumatoid arthritis.
Nutrients Omega-3 fatty acids.

BERRIES
PAGE 82

Benefits Include vitamins involved in the production of adrenal hormones and regulation of the pituitary gland, which activates the thyroid gland.
Useful for Thyroid problems.
Nutrients Vitamin C.

SEAWEEDS
PAGE 70

Benefits The richest-known sources of iodine, needed for the production of thyroid hormones.
Useful for Those with an underactive thyroid gland caused by iodine deficiency.
Nutrients Iodine.

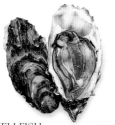

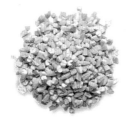

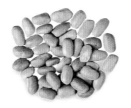

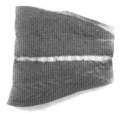

SHELLFISH
PAGE 120

Benefits Oysters, in particular, are useful for encouraging the smooth working of the pituitary gland, which controls growth.
Useful for The regulation of growth and metabolism.
Nutrients Zinc, selenium.

OATS
PAGE 95

Benefits These carbohydrate-rich foods help to slow down the absorption of sugar into the blood after a meal, thus reducing the amount of insulin needed.
Useful for People with diabetes.
Nutrients Carbohydrates, zinc.

LEGUMES
PAGE 58

Benefits Rich source of soluble fiber; help in the regulation of blood sugar levels.
Useful for Those people with either type I or II diabetes.
Nutrients Carbohydrates, protein.

SALMON
PAGE 118

Benefits Can help in the production of hormones released by the thyroid gland.
Useful for Helping to promote good metabolism.
Nutrients The amino acid tyrosine, omega-3 fatty acids.

OTHER BENEFICIAL FOODS

BRAZIL NUTS
PAGE 100

Benefits May play a role in sustaining the health of the thyroid gland.
Useful for Maintaining a steady metabolic rate in the body.
Nutrients Selenium.

PASTA
PAGE 97

Benefits Has a low glycemic index (*see page 19*) for a carbohydrate.
Useful for Those who have to control blood sugar levels, such as athletes and people with diabetes.
Nutrients Carbohydrates.

APPLES
PAGE 74

Benefits May reduce amount of insulin needed to restore normal blood sugar levels after a meal.
Useful for People with fluctuating blood sugar levels.
Nutrients Carbohydrates.

WHOLEGRAIN BREAD
PAGE 98

Benefits Could help to improve the body's sensitivity to insulin.
Useful for Reducing the amount of insulin needed to regulate blood sugar levels.
Nutrients Vitamin E, folate.

FOODS TO AVOID

COFFEE & SODAS
Caffeine, in carbonated drinks and coffee, when consumed in large amounts over time, is thought capable of overloading the endocrine system. In later life this could contribute to underactivity of the thyroid gland. Avoid drinking more than two caffeine-rich drinks a day.

SUGARY FOODS
Candy and foods rich in sugar require increased amounts of insulin to restore blood sugar levels to normal after ingestion. This can put a strain on the pancreas and may lead to increased fat deposition. In people with diabetes, a diet high in sugar can cause sustained high blood sugar levels, which may damage the eyes and nerves and increase the risk of heart disease.

LEGUMES & CABBAGE
People with underactive thyroid glands may be advised by their doctor to avoid eating cabbage, soybeans, and peas, which contain substances capable of inhibiting the thyroid gland.

SODIUM (SALT)
Large amounts of sodium, usually as salt, in the diet can lead to excessive urine production as the body works to eliminate the excess. Overproduction of urine puts a strain on the hormones involved in maintaining the body's water balance. Avoid using salt during cooking and adding salt to foods at the table, and reduce intakes of processed foods that may contain high sodium levels, such as soups, ready-made meals, and anything preserved in brine.

FOODS & WEIGHT

Excessive loss or gain of weight both affect hormone production. Weight gain in men can lead to feminization as estrogen production increases. In women, weight loss can reduce reproductive hormone production, causing menstruation to stop. Avoid sudden and rapid weight fluctuations to help maintain a healthy endocrine system.

DIABETES

KEY FOODS

OATS
page 95

LEGUMES
pages 58–60

FRUITS
pages 72–91

WHOLE GRAINS
pages 92–99

LOW-FAT
DAIRY
PRODUCTS
pages 126–128

MEATS
page 122

POULTRY
page 124

OILY FISH
page 118

SEEDS
pages 103–105

VEGETABLES
pages 44–71

IN PEOPLE WHO HAVE DIABETES, the amount of glucose (or "sugar") in the blood becomes abnormally high, due either to the failure of the pancreas to produce enough of the hormone insulin, or to the lack of insulin action. Type I diabetes usually affects young adults and is due to a lack of insulin normally produced by the pancreas. In type II diabetes, which usually starts after the age of 40, the pancreas produces inadequate amounts of insulin, causing a reduction in the sensitivity of the body cells to the action of insulin. Type II diabetes is often triggered by obesity.

SYMPTOMS

Diabetes results in the production of large amounts of urine, which causes dehydration and leads to excessive thirst. In type I diabetes weight loss often occurs and a person may experience extreme hunger.

CONVENTIONAL TREATMENT

Type I diabetes is treated with injections of insulin. Tailor-made dietary advice and counseling are an essential part of the treatment. Type II diabetes needs to be managed on an individual basis. Weight loss can be enough to get this type of diabetes under control, but in some cases, tablets may be required to increase insulin production and to regulate the absorption of glucose. In others cases, insulin injections may be necessary.

BENEFICIAL FOODS

People who are being treated for diabetes with insulin need to be particularly careful to eat regular meals that contain carbohydrates.

Oats contain soluble fiber, which slows the rate at which sugar is absorbed into the blood and results in less insulin being required. Oats may also reduce blood cholesterol. High cholesterol levels are a risk factor associated with diabetes.

Beans, chickpeas, and lentils are rich in soluble fiber and raise blood sugar levels slowly. They are good sources of carbohydrates, protein, and fiber.

Apples, pears, apricots, bananas, grapefruits, oranges, peaches, and plums also provide soluble fiber and release sugar into the bloodstream slowly. These fruits can make excellent snacks.

Pasta, sweet potatoes, and rye bread provide a slow, steady release of energy, so they are good sources of carbohydrates.

Wholewheat bread, brown rice, wholewheat pasta, and whole-grain cereals are rich in insoluble fiber. They supply zinc and chromium, which enhance the action of insulin.

Low-fat yogurt and skim milk are low in total and saturated fats. These products provide carbohydrates, protein, and calcium.

Lean red meats, poultry without the skin, fish, and tofu are low-fat sources of protein. Limiting fat can help to prevent weight gain and reduce the risk of increasing blood cholesterol.

Mackerel, salmon, sardines, and pilchards supply omega-3 fatty acids, which are believed to help reduce the risk of heart disease.

Flax, hemp, and pumpkin seeds supply omega-3 fatty acids. A mixture of these seeds can be sprinkled onto breakfast cereals or desserts.

Fruits and vegetables are excellent sources of potassium, a deficiency of which is associated with glucose intolerance. They are low in calories and supply a variety of antioxidant vitamins, minerals, and phytonutrients.

FOODS TO AVOID

Sausages, burgers, meat pies, and other fatty meat products, and butter, cheese, and other whole-milk dairy products contain significant amounts of saturated fats, which can raise blood cholesterol levels. Consumption of these foods needs to be kept to an absolute minimum.

Soft margarines that do not state they are low in "trans fats" are best avoided. Trans fats have a similar cholesterol-raising effect to saturated fats.

Sweets and sugar-rich foods need to be restricted. The exception to this advice is when someone with type I diabetes has a sudden drop in blood sugar levels. Fast-releasing sugar is then needed to restore blood sugar levels quickly.

OTHER MEASURES

❑ Exercise is important. As well as helping to control body weight, physical activity may help the body to process sugar more efficiently. People with type I diabetes need to balance exercise with insulin injections and food intake.

❑ Brewer's yeast is a rich source of chromium, which improves the action of insulin.

❑ Guar gum is extracted from a seed. When added to foods such as bread it helps to slow the rate at which blood sugar levels are raised.

❑ Pectin can be extracted from fruits. When taken in drinks such as skim milk shakes, it may reduce the amount of insulin required to lower blood sugar levels.

❑ Psyllium seeds are small, dark reddish-brown seeds that form a sticky mass when mixed with water. Taken just before a meal, psyllium seeds may reduce levels of glucose in the blood.

See Also Heart Disease, page 152, Obesity, page 178

EATING PLAN FOR DIABETES

The following are suggestions for the types of meal that might be appropriate for a person who has diabetes. For each individual case, especially for people who need to take insulin, it is important to discuss appropriate quantities of suitable foods with a nutritionist or doctor.

BREAKFASTS	LIGHT MEALS	MAIN MEALS	SNACKS
Cooked cereal with chopped, ready-to-eat apricots	Lean bacon, broiled and made into a sandwich using 100 percent wholewheat bread with slices of tomato	Fisherman's stew with new potatoes in their skins	Whole-grain cereal with skim milk
Glass of orange juice	Fresh cherries	Low-fat, sugar-free mousse with fresh fruits	
♦		♦	Low-fat yogurt with an apple
Grapefruit	♦	Salmon pasta bake with broccoli florettes	♦
Whole-grain cereal with skim milk and chopped pear	Salad niçoise with low-fat dressing and hot wholewheat roll	Mango and strawberry fruit salad	Fruit salad with apple, oranges, and cottage cheese
Wholewheat bread and yeast extract spread	Pear	♦	
♦	♦	Broiled chicken breasts with baked sweet potatoes	Oatcakes with cottage cheese
Broiled tomatoes, broiled mushrooms, and baked beans	Baked potato with barbecue beans	Peach or blueberry compote	
Glass of grapefruit juice	Plums		

THYROID DISORDERS

KEY FOODS

CITRUS FRUITS
pages 86–88

GREEN VEGETABLES
pages 44–51

WHOLE GRAINS
pages 92–99

RED MEATS
page 122

DAIRY PRODUCTS
pages 126–128

THE THYROID GLAND SECRETES hormones that help to maintain body processes and control carbohydrate and fat metabolism. They also affect levels of cholesterol and vitamins in the blood, heart rate, digestion, muscular function, and normal sexual development. Problems may arise from thyroid underactivity or overactivity.

✪ SYMPTOMS An underactive thyroid causes fatigue, muscular and mental slowness, reduced heart rate, decreased hair growth, increased weight, and constipation. An overactive thyroid can increase the rate of metabolism. Symptoms include weight loss, palpitations, diarrhea, muscle weakness, nervousness, extreme tiredness but inability to sleep, and tremor of the hands.

✚ CONVENTIONAL TREATMENT Thyroid problems must be treated by a specialist. Drug therapy or surgery are possible treatments. For an underactive thyroid due to iodine deficiency, treatment may simply be iodine therapy.

✔ BENEFICIAL FOODS

Citrus fruits, berries, peppers, and green leafy vegetables supply vitamin C, which is involved in the production of thyroid hormones.

Whole-grain foods and red meats provide the body with zinc, a mineral that is important for the correct functioning of the thyroid.

Milk, eggs, beef, and wholewheat flour contain the amino acid tyrosine, which is needed for the production of thyroid hormones.

Fruits and vegetables, cereals, low-fat dairy products, lean meats, poultry, fish, and legumes are helpful if there is a need to maintain weight.

Seaweeds are particularly rich sources of iodine, but stewing or boiling can reduce iodine by half.

✖ FOODS TO AVOID

Milk produced by cattle that are fed large amounts of kale may cause thyroid deficiencies.

Peanuts, soybeans, and cassava may have an adverse effect on the thyroid.

✪ OTHER MEASURES

❑ For an underactive thyroid, supplements of L-tyrosine are sometimes recommended.

❑ Bayberry, black cohosh, and goldenseal are herbal remedies believed to be beneficial for the condition of an underactive thyroid gland.

See Also Fatigue, page 235; Obesity, page 178

WOMEN'S & MEN'S HEALTH

TRADITIONALLY, women have often had a greater awareness of their bodies and their state of health than men. Possibly for this reason, a wealth of anecdotal, dietary-based remedies for female problems has accumulated over the years. Men are, however, showing increasing interest in the effect of nutrition on health. Many of the health concerns of men and women concern their reproductive systems.

THE INFLUENCE OF DIET
Studies have revealed that increasing intakes of essential fatty acids and various vitamins and minerals may help ease the symptoms of certain female ailments. Candida, breast and cervical cancer, and menopausal problems may all be helped by dietary manipulation. Recent studies of men's health have highlighted the benefits of diet for the prevention and treatment of infertility, impotence, prostate problems, and heart disease.

MAINTAINING GOOD HEALTH
A balanced diet is the cornerstone to good health in women and men, but ensuring that the specific nutritional needs of the sexes are met at various times throughout life is also essential. Young women must be particularly vigilant with regard to calcium and iron intakes, while men are advised to make sure that they select foods rich in zinc and selenium.

MALE REPRODUCTIVE SYSTEM

The male reproductive organs are responsible for producing sperm, which can then be ejaculated in semen into a female to fertilize eggs produced by the ovaries of her reproductive system.

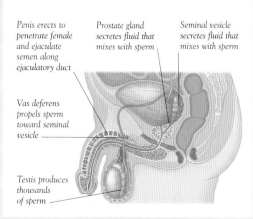

Penis erects to penetrate female and ejaculate semen along ejaculatory duct

Prostate gland secretes fluid that mixes with sperm

Seminal vesicle secretes fluid that mixes with sperm

Vas deferens propels sperm toward seminal vesicle

Testis produces thousands of sperm

Uterus holds egg for fertilization by sperm, or sheds it with menstrual flow each month

Each ovary produces one egg per month in an adult female

Vagina receives erect penis during sexual intercourse, and provides external passage for menstrual blood and for babies

Fallopian tube carries egg to uterus for fertilization

TOP HEALING FOODS

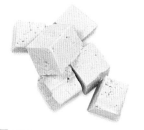

TOFU   PAGE 60

Benefits A rich source of isoflavones, plant nutrients that can mimic human estrogen.
Useful for Those at risk from breast, endometrial, and ovarian cancers, and also prostate cancer.
Nutrients Isoflavones, protein.

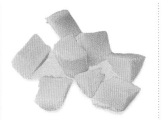

OYSTERS   PAGE 120

Benefits May help to improve fertility and reduce impotence that is caused by zinc deficiency.
Useful for Men with fertility and impotence problems.
Nutrients Zinc, iron, magnesium, copper, protein.

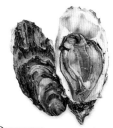

MANGOES   PAGE 91

Benefits Protect sperm from free-radical damage and may protect the cervix against cancer.
Useful for Men with fertility problems, and women with any signs of cervical dysplasia.
Nutrients Beta carotene.

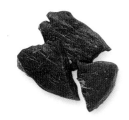

LEAN RED MEATS   PAGE 122

Benefits Reduce the risk of anemia, especially in women, and supply minerals needed for general reproductive health.
Useful for Women and men of all ages.
Nutrients Iron, selenium, zinc.

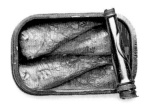

SARDINES   PAGE 119

Benefits Help to maintain healthy blood circulation and may reduce impotence.
Useful for Women of child-bearing age and all men.
Nutrients Omega-3 fatty acids, and, when canned, calcium.

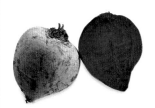

BEETS   PAGE 57

Benefits May reduce incidence of spinal defects in babies and lower homocysteine levels in the blood.
Useful for Women of child-bearing age and postmenopausal women at risk of heart disease.
Nutrients Folate.

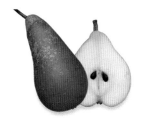

PEARS   PAGE 75

Benefits May help to reduce levels of blood cholesterol and to regulate blood sugar levels.
Useful for Those prone to heart disease and people with diabetes.
Nutrients Carbohydrates, potassium.

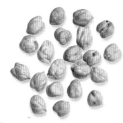

CHICKPEAS   PAGE 59

Benefits A source of isoflavones, which act as weak estrogens.
Useful for May help to reduce hormone-related cancers and reduce menopausal symptoms.
Nutrients Isoflavones, protein, calcium, iron.

OTHER BENEFICIAL FOODS

FLAX SEEDS   PAGE 105

Benefits Supply fatty acids, which may relieve PMS.
Useful for Men with benign prostate enlargement and women, notably before menopause.
Nutrients Essential fatty acids.

AVOCADOS   PAGE 51

Benefits Supply a rich source of vitamin E, needed for healthy skin and for male fertility.
Useful for Men and women of all ages.
Nutrients Vitamin E.

GARLIC   PAGE 66

Benefits Supplies phytonutrients capable of antifungal activity.
Useful for Women who have a tendency to develop fungal infections such as candidiasis.
Nutrients Phytonutrient allicin.

BLACK CURRANTS   PAGE 82

Benefits A particularly rich source of antioxidants.
Useful for Reducing the risk of certain cancers and boosting the immune system.
Nutrients Vitamin C.

FOODS TO AVOID

SATURATED FATS

Found in meat products, cream, cakes, and cookies, saturated fats tend to raise blood cholesterol levels and so may increase the risk of heart disease in men and postmenopausal women.

SUGAR

Women prone to candida infections may find that their symptoms improve if they severely restrict their intake of sugar, sugary foods, and even fruits. Restricting sugar in the diet helps to starve the fungi that cause candidiasis.

YEAST

Foods that contain yeast, including breads, yeast extracts, beer, and dried fruits, should also be excluded by those susceptible to candida infections.

SODIUM (SALT)

People with high blood pressure, especially men with impotency problems, should avoid adding extra salt to foods at the table. They should also avoid, or at least greatly restrict, processed foods, which tend to have high levels of sodium. These include cured meat; meat products such as burgers; corned beef; fish and vegetables canned in brine; soups; sauces; and savory snacks such as salted nuts and potato chips.

BEER

There is increasing evidence that beer may contain xenoestrogens. These estrogen-like compounds, derived for example from pesticides, may decrease male fertility. Men planning a family may be advised to avoid beer and beer products.

ALCOHOL

Alcohol is particularly toxic to the male reproductive tract and may be responsible for up to 40 percent of male fertility problems, seemingly through its ability to decrease levels of testosterone, lower the sperm count, and reduce sex drive. Even at fairly low levels, alcohol has been linked to an increased risk of breast cancer in women.

PREMENSTRUAL SYNDROME (PMS)

KEY FOODS

NUTS &
SEEDS
pages 100–105

POULTRY
page 124

MEATS
page 122

FISH
pages 118–121

DAIRY
PRODUCTS
pages 126–128

WHOLE GRAINS
pages 92–99

FRUITS
pages 72–91

PRUNES &
FIGS
pages 79–80

AVOCADOS
page 51

GREEN
VEGETABLES
pages 44–51

PREMENSTRUAL SYNDROME (PMS) is a group of physical and mental changes that typically start between seven and ten days before menstruation. The cause is considered to be associated with hormonal changes. Symptoms are relieved after a period starts.

⊙ SYMPTOMS Physical symptoms of PMS include weight gain due to fluid retention, painful breasts, headaches, migraines, backache, and skin disorders. Psychological symptoms include tension, irritability, depression, lethargy, food cravings, and poor concentration.

✚ CONVENTIONAL TREATMENT Drugs prescribed for PMS include diuretics for fluid retention, antidepressants for psychological problems, hormones such as progesterone to relieve all symptoms, and bromocriptine for breast pain. Tranquilizers are still occasionally prescribed for some patients.

✔ BENEFICIAL FOODS
Sunflower, pumpkin, and sesame seeds, hemp-seed oil, and evening primrose oil are all rich sources of omega-6 fatty acids. It is possible that women with PMS may be deficient in these fats.
Chicken, pork, fish, milk, eggs, brown rice, whole grains, soybeans, potatoes, beans, walnuts and other nuts, seeds, and green leafy vegetables all provide vitamin B_6. This vitamin is thought to help relieve depression because it helps to raise levels of the mood-enhancing chemical serotonin in the brain.
Rye bread, pasta, oatmeal, basmati rice, legumes, and fruits contain sugars that are broken down slowly and released gradually into the blood. A slow and steady release of sugar into the blood may help to control sugar cravings.
Figs, prunes, bananas, black currants, potatoes, brussels sprouts, broccoli, cauliflower, mushrooms, onions, parsnips, kale, sweet potatoes, and tomatoes are good sources of potassium. This mineral can help to reduce bloating and swelling due to water retention.
Turkey, game, and cottage cheese supply the body with tryptophan, an amino acid that is converted in the body into the brain transmitter serotonin, which can help to relieve depression.
Avocados, dates, bananas, blue and red plums, eggplants, papayas, passion fruits, plantains, pineapples, and tomatoes contain serotonin, which binds to receptor sites in the stomach and may trigger serotonin-like reactions in the brain.
Carbohydrate-based foods encourage serotonin production in the brain and may be eaten as snacks for reducing PMS-related low moods.
Green vegetables, breads, breakfast cereals, pasta, and potatoes are good sources of the mineral magnesium, which is needed for normal hormone function and smooth muscle control. A lack of magnesium may contribute to muscle cramps and aches.

✖ FOODS TO AVOID
Meat products, cakes, whole-milk dairy products, and savory foods made with saturated fats are best eaten in strict moderation. All these foods can interfere with the metabolism of the omega-6 fatty acids and may lead to weight gain.
Caffeine stimulates the nervous system and may worsen symptoms such as irritability. Try to limit coffee, tea, cola drinks, and cold remedies that contain caffeine to no more than six cups a day.
Ready-made meals and prepackaged foods tend to be high in salt and need to be restricted since they can make water retention worse.

⊘ OTHER MEASURES
❑ Evening primrose oil capsules taken daily have been shown to help reduce breast discomfort associated with PMS. Evening primrose oil may also help symptoms such as a swollen abdomen, irritability, swollen fingers and ankles, and anxiety. Six 500mg capsules daily are advised.
❑ Vitamin B_6 supplements, in doses of 100–200mg a day throughout the cycle, benefit some women who experience premenstrual depression, irritability, and fatigue.
❑ Chromium supplements may help to stabilize blood sugar levels and reduce sugar cravings.

See Also Carbohydrates, page 16; Depression, page 233; Women & Nutrition, page 140

CASE STUDY

Belinda Scadafi, 32, first took evening primrose oil supplements when her husband threatened to leave her because of her dramatic mood swings. She had not linked her bad moods with her menstrual cycle. Belinda now takes six evening primrose oil capsules a day throughout the month and has recently begun to reduce her intake of tea and coffee. Once she became interested in helping herself, she read about PMS and discovered that too much caffeine may have adverse effects. Her symptoms have been greatly relieved and her relationship is running much more smoothly.

MENOPAUSAL PROBLEMS

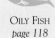
AROUND THE AGE OF 50, most women have their last menstrual cycle. Menopause occurs when the production of the hormones estrogen and progesterone by the ovaries decreases.

☣ SYMPTOMS

Menopausal symptoms vary but can include mood changes, headaches, hot flashes, anxiety, irritability, night sweats, dry vagina, loss of interest in sex, painful sex, and genital itching. After the last menstrual cycle, women may experience difficulty in controlling urination or the need to pass urine urgently. There may be thinning of the skin and hair. Long-term symptoms include an increased risk of heart disease and brittle bones (osteoporosis).

✚ CONVENTIONAL TREATMENT

Hormone replacement therapy (HRT) is the main form of treatment. Symptoms may be alleviated by taking estrogen and progesterone in the form of tablets, creams, suppositories, gels, patches, or subcutaneous implants. Nonhormonal treatments include drugs to treat hot flashes, high blood pressure, and spinal osteoporosis.

✔ BENEFICIAL FOODS

Soybeans and products made from soy contain plant estrogens. Research has shown that soy in the diet may reduce hot flashes, vaginal dryness, and loss of bone density. It may also lower blood cholesterol levels.

Alfalfa seeds and sprouts, flaxseeds, and red clover sprouts supply plant estrogens that may help to reduce thinning of the vaginal tissues.

Broccoli, watercress, cauliflower, kale, and cabbage contain phytonutrients that have weak estrogenlike activity. They also help to keep the skin, arterial walls, capillaries, and joints flexible and protect blood vessels from oxidation, which may help to guard against heart disease.

Oranges, grapefruits, berries, papayas, green leafy vegetables, peppers, sweet potatoes, and potatoes provide vitamin C. Avocados, whole-grain foods, nuts, and seeds supply vitamin E. Both of these vitamins are antioxidants and may protect the skin against loss of flexibility, as well as guarding internal organs against degenerative changes.

Fortified breads, breakfast cereals, and yeast extract are excellent sources of folic acid, one of the B vitamins. Folic acid is believed to help to reduce the risk of heart disease.

Beets, brussels sprouts, asparagus, kale, black-eyed peas, chickpeas, peas, green beans, and bean sprouts are rich sources of folate, the form that folic acid takes in foods.

Garlic supplies the body with sulfurous compounds that help to lower cholesterol and may help to reduce the risk of heart disease.

Sardines and pilchards, canned and eaten with their softened bones, are excellent sources of calcium. They also provide vitamin D and omega-3 fatty acids, both of which help to improve calcium absorption and decrease its excretion in the urine and stools.

Oily fish, such as mackerel, salmon, sardines, and kippers are considered to be a useful protection against heart disease.

Low-fat dairy foods, sesame seeds, nuts, and legumes supply calcium and should be eaten as a regular part of the diet.

✖ FOODS TO AVOID

Margarine, butter, lard, and oils are highly concentrated sources of fat and should be eaten sparingly in order to avoid weight gain.

Cookies, cakes, pies, meat products, and whole-milk dairy foods contain a high proportion of fats, and are best eaten in moderation.

Carbonated drinks and foods containing phosphates need to be avoided. Phosphorus is required for strong bones, but when consumed in large quantities, calcium retention may be retarded and the bones may begin to lose strength.

Ready-made soups and meals, savory snacks, and processed meats, such as sausages, burgers, salami, and meat pies, should be eaten in strict moderation as they are rich in salt, which is thought to increase the risks of high blood pressure and heart disease.

Alcohol consumed regularly is associated with an increased risk of breast cancer. Drinking alcohol can also lead to mood swings and weight gain.

⊘ OTHER MEASURES

❑ Supplements with standardized extracts of hypericum (St. John's Wort) have been tested in clinical trials and appear to improve the sex lives of women in menopause.

❑ Regular exercise can help in weight-loss programs. It can also contribute to providing a general sense of well-being and help to prevent loss of bone density.

❑ Relaxation techniques such as yoga, and alternative health therapies, can help to relieve both psychological and physiological symptoms associated with menopause.

See Also Heart Disease, page 152; Osteoporosis, page 199; Women & Nutrition, page 140

KEY FOODS

GARLIC
page 66

RED MEATS
page 122

SHELLFISH
page 120

NUTS &
SEEDS
pages 100–105

MILK
page 126

CITRUS
FRUITS
pages 86–88

BERRIES
pages 82–85

GREEN
VEGETABLES
pages 44–51

EGGS
page 129

CANDIDIASIS

CANDIDA ALBICANS is a yeast that is present in the intestines and normally has no adverse effects. Candida becomes a problem when it replicates and grows excessively. This can occur in the gut and the vagina but may also affect the throat and mouth. Candida can be a problem for those with very depressed immune systems.

ⓧ SYMPTOMS
In the vagina, candida leads to painful itching and a creamy discharge, a condition known as a yeast infection. In the bladder and urinary tract, it causes a burning sensation when passing urine. In the mouth, it can cause white, sticky deposits on the tongue.

✚ CONVENTIONAL TREATMENT
Doctors may prescribe the antifungal drug nystatin. Other drugs prescribed are clotrimazole, miconazole, fluconazole, and itraconazole. Doctors may also suggest a low-sugar, low-yeast diet, as sugar and yeast in foods may make symptoms worse.

✔ BENEFICIAL FOODS
Garlic contains a natural antifungal substance, allicin. Garlic is also known to help fight bacterial and viral infections, both of which can lower the resistance of the immune system. It should be included regularly in the diet.
Red meats, shellfish (especially oysters), nuts, seeds, milk, and milk products are good suppliers of zinc, which is essential for the optimal functioning of the immune system. Eating these foods on a regular basis is recommended.
Citrus fruits and berries are good sources of vitamin C, as are red, green, and yellow peppers, green leafy vegetables, and potatoes. Vitamin C and other phytonutrients in these foods are needed for a strong immune system.
Fruit drinks containing "pro-biotic" bacteria, such as *Lactobacillus plantarum*, may help to restore the balance of microorganisms in the intestine. These drinks can be taken daily.
Red meats, fish, eggs, nuts, seeds, and green leafy vegetables supply the mineral iron. A deficiency of iron may make certain people susceptible to candida infections. Replenishing iron stores by eating these foods regularly may contribute to the healing of candidiasis.

✖ FOODS TO AVOID
Breads, buns, doughnuts, yeast extract, stock cubes, hydrolyzed vegetable protein, beer, wine and cider, vinegars and pickles, and sauerkraut are the main sources of yeast in the diet and need to be excluded by those on a low-yeast diet.

CASE STUDY

Karen Brown, 28, had experienced candida, which caused chronic yeast infections, beginning in her mid-twenties. It was painful, embarrassing, and depressing. Eventually, she consulted a specialist in food allergies and intolerances. He recommended a yeast-free, sugar-free diet and prescribed the drug nystatin. At first, she found the diet very difficult to follow. She had to exclude all her favorite foods, including those that she felt she relied on, such as bread and rolls. She also had to cut out all sugary foods and wine. At times she wondered if it was worth all the deprivation. But she persevered and the change in her diet was a success. After a few months, the yeast infectons had almost cleared up.

Dried fruits, overripe fruits, and fruits with their skins on, commercial fruit juices, malted products, yogurt, buttermilk, sour cream, synthetic cream, soy sauce, tofu, leftover food, whisky, vodka, gin, and other spirits are secondary sources of yeast and are best avoided by anyone following a strict yeast-free diet.
Mushrooms and other edible fungi, and cheese, especially brie and camembert, may make symptoms worse in some people.
Sugar, honey, golden syrup, molasses, maple syrup, malt, all jams, chutneys and pickles, cakes, cookies, ice cream, chocolate, candy, carbonated and artificial fruit-flavored drinks, and any foods containing corn syrup, dextrose, fructose, glucose, maltose, sucrose, or sugar need to be avoided by those following a low-sugar diet.
Baked beans, including low-sugar versions, dried fruits, some processed meat products, and some medicines are rich in sugar and are best avoided.

❂ OTHER MEASURES
❑ Grapefruit seed extract, called citricidal, is recommended by some nutritionists for the treatment of candidiasis because of its apparently powerful antifungal effects and ability to leave beneficial intestinal bacteria intact. It comes in drops and can be swallowed or, for those with candida in the mouth, it may be gargled.
❑ Caprylic acid is recommended by some nutritionists. Derived from coconuts, it is thought to have strongly antifungal effects and may eliminate candida and yeast infections. The correct dosage is essential since it can be toxic.

See Also Immune System, page 208; Infections, page 212; Urinary System, page 188

KEY FOODS

GREEN
VEGETABLES
pages 44–51

ROOT
VEGETABLES
pages 54–57

CITRUS
FRUITS
pages 86–88

AVOCADOS
page 51

CERVICAL DYSPLASIA

THE DEVELOPMENT of abnormal cells in the cervix is known as cervical dysplasia. Left untreated, it may lead to cancer. Infection with the sexually transmitted human papillomavirus (HPV) is the primary risk factor. Other contributory factors include a history of multiple sexual partners and promiscuous male partners.

✪ SYMPTOMS
There are no physical symptoms associated with early cervical dysplasia. Screening programs in which women undergo regular cervical smears are the only way to detect symptoms at a cellular level.

✚ CONVENTIONAL TREATMENT
If dysplastic cells are found in the cervix, a laser scalpel is used to remove the affected part of the cervix under general anesthetic. Other surgery may be carried out under local anesthetic.

✔ BENEFICIAL FOODS
Cabbage, spinach, squashes, and sweet potatoes, eaten regularly in good amounts, are associated with a lower risk of cervical cell dysplasia than in people with low intakes of these vegetables.

Carrots, sweet potatoes, and green leafy vegetables supply beta carotene, which has been associated with a decreased risk of dysplasia. **Citrus fruits, berries**, papayas, peppers, green leafy vegetables, and potatoes are all rich in vitamin C. High dietary intakes of vitamin C may help to reduce the risk of cervical cancer. **Avocados, wheatgerm**, and whole-grain wheat products contain vitamin E, which may help to lessen the risk of cervical cancer.

✖ FOODS TO AVOID
Highly processed, manufactured foods need to be limited, since they can be low in essential vitamins and protective phytonutrients.

◐ OTHER MEASURES
❑ Smokers are advised to give up the habit, because there is strong evidence that it increases the risk of cervical cancer.
❑ Regular pap smears are important as a screening process to detect dysplasia as early as possible.

See Also Cancer, page 214

KEY FOODS

SEEDS
pages 103–105

AVOCADOS
page 51

WHOLE GRAINS
pages 92–99

GREEN
VEGETABLES
pages 44–51

BENIGN BREAST DISEASE

THE TERM BENIGN BREAST DISEASE covers breast pain (mastalgia), tenderness, and noncancerous lumps and cysts. Any tenderness or lump in the breast must be investigated by a doctor in order to determine whether it is benign or malignant.

✪ SYMPTOMS
The symptoms of benign breast disease range from small to larger lumps and from mild discomfort to extreme pain. The pain may extend into the upper arm or elbow.

✚ CONVENTIONAL TREATMENT
Doctors may prescribe hormone-based drugs, such as danazol or bromocriptine. Diuretics may also be prescribed. Doctors are now also prescribing the omega-6 fatty acid gamma linolenic acid (GLA).

✔ BENEFICIAL FOODS
Pumpkin, sunflower, and sesame seeds are good sources of omega-6 unsaturated fatty acids, which are recognized as being beneficial to breast tissue. **Avocados, wheat germ**, whole-grain cereals, and green leafy vegetables all provide vitamin E. Studies have shown that supplements of this vitamin can help to alleviate breast tenderness.

Wholewheat pasta, breads, and rice can improve bowel function. Regular bowel movements may help hormone-related breast discomfort.

✖ FOODS TO AVOID
Coffee, chocolate, and cocoa contain substances known as methylxanthines, which include caffeine. Women may find that breast pain is reduced by lowering intakes of these products. **Sausages, burgers, meat pies** and other processed meat products, and milk and whole-milk dairy products contain large amounts of saturated fats and are therefore best avoided. Large intakes of saturated fats appear to disturb the sensitivity of breast cells to circulating hormones.

◐ OTHER MEASURES
❑ Evening primrose oil can be taken as a food supplement to provide omega-6 fatty acids. It is also available on prescription.
❑ Vitamin E supplements have been found to help relieve symptoms of breast tenderness.

See Also Women & Nutrition, page 140

KEY FOODS

FRUITS
pages 72–91

VEGETABLES
pages 42–71

WHOLE GRAINS
pages 92–99

POULTRY
page 124

LEAN MEATS
page 122

OILY FISH
page 118

**NUTS &
SEEDS**
pages 100–105

**CITRUS
FRUITS**
pages 86–88

BERRIES
pages 82–85

LEGUMES
pages 58–60

INFERTILITY IN WOMEN

THE INABILITY TO CONCEIVE A CHILD after a year or more of regular, unprotected sexual activity is defined as infertility. Female infertility can be due to various factors. Failure to ovulate may be caused by a hormonal disorder, an underactive or overactive thyroid gland, a problem with the pituitary gland, weight loss or weight gain, chronic illness, stress, or excessive physical activity. Anticancer drugs and drugs for high blood pressure can also be a cause. Infertility may also be due to a blockage in one or both fallopian tubes, or a deformity of the uterus or vagina. In some cases, the woman may produce antibodies that attack the man's sperm. In many cases, the actual cause of infertility is not known.

✪ SYMPTOMS An inability to become pregnant can cause a great deal of emotional stress. If conception has not occurred within one year of trying, medical advice should be sought.

✚ CONVENTIONAL TREATMENT Failure to ovulate may be treated by correcting an underlying hormonal abnormality or by giving drugs to stimulate ovulation. Ovarian cysts and diseases of the fallopian tubes may be treated by surgical intervention. Some women may be suitable candidates for assisted reproduction techniques, such as in-vitro fertilization (IVF).

✔ BENEFICIAL FOODS
Fruits, vegetables, whole-grain breads, pasta, rice, and lean sources of protein, such as chicken, fish, lean meats, and legumes, should form the basis of the diet. These foods are low in fat and can help those who are trying to lose weight. Women who are obese can have ovulatory dysfunction (a failure to ovulate).
Lean red meats, oily fish, nuts, seeds, green leafy vegetables, and legumes supply the body with iron. Infertile women with depleted reserves of this mineral have been shown to become fertile once again on increasing their iron intakes.
Citrus fruits, berries, and green leafy vegetables are good sources of vitamin C. For women whose diet may be low in iron, vitamin C is essential because it enhances the absorption of iron.
Rye bread, pasta, basmati rice, legumes, fruits, and vegetables are all sources of slow-releasing energy that feeds sugar into the blood in a very slow and controlled way. These foods help people who have diabetes to control their levels of blood sugar to within as normal a range as possible. It is particularly important when trying for a baby to keep blood sugar levels under control.

CASE STUDY

Joanne Posser became pregnant for the first time when she was 23 and just married. During her pregnancy, Joanne put on 35lb in weight, and after the baby was born she could not lose the weight. Two years later, when Joanne was 25, she and her partner began to try for another baby. In the three years that followed they had no success. Joanne consulted her doctor, who said that her inability to conceive could be due to the fact that she was overweight. He suggested a low-fat eating plan and regular exercise. Now that Joanne had a good reason to lose weight, she made a concerted effort and within a year had returned to her normal weight. Possibly as a result, she later became pregnant and had a second child.

✖ FOODS TO AVOID
Sausages, burgers, ready-made meat products, cakes, cookies, and chocolate are rich in fat and are best kept to a minimum. High-fat foods are high in calories and appear to fail to let the body know that it has had enough to eat. Passive overconsumption of fatty foods and subsequent weight gain is therefore common.
Margarine, butter, and oils are rich in fats and these foods need to be strictly moderated.
Coffee, tea, and cola drinks contain caffeine, which may contribute to infertility if it is consumed in excessive amounts. This is possibly because caffeine reduces the circulating levels of the pituitary hormone prolactin. Low levels of prolactin are associated with infertility.
Alcohol may cause excessive production of prolactin if it is consumed in large amounts on a regular basis. This can lead to menstrual cycle abnormalities and therefore to infertility.

✐ OTHER MEASURES
❑ Daily folic acid supplements have been shown to be beneficial to some women if they originally had depleted levels of this B vitamin.
❑ Supplements of vitamin B_6 seem to improve fertility in women with premenstrual syndrome. About 100–800mg a day may be useful.
❑ Regular exercise is important.
❑ Stress management and relaxation are essential for those having problems conceiving.
❑ Smokers are advised to give up the habit, because smoking can cause infertility.

See Also Stress & Anxiety, page 231; Vitamins, page 26; Women & Nutrition, page 140

INFERTILITY IN MEN

KEY FOODS

BRAZIL NUTS
page 100

RED MEATS
page 122

BERRIES
pages 82–85

CARROTS
page 56

THE CAUSES OF INFERTILITY in men include problems in the development of sperm, with erection and ejaculation, and in the sperm's ability to fertilize the ovum once attached.

✪ SYMPTOMS Inability to fertilize and lack of ability to achieve erection or ejaculation are the only physical symptoms of male infertility.

✚ CONVENTIONAL TREATMENT The treatment can be as simple as making lifestyle changes, such as reducing smoking and alcohol intake, reducing heat around the testicles, and treating infections and testicular problems.

✔ BENEFICIAL FOODS
Brazil nuts, sesame seeds, eggs, meats, and cereals are good sources of the trace element selenium, which is essential for the male reproductive system. **Red meats, seafood,** wholewheat breads, brown rice, and brown pasta are all sources of zinc. This mineral is necessary for male sexual maturation. **Berries, peaches, avocados,** papayas, peppers, and green vegetables are all rich in vitamins C and E, which may help increase sperm count and mobility.

Carrots, sweet potatoes, mangoes, apricots, and green leafy vegetables supply beta carotene, which is needed for the maturation of sperm.

✘ FOODS TO AVOID
Alcohol can damage the male reproductive tract. It appears to decrease testosterone levels, lower sperm count, and negatively affect sex drive. **Dairy products** and zinc-rich foods should not be eaten together, as calcium reduces zinc absorbtion.

⊘ OTHER MEASURES
❑ Smokers are advised to give up the habit, since it may cause genetic damage to sperm.
❑ Supplements of vitamins E and B_{12} have been shown to improve sperm count.
❑ Zinc supplements may improve sperm count.
❑ Selenium supplements have been proven to significantly improve the activity of sperm.
❑ Losing any excess weight, if overweight, may help to improve sperm count.
❑ Reducing stress can enhance sperm count.

See Also Men's & Women's Health, page 220

MALE IMPOTENCE

KEY FOODS

RED MEATS
page 122

SHELLFISH
page 120

WHOLE GRAINS
pages 92–99

OILY FISH
page 118

IMPOTENCE REGULARLY AFFECTS about 25 percent of all men and can occur at any age. In nearly half of all cases there is a physical cause, and most of these can be treated. In many cases of impotence, the problem is of psychological origin.

✪ SYMPTOMS Impotence describes the inability to achieve and sustain an erection.

✚ CONVENTIONAL TREATMENT Oral drugs or patches can improve erection. Plastic cylinders placed over the penis can create a vacuum-induced erection. Surgical implants can give rigidity to the penis. If the cause is not physical, psychotherapy can be extremely helpful.

⊘ BENEFICIAL FOODS
Red meats, oysters and other shellfish, and whole-grain cereals supply the mineral zinc. A lack of zinc in the diet can lead to impotence. **Mackerel, herrings, tuna,** salmon, sardines, anchovies, and other oily fish need to be consumed regularly. The fatty acids in these fish may help to improve blood flow around the body, including the groin area.

✘ FOODS TO AVOID
Butter, margarine, lard, and oils are rich in fat and calories and need to be limited by those wishing to lose weight.
Salt added at the table, prepackaged foods, cured meats, and foods canned in brine are best avoided by men with high blood pressure.
Alcohol can be a cause of impotence and intake needs to be strictly moderated.

⊘ OTHER MEASURES
❑ Ginseng and gotu kola are herbs that help to improve blood flow and may be useful.
❑ Evening primrose oil supplements may help to delay the onset of diabetic erectile dysfunction.
❑ Regular exercise can help to keep the body in good shape and improve self-confidence.
❑ Alternative therapies to help relaxation, such as aromatherapy, reflexology, and yoga, may help.
❑ Male hormone replacement therapy could be a consideration for men who lose potency during "male menopause."

See Also Obesity, page 178

NERVOUS SYSTEM

THIS COMPLEX SYSTEM is responsible for gathering and analyzing information from the body's external and internal environment, storing experiences, and regulating body systems. It connects with all parts of the body, controlling every conscious and unconscious action within it on a second-by-second basis, from involuntary processes such as blood circulation and digestion to the thoughts, emotions, sensory perceptions, and actions that a person feels or makes.

DIET & THE NERVOUS SYSTEM

Scientific research indicates that good nutrition is essential for the correct development and functioning of the nervous system. A lack of folic acid in pregnancy, for example, may increase the risk of the baby's spinal cord not forming correctly, while a lack of vitamin B_{12} may lead to nervous disorders in both mother and child. Dietary manipulation has been found to relieve symptoms of some nervous-system disorders and improve emotional well-being.

MAINTAINING HEALTHY NERVES

Adequate amounts of sleep and relaxation, together with regular exercise, are important for the maintenance of a healthy nervous system. Specific nutrients, as well as a steady supply of energy, are needed to maximize the health of nerves throughout the body and keep them functioning at optimum levels.

STRUCTURE OF A NERVE CELL

A nerve cell, or neuron, consists of a cell body and branching projections, or dendrites. Extending from each cell body is a nerve fiber called an axon, which can vary from a fraction of an inch to a yard in length. Axons transmit electrical signals to and from the brain.

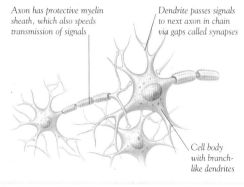

Axon has protective myelin sheath, which also speeds transmission of signals

Dendrite passes signals to next axon in chain via gaps called synapses

Cell body with branch-like dendrites

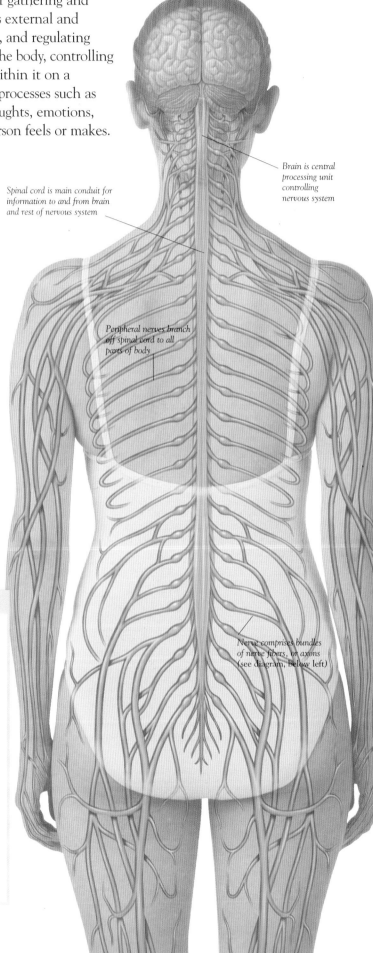

Spinal cord is main conduit for information to and from brain and rest of nervous system

Brain is central processing unit controlling nervous system

Peripheral nerves branch off spinal cord to all parts of body

Nerve comprises bundles of nerve fibers, or axons (see diagram, below left)

TOP HEALING FOODS

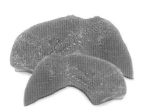

TURKEY — PAGE 124

Benefits May boost the brain's levels of serotonin, which plays a role in improving mood.
Useful for Those prone to SAD (seasonal affective disorder).
Nutrients The amino acid tryptophan.

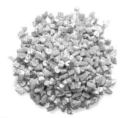

OATMEAL — PAGE 95

Benefits Oatmeal and other cooked cereals are known for their antidepressant qualities.
Useful for Those who are prone to low spirits and depression.
Nutrients Saponins and B vitamins.

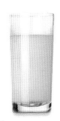

SKIM MILK — PAGE 126

Benefits Can help produce the enzymes involved in the functioning of the nervous system.
Useful for Growth and general maintenance and good health of the nervous system.
Nutrients Calcium.

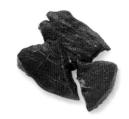

RED MEATS — PAGE 122

Benefits Provides a B vitamin that is essential in forming and maintaining the nervous system.
Useful for Building robust nerves and the prevention of neuropsychiatric disorders.
Nutrients Vitamin B_{12}.

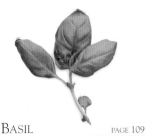

BASIL — PAGE 109

Benefits Has long been prescribed by western herbalists for the treatment of depression.
Useful for Those who experience depression, especially with the onset of the winter months.
Nutrients Volatile oils.

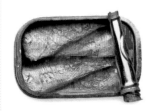

SARDINES — PAGE 119

Benefits Provide fatty acids crucial to the development of the nervous system and for the health of brain and nerves.
Useful for Pregnant and breast-feeding women.
Nutrients Omega-3 fatty acids.

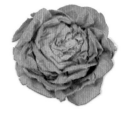

LETTUCES — PAGE 62

Benefits Supply a mild sedative, lactucarium, in the white sap that oozes mainly from the stalk.
Useful for Those who are over-stimulated and those affected by insomnia.
Nutrients Calcium, potassium.

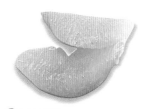

ORANGES — PAGE 88

Benefits May help to protect the nerves from free-radical damage.
Useful for The relief of stress, nervous anxiety, and general sleeping difficulties.
Nutrients Vitamin C, alpha and beta carotenes, folate.

OTHER BENEFICIAL FOODS

BEETS — PAGE 57

Benefits May help to alleviate symptoms of depression.
Useful for Those affected by low spirits linked to low folate levels.
Nutrients Folate, vitamin C, beta carotene, carbohydrates.

SESAME SEEDS — PAGE 103

Benefits Supply essential fats needed for the transmission of nerve impulses.
Useful for Improving the functioning of the memory.
Nutrients Omega-6 fatty acids.

CHAMOMILE TEA — PAGE 108

Benefits Infusions are well known for their sedative effects.
Useful for Those with insomnia and general sleeping difficulties, or for relaxation purposes.
Nutrients Volatile oils.

WHOLE-GRAIN BREAD — P 98

Benefits Supplies B vitamins.
Useful for Maintaining the health of the nervous system. May be useful for women with stress-related PMS.
Nutrients B vitamins.

FOODS TO AVOID

CHEESE

People who are affected by migraines may be advised by a doctor to avoid foods such as cheese that are rich in tyramine. Chocolate, alcohol, and foods containing cheese should also be avoided.

SWEETS

Sugary foods and other carbohydrates that are absorbed very quickly may lead to surges in blood sugar. Such surges can cause nervousness and over-stimulation, or hyperactivity, in some children and adults.

ORANGE SODA

Foods colored with the orange coloring tartrazine may cause hyperactivity in some children and should be avoided by those who appear to be affected.

COFFEE, TEA & SODAS

Large amounts of coffee, soda, strong tea, and cold remedies should be avoided by those with insomnia and sleeping difficulties. Excessive amounts of caffeine in these drinks directly stimulate the nervous system and can lead to sweats, heart palpitations, and high blood pressure. It has been suggested that drinks containing caffeine should be limited to two a day. Any reduction in caffeine consumption should be made gradually to reduce the risk of withdrawal symptoms.

PROCESSED FOODS

Cakes, cookies, candy, and ready-made meals are highly processed and can lack the essential nutrients needed for a healthy nervous system. In preference, prepare as many meals as possible from fresh produce.

ALCOHOL

Alcohol inhibits the transmission of nerve impulses, reducing the speed of movement, thought, and speech. Alcohol also acts as a depressant on the nervous system and may even cause seizures. It should be particularly avoided by people who experience epileptic fits and those susceptible to low spirits, depression, or the effects of stress.

ALCOHOLISM

KEY FOODS

WHOLE GRAINS
pages 92–99

OILY FISH
page 118

GREEN VEGETABLES
pages 44–51

NUTS & SEEDS
pages 100–105

AVOCADOS
page 51

CITRUS FRUITS
pages 86–88

DAIRY PRODUCTS
pages 126–128

SHELLFISH
page 120

RED MEATS
page 122

ADDICTION TO ALCOHOLIC DRINKS is a form of psychological and physical dependence. Alcoholism is one of the most serious public health problems in the West. The condition is characterized by the need for alcohol and a difficulty in performing routine activities without it. An alcoholic person may consume increasing amounts of alcohol without becoming incapacitated, and experiences unpleasant symptoms when the alcohol is withdrawn.

⊗ SYMPTOMS Behavioral changes may include an inability to cope with normal activities, sleeplessness, and uncharacteristic emotional outbursts. Alcoholism carries with it an increased risk of liver disease, high blood pressure, brain damage, heart disease and heart-rhythm disturbance, stroke, pancreatitis, peptic ulcers, and cancer. Factors affecting symptoms include genetic disposition, nutritional status, and pre-existing health conditions.

✚ CONVENTIONAL TREATMENT This usually involves periodic admissions to a hospital followed by medical and local advisory service support. Withdrawal symptoms may be treated with drugs such as phenothiazines, diazepam, haloperidol, or chlormethiazole. In severe cases of nutritional deficiencies due to alcoholism, nutritional advice may be given.

✔ BENEFICIAL FOODS
Rye bread, legumes, basmati rice, unsweetened muesli, apples, pears, grapefruits, cherries, oranges, peaches, and yogurt have medium to low glycemic indexes, or GIs (*see page 18*). These foods release sugar into the bloodstream gently and are useful for those with cirrhosis of the liver, who have a high risk of developing diabetes.
Herrings, mackerel, salmon, sardines, and trout supply vitamin D, as do eggs, fortified breakfast cereals, margarines, and butter. Chronic liver disease caused by alcoholism can result in vitamin-D deficiency.
Cabbage, brussels sprouts, cauliflower, and spinach provide vitamin K. Liver, butter and other whole-milk products, and fortified margarine contain "preformed" vitamin A. Carrots and other orange fruits and vegetables, and green vegetables provide beta carotene. Liver disease can cause the poor absorption of fat and a shortage of vitamins A and K.
Nuts, seeds, avocados, and whole-grain cereals provide vitamin E, which may be poorly absorbed by those with liver disease.

Beetroots, brussels sprouts, spinach, asparagus, kale, and black-eyed peas are good sources of the B vitamin folate, while fortified breakfast cereals and yeast extracts supply folic acid. The absorption of these may be reduced by alcohol.
Citrus fruits, citrus fruit juices, papayas, berries, peppers, and sweet potatoes supply vitamin C, which may be low in alcoholics. High intakes of this vitamin may improve the rate at which alcohol can be cleared from the system.
Breakfast cereals, breads, and whole grains supply a range of B vitamins, which may be low in those with high alcohol intakes. Vitamin-B deficiency can worsen symptoms of alcoholism.
Dairy products, nuts, seeds, green leafy vegetables, calcium-fortified soy milk, and tofu are good sources of calcium. Poor absorption of calcium is common in alcoholics. In women, poor intakes can increase the risk of osteoporosis.
Milk, breads, cereal products, and potatoes provide magnesium, which is often poorly absorbed and excreted in excessive amounts by those with high alcohol intakes. Low magnesium levels can cause disorders of the heart.
Fruits, vegetables, and fruit juices are rich in potassium, intakes of which are frequently poor in alcoholics. Low potassium levels can lead to symptoms similar to those of delirium tremens.
Shellfish, red meats, and whole-grain cereals supply zinc. Adequate intakes of zinc may be beneficial in preventing alcohol toxicity.

✖ FOODS TO AVOID
Meats, poultry, fish, eggs, and dairy products are rich in protein. In cases of severe liver damage due to alcoholism, protein should be restricted, under the supervision of a doctor and a dietician.
Bony fish and foods that are rough in texture must be avoided by those with esophageal varices. These dilated veins in the throat could burst if scratched or pierced, causing large blood loss.

⊘ OTHER MEASURES
❑ Vitamin-B-complex supplements including vitamin B_1 can prevent Wernicke-Korsakoff syndrome, a disorder caused by the malnutrition that may result from alcohol dependence.
❑ General vitamin and mineral supplements may help with the process of detoxification.
❑ Evening primrose oil contains omega-6 fatty acids, which may reduce the severity of symptoms of alcohol withdrawal.

See Also Depression, page 233

STRESS & ANXIETY

aKEY FOODS

WHOLE GRAINS
pages 92–99

FRUITS
pages 72–91

VEGETABLES
pages 42–71

LEAN MEATS
page 122

POULTRY
page 124

EGGS
page 129

LOW-FAT DAIRY PRODUCTS
pages 126–128

LEGUMES
pages 58–60

LEVELS OF ANXIETY that remain high over a long period are a sign of stress. Bereavement, financial worries, too much work, job loss, and poor relationships can all cause stress. For children and teenagers, parental breakup, the pressure of school work, and worries associated with growing up are common factors. An overactive thyroid gland may cause anxiety, as may drug addiction.

☻ SYMPTOMS

Stress may weaken the immune system, resulting in frequent minor illnesses such as coughs, colds, and cold sores. Sleep disturbances may develop, leading to daytime tiredness. Headaches, indigestion, panic attacks, irritability, and a rapid heartbeat may occur. Stress may induce loss of appetite or trigger overeating. Children are particularly prone to eating disorders if under stress.

✚ CONVENTIONAL TREATMENT

If other causes are ruled out, the root of the problem needs to be found and addressed. This may involve counseling, time away from the source of the pressure, drug treatments, relaxation techniques, or exercise programs.

✔ BENEFICIAL FOODS

Wholewheat breads, pita bread, scones, wholegrain breakfast cereals and pasta, and brown rice are rich in a range of B vitamins, which help to nourish the nervous system. The insoluble fiber in these foods helps to prevent constipation and other bowel-related disorders triggered by stress. Approximately 60 percent of calorie intake should come from these starchy foods, with some incorporated at each meal.

Fruits and vegetables contain vitamins C, E, and the B group, calcium, iron, zinc, potassium, and copper, and phytonutrients such as carotenoids and bioflavonoids. These substances help to boost the body's ability to fight infections, certain forms of cancer, and heart disease. Five servings of fruits and vegetables a day, with as much variety as possible, are recommended.

Lean meats, chicken and turkey without the skin, white and oily fish, eggs, low-fat milk and dairy products, legumes, tofu, and textured vegetable protein are all good sources of lean protein. Two to three servings of protein-rich foods are needed daily for good health.

✘ FOODS TO AVOID

Fats and oils should be consumed in moderation. Foods that are rich in saturated fats should be monitored strictly. These include fatty meat cuts,

CASE STUDY

David Chen, aged 26, had anxiety attacks when under pressure at work. At times he sweated profusely and felt a tightness in his chest. His hair began to fall out, which his doctor attributed to stress. David was referred to a nutritionist, who advised him to stop drinking alcohol for several weeks, to reduce his coffee intake, and to drink herbal teas instead. The nutritionist also recommended eating slow-releasing carbohydrates and avoiding sugary snacks. After a month of this eating plan and a course of hypnotherapy, David began to feel better able to deal with stressful situations.

meat products such as hamburgers and sausages, whole-milk dairy products, cookies, cakes, and ready-made desserts. These foods can raise cholesterol, increasing the risk of heart disease. A high proportion of fatty foods also increases the chances of weight gain. Carrying excess weight can lead to many physical and psychological problems that exacerbate stress. **Alcohol** acts as a depressant on the nervous system. It can increase "down" feelings, and there is a risk of increasing dependence in order to escape rather than deal with the causes of stress. **Colas, coffee, tea**, and cold remedies contain caffeine, which stimulates the nervous system. Taken in excess, caffeine can lead to tremors, sweating, palpitations, rapid breathing, and sleep disturbances. Any reductions in intake should be made gradually to avoid withdrawal symptoms such as headaches and fatigue. Reducing daily intake of caffeine-containing drinks to one cup or less may relieve symptoms.

⊘ OTHER MEASURES

❏ A tincture or infusion of vervain may help relaxation. Vervain is an herb that has a relaxing effect on the nervous system.

❏ Wood betony is an herb with known calming effects on the nervous system and is particularly recommended for exhaustion. The powdered herb is available in capsule form.

❏ The damask rose has gentle sedative effects. Damask rose water can be added to the evening meal in order to assist with sleep.

❏ Chamomile tea may help to calm the nerves and improve sleep when drunk at nighttime.

❏ Vitamin and mineral supplements may help to fortify the body against the effects of stress.

See Also Depression, page 233; Fatigue, page 235

INSOMNIA

KEY FOODS

WHOLE GRAINS
pages 92–99

TURKEY
page 124

FIGS
page 80

BANANAS
page 90

LOW-FAT MILK
page 126

OILY FISH
page 118

SEEDS
pages 103–105

GREEN VEGETABLES
pages 44–51

CHAMOMILE TEA
page 108

AN INABILITY TO SLEEP at night is classified as insomnia. The condition may be temporary, and possibly caused by stressful situations or events; or it may be long-term, which tends to result from chronic stress or more serious psychological or emotional problems. There may also be physical causes for insomnia, such as indigestion, asthma, apnea, or hypoglycemia, or it could be a side effect of certain drugs or excessive alcohol consumption.

✪ SYMPTOMS Insomnia is characterized by an inability to fall asleep and also frequent wakefulness during the night. Restlessness and vivid dreams are also common. All of these problems result in a feeling of listlessness, irritability, and being unrefreshed on waking.

✚ CONVENTIONAL TREATMENT When treating insomnia, underlying medical problems must be eliminated first. Thyroid problems, depression, diabetes, infections, and hemoglobin levels that reflect iron intake need to be checked. Advice on when to eat and drink, alcohol consumption, and lifestyle may be given. In the short term, sleeping pills may be prescribed to break the pattern of insomnia. If depression is the underlying cause, this must also be treated.

✔ BENEFICIAL FOODS
The careful choice of foods and drinks and the timing of their consumption, in conjunction with advice from a doctor, may help to prevent insomnia or relieve the symptoms.
Breads, pasta, potatoes, and rice are rich in carbohydrate, which the body burns slowly. An evening meal high in carbohydrate and low in protein can help to prepare the body for sleep.
Turkey, figs, bananas, dates, yogurt, and tuna all supply tryptophan, which helps to promote sleep. These foods could be included in an evening meal to help combat insomnia.
Lean meats and low-fat milk supply vitamin B_6 needed for serotonin production from the amino acid tryptophan. Low vitamin B_6 intakes are associated with insomnia.
Mackerel, salmon, sardines, and other oily fish, along with flax seeds and pumpkin seeds, are good sources of omega-3 fatty acids.
Sunflower, sesame, and pumpkin seeds supply omega-6 fatty acids. Research suggests that these fatty acids have a direct effect on nerve membranes in the brain and an indirect effect on prostaglandins, neurotransmitters, amino acids, and substances called interleukins, which

CASE STUDY

Beverley Chandler, aged 48, began to experience insomnia as a result of stress when her daughter was going through marital difficulties. Beverley's doctor recommended that she eat foods high in carbohydrate, such as potatoes, cereals, and breads, and drink chamomile tea in the evenings. He also suggested taking up yoga as a way of relaxing. After taking these steps to deal with the insomnia, Beverley soon began to feel less anxious about going to sleep. The combination of approaches worked, and she gradually became more relaxed at bedtime and was able to fall asleep naturally, without having to resort to taking sleeping pills.

initiate and help to maintain sleep.
Red meats, dark poultry, fish, fortified breakfast cereals, and green leafy vegetables all provide iron. There is some evidence that a lack of iron or low iron stores can lead to insomnia.
Lettuce, especially wild lettuce, contains a sedative known as lactucarium. Eating a salad that includes lettuce before bed may be helpful.
Chamomile tea may help to calm the nervous system, thereby preparing it for sleep.

✖ FOODS TO AVOID
Butter, margarine, lard, oils, cakes, cookies, meat products, and fried foods should be avoided by those with apnea, a breathing disorder that occurs during sleep. Rich in fat and calories, these foods should be kept to a minimum by those who are obese, since there is an association between apnea and obesity. Studies find weight loss to be a significant factor in improving apnea.
Coffee, tea, cola drinks, and cold remedies contain caffeine. Large intakes can overstimulate the nervous system and lead to sleep disturbances. Avoid caffeine drinks before bedtime.

◷ OTHER MEASURES
❑ Eating late at night and going to bed on a full stomach can cause indigestion and sleeplessness.
❑ Drinking late at night increases the need to interrupt sleep in order to urinate.
❑ Regular exercise, at least four or five times a week, is recommended.
❑ Tinctures of Californian poppy, hops, or passionflower may help when taken at night. Herbal remedies should be taken only on the advice of a medical herbalist.

See Also Asthma, page 187; Depression, page 233; Heartburn, page 170; Stress & Anxiety, page 231

KEY FOODS

OATS
page 95

BASIL
page 109

GREEN
VEGETABLES
pages 44–51

LEAN MEATS
page 122

LOW-FAT MILK
page 126

DEPRESSION

THIS DISORDER IS CHARACTERIZED by intense and persistent feelings of sadness, pessimism, and loss of interest in life so pervasive that it may be impossible to continue normal daily activities. Added to this may be disturbed sleep, a lack of appetite, and a reduced sex drive. When severe, depression may also be associated with suicidal thoughts. Causes include stressful life events such as bereavement, job loss, retirement, or financial worries, but depression can also be present without any apparent cause. Depression often goes unrecognized, and it is estimated that one in five people experiences depression in their lives.

✪ SYMPTOMS
The symptoms of depression are sustained and go beyond simply feeling down. They can include anxiety, poor concentration, loss of enjoyment, fatigue, low energy levels, lack of self-confidence and low self-esteem, feelings of guilt, and pessimism about the future. Self-harm or suicide in thought, word, or deed may arise. Sleep may be disturbed and appetite reduced.

✚ CONVENTIONAL TREATMENT
It is essential that medical advice is sought. Any dietary changes should be discussed with a doctor and incorporated into a holistic treatment. Antidepressant drugs are frequently prescribed and include tricyclic antidepressants, monoamine oxidase inhibitors, and selective serotonin reuptake inhibitors (SSRIs).

✔ BENEFICIAL FOODS
Foods may not cure depression, but they can be useful in conjunction with therapies suggested by a doctor. Dietary changes prove most helpful to those with mild to moderate depression.
Oats, known for their antidepressant actions, are rich in saponins, alkaloids, B vitamins, and flavonoids. Eaten in the form of oatmeal, oats are a useful remedy for those with low moods.
Basil leaves added to salads have long been prescribed by herbalists for their antidepressant actions. Active constituents of this herb include volatile oils and basil camphor.
Brussels sprouts, cabbage, broccoli, beets, asparagus, spinach, kale, and black-eyed peas are all rich sources of the B vitamin folate. Depression is a common symptom of folate deficiency. Low levels of folate have been linked to a poor response to antidepressant drugs, such as serotonin inhibitors.
Breakfast cereals, breads, and yeast extracts that are fortified with folic acid help to increase blood levels of this B vitamin.

CASE STUDY

George Olsen, aged 56, began to feel increasingly isolated and depressed following his divorce. He socialized less and less, and his diet consisted mainly of take-out foods low in nutrients. Within six months, George had put on 26lbs in weight. A work colleague recognized that he was mildly depressed and suggested he consult a nutritionist. She recommended taking hypericum (St. John's Wort), a low-fat diet, and a 40-minute daily walk. The diet included turkey and cottage cheese, which help increase levels of serotonin in the brain. Within two months, George had regained his normal weight and had begun to feel more positive.

Lean meats, turkey, and low-fat milk are good suppliers of vitamin B_6, needed for converting the amino acid tryptophan into the neurotransmitter serotonin, which is responsible for lifting moods. In some tests, depressed people have been found to have significantly lower levels of vitamin B_6 than those who are not depressed.

✖ FOODS TO AVOID
Sugar, honey, candy, cookies, cakes, and sweet drinks cause sudden increases in blood sugar levels, which are often followed by sugar "lows." These foods may accentuate feelings of despondency, and should be eaten in strict moderation by those who have depression.
Cheese, especially blue cheese, aged or processed cheese, game, meat extracts and foods containing them, pickled herrings, flavored, textured vegetable protein, and alcoholic drinks contain biologically active amines, such as tyramine, histamine, and dopamine. They should be avoided by people taking monoamine oxidase inhibitor drugs. Failure to do so can cause unpleasant and even life threatening reactions, especially headaches and increased blood pressure.

⊘ OTHER MEASURES
❑ Oat tincture, basil juice, or damiana tincture are well-known herbal remedies that may be advised for use by medical herbalists.
❑ Hypericum (St. John's Wort) is available as a supplement in tablet form and can be obtained from pharmacies and health-food stores. In Germany, this herb is often prescribed for people with mild to moderate depression.

See Also Fatigue, page 235; Seasonal Affective Disorder, page 234; Stress & Anxiety, page 231

Seasonal Affective Disorder (SAD)

Key Foods

Poultry
page 124

Whole Grains
pages 92–99

Legumes
pages 58–60

Fruits
pages 72–91

Fish
pages 118–121

Avocados
page 51

Dairy
Products
pages 126–128

Citrus
Fruits
pages 86–88

Green
Vegetables
pages 44–51

Diagnosis of seasonal affective disorder, or SAD, can be made when depressive symptoms start in winter and occur for three winters, at least two of which are consecutive. The onset of this condition usually occurs between the ages of 22 and 35. Several biological abnormalities have been demonstrated in SAD relating to the secretion of the hormone serotonin in the brain.

Symptoms Depression, guilt, irritability, low self-esteem, apathy, anxiety, a desire to be alone, paranoia, obsession, elation, and hyperactivity are all associated with SAD. Other symptoms are fatigue, sleep problems, constant eating, weight gain, decreased libido, low body temperature, and muscle aches and pains. There may also be reduced resistance to illness and menstrual problems in women.

Conventional Treatment

Conditions such as nonseasonal and recurrent depression need to be ruled out, as well as hypothyroidism, hypoglycemia, and chronic fatigue syndrome. Light therapy is successful in 85 percent of diagnosed cases. Antidepressant drugs may alleviate symptoms of depression.

Beneficial Foods

Diet can help to increase the amount of the mood-enhancing neurotransmitter serotonin in the brain and help to control the weight gain that sometimes accompanies SAD.

Turkey, pheasant, partridge, and cottage cheese are particularly good sources of the amino acid tryptophan, which is a precursor of serotonin. Lean meat, fish, eggs, low-fat dairy products, and legumes also supply tryptophan.

Cooked cereals, unsweetened muesli, and bran-flake breakfast cereals have low glycemic indexes, or GIs (*see page 18*). This means that they release sugar into the bloodstream slowly. This steady supply of blood sugar to the brain helps to raise serotonin levels for sustained periods. As a result, these foods may help to relieve mild depression.

Basmati rice, rye bread, and pasta have low glycemic indexes and should form the basis of meals. These foods help to prevent big "highs" and subsequent dips in blood sugar levels, which tend to increase the risk of weight gain.

Legumes have low glycemic indexes and should be included in meals to help maintain a steady serotonin supply throughout the day and night.

Apricots, apples, pears, grapes, plums, grapefruits, and oranges raise blood sugar and serotonin levels gradually and help to maintain them.

Fish, shellfish, chicken and turkey without the skin, cottage cheese, very lean ham, pork, bacon, lamb, tofu, plain yogurt, skim milk, and eggs all supply the brain with the amino acid tyrosine. Tyrosine is used to make the chemicals dopamine and noradrenaline. These appear to act on brain cells to improve concentration and alertness.

Avocados, dates, bananas, plums, eggplant, papayas, passion fruits, plantains, pineapples, and tomatoes contain a natural supply of "preformed" serotonin. This serotonin seems to attach itself to receptor sites in the stomach, which send signals to the brain to suppress appetite.

Cottage cheese, turkey, chicken, very lean meats, textured vegetable protein, and low-fat dairy products are protein foods with a low calorie and fat contents. Protein foods can help to reduce hunger and the tendency to overeat.

Oranges, grapefruits, berries, sweet potatoes, and green leafy vegetables are rich sources of vitamin C, which is needed to help maintain a robust immune system.

Foods To Avoid

Sugar, honey, sweets, sweet drinks, cookies, and cakes raise blood sugar levels quickly, providing a short, sharp burst of sugar to the brain and a quick, but poorly maintained, boost in serotonin. The boost is followed by a dip, which triggers a desire for more quick, sugar-based "fixes."

Croissants, crumpets, bagels, bread, cornflakes, sugar-coated cereals, and potatoes all bring about a rapid release of blood sugar. These foods are best replaced with slow-releasing options.

Butter, margarine, lard, and fried and fatty foods should be avoided or eaten in strict moderation. These foods may cause weight gain, which can lead to low self-esteem and depression.

Other Measures

❏ Hypericum (St. John's Wort) increases the production of serotonin, which helps to improve moods and decrease hunger. The standardized active extract of this herb can be bought in tablet form from chemists and health-food stores.

❏ Vitamin D_3 supplements, with doses of 400mcg a day taken over a five-day period, have been shown to have a powerful effect on mood. It is thought that a decrease in vitamin D_3 during winter months due to lack of sunshine may cause variations in mood by affecting serotonin levels.

See Also Depression, page 233; Fatigue, page 235; Stress & Anxiety, page 231

CHRONIC FATIGUE SYNDROME (CFS)

KEY FOODS

WHOLE GRAINS
pages 92–99

BANANAS
page 90

APPLES &
PEARS
pages 74–75

LEGUMES
pages 58–60

ALSO KNOWN AS myalgic encephalomyelitis (ME), postviral fatigue syndrome, or chronic fatigue and immune dysfunction syndrome (CFIDS), CFS is a potentially severe and disabling illness. It most commonly affects people between the ages of 20 and 40. The cause of this condition is not known.

⊕ SYMPTOMS The key symptoms are exercise-induced muscle fatigue, flu-like malaise, clumsiness, and poor memory, concentration, and balance. Muscle pain, nonrefreshing sleep, sore throats, enlarged glands, joint pains, and alcohol intolerance may also occur. About 25 percent of people with CFS also experience depression.

⊕ CONVENTIONAL TREATMENT Drugs are prescribed to relieve symptoms. Low doses of antidepressants may relieve sleep disturbance and muscle pain. Adequate rest and careful pacing of physical and mental activities are very important.

✔ BENEFICIAL FOODS
Cooked oats, basmati rice, unsweetened muesli, pasta, and rye bread are all digested slowly, releasing sugar into the bloodstream gradually. By keeping blood sugar levels steady, these foods reduce the likelihood of extreme tiredness.
Medium-ripe bananas, apples, pears, apricots, oranges, grapefruits, plums, and peaches help to maintain steady blood sugar levels.
Chickpeas, kidney beans, lentils, soybeans, and baked beans are sources of low-fat protein that help to keep blood sugar levels steady.

✘ FOODS TO AVOID
Sugar, candy, honey, soft drinks, and cakes raise blood sugar levels quickly. These "highs" may be followed by sugar "lows," which causes tiredness.
Alcohol should be avoided because many people with CFS have alcohol intolerance.

⊘ OTHER MEASURES
❑ Evening primrose oil and fish oil supplements provide a combination of omega-6 and omega-3 fatty acids and can improve some symptoms.
❑ Multivitamin and mineral supplements may be useful, especially for anyone on a restricted diet.

See Also Depression, page 233

FATIGUE

KEY FOODS

MEATS
page 122

FISH
pages 118–121

VEGETABLES
pages 42–71

CITRUS
FRUITS
pages 86–88

MILD TO SEVERE FATIGUE can result from poor sleep, stress, too much work, poor fitness, dietary deficiencies, and certain illnesses.

⊕ SYMPTOMS Tiredness, lethargy, feeling "down," and an inability to concentrate are the main symptoms of fatigue.

⊕ CONVENTIONAL TREATMENT Any underlying illness can be diagnosed by a doctor through a physical examination, blood tests, and biochemical tests to check on kidney, liver, and thyroid function, and to reveal mineral imbalances.

✔ BENEFICIAL FOODS
Red meats, oily fish, poultry, fortified breakfast cereals, green leafy vegetables, seeds, and legumes supply iron. A lack of iron can cause anemia, which leads to severe tiredness.
Oranges, grapefruits and their juices, papayas, berries, green leafy vegetables, sweet potatoes, and peppers are rich in vitamin C. This vitamin helps the body to absorb iron.
Carrots, sweet potatoes, mangoes, and apricots supply beta carotene and enhance iron absorption.
Milk, breads, and cereals are good sources of magnesium. Low levels lead to muscle weakness.
Meats, poultry, fish, eggs, dairy products, soy milk, and fortified cereals provide vitamin B_{12}. Deficiency of this vitamin causes fatigue.
Shellfish, meats, milk, bread, and whole-grain cereals supply zinc. Zinc can help to fight infections, which tend to exacerbate fatigue.
Meats, fish, and other foods rich in protein stimulate the brain and improve mental alertness.

✘ FOODS TO AVOID
Refined and fast foods tend to be low in the B vitamins needed for energy metabolism.
Coffee, tea, colas, and some cold remedies contain caffeine and are best avoided at bedtime.

⊘ OTHER MEASURES
❑ Two liters of water or other fluid are needed daily, plus one liter for each hour of exercise, since dehydration can lead to fatigue.

See Also Depression, page 233; Insomnia, page 232; Stress & Anxiety, page 231

KEY FOODS

WHOLE GRAINS
pages 92–99

YOGURT
page 128

PRUNES
& FIGS
pages 79–80

FRUITS
pages 72–91

PARKINSON'S DISEASE

FIRST DESCRIBED BY the English physician James Parkinson nearly two centuries ago, the underlying origin of this brain disorder still remains unknown. Parkinson's disease occurs in every culture throughout the world. It tends to start after the age of 40 and is more likely to affect men than women. Parkinson's disease slowly destroys a tiny part of the brain called the substantia nigra, which produces dopamine, a neurotransmitter that controls movement.

⊕ SYMPTOMS
As dopamine production decreases, movements slow down and become erratic. Muscles become overtense, causing stiffness and rigidity in the joints. Trembling occurs, even at rest. Speech can be impaired and a fixed facial expression can occur. Weakness, drooling, loss of appetite, and a stooped, shuffling gait are all characteristic of Parkinson's disease.

⊕ CONVENTIONAL TREATMENT
Parkinson's disease cannot be cured, but the symptoms can be treated and minimized by the use of the drug levodopa, which the body transforms into dopamine. Levodopa is often combined with carbidopa, a drug that prolongs the effects of levodopa. Reduced doses of levodopa are needed, lessening the risks of side effects. If the effects of levodopa wear off, the drugs bromocriptine and amantadine can be used, with levodopa being reintroduced later. The slow, steady release of levodopa through special drug-delivery systems can help to slow the progression of symptoms.

✔ BENEFICIAL FOODS
Wholewheat breads, brown rice, and whole-grain pasta and cereals are recommended to help people with Parkinson's disease who frequently experience constipation.
Yogurt, cooked lentils, milk powder, and puréed peas can be used to thicken runny foods that are puréed for those with swallowing difficulties.
Prunes directly stimulate the smooth muscle of the colon wall and help to speed the movement of the stools. Prunes can therefore be a useful part of the diet for dealing with constipation.
Figs and other dried and fresh fruits can help people to overcome constipation associated with Parkinson's disease, and these foods should be included in the diet wherever possible.
Fluids are important. About eight to ten cups or glasses of water or other drinks should be consumed each day in order to maintain hydration and help to prevent constipation.

✖ FOODS TO AVOID
Protein-rich foods, such as meats, poultry, fish, eggs, milk, cheese, and other dairy products, should be consumed in very small amounts. Doctors and researchers are still divided on this issue, but it is believed that protein can interfere with the absorption of the drug levodopa by the brain and it may therefore be less effective when taken with or after a protein-rich meal.

Severe restriction of protein intakes during the daytime has been tried in people with serious symptoms of Parkinson's disease and, in some tests, people have shown a marked improvement in response to their levodopa medication. These people were restricted to 10g of protein during the day. The rest of the day's protein (0.4–0.5g per lb [$^1/_2$kg] of body weight) was then given in the evening meal and as a bedtime snack. For a man weighing 155lbs (70kg), this is about 60g of protein per day. This diet is not of benefit to everyone, since restricting protein may also lead to excessive weight loss. Any changes to the diet regarding protein should be made in consultation with the doctor in charge of treatment.
Legumes of all types can lead to flatulence in certain individuals. These foods should be excluded from the diets of people with Parkinson's disease who experience problems with excessive wind as the disease progresses.
Nuts, crisp toast and cookies, and flaky and dry foods can be a problem for those experiencing swallowing difficulties.
Soups and stews, custards, and yogurt can be difficult to eat for people with Parkinson's disease since they are likely to be spilled due to tremor.

⊘ OTHER MEASURES
❑ Nutritional supplements containing vitamin B$_6$ need to be avoided, since excessive amounts of this vitamin can break down the drug levodopa before it reaches the brain.
❑ Small, frequent meals will lessen the problem of slowness in eating due to tremor.
❑ There are special plates available that keep food warm, and dishes and cutlery that are designed to improve grip and thereby reduce the chance of spilling.
❑ Speech therapy can help to deal with swallowing problems. Good posture, taking time over meals, and lowering the chin toward the chest before swallowing can also be helpful.

See Also Constipation, page 175; Flatulence, page 176; Muscles, Bones & Joints, page 194

SCHIZOPHRENIA

KEY FOODS

OILY FISH
page 118

WHOLE GRAINS
pages 92–99

A PERSON WITH SEVERE schizophrenia periodically loses touch with reality and has bizarre ideas and behavior. Medical opinion is divided as to the causes of the disease.

✪ SYMPTOMS Typical symptoms include delusions, hallucinations, a lack of real meaning to conversation and speech, the loss of rational thinking, and a breakdown of associations between words and ideas. Speech may become impaired or incomprehensible.

✚ CONVENTIONAL TREATMENT Tranquilizers and antipsychotic drugs are commonly used. Recently, psychological therapies have been used in combination with drug treatment, with some benefit.

✔ BENEFICIAL FOODS
Sardines, mackerel, and salmon are rich in omega-3 fatty acids, which may be depleted in people with schizophrenia.
Low-calorie fruit drinks are preferable to soft drinks for those in whom drugs stimulate thirst through a drying effect in the mouth.

Cereals, breads, rice, and pasta provide a range of B vitamins needed for good general neurological functioning. Deficiencies of these vitamins can exacerbate schizophrenic symptoms.

✘ FOODS TO AVOID
Wheat and dairy products may be avoided, since some people who have schizophrenia may show improvement of symptoms with the removal of these foods from their diet.
Lard, butter, margarine, and oils should be eaten in strict moderation by those taking phenothiazine and dibenzodiazepine drugs, since these make a person prone to weight gain.

⊘ OTHER MEASURES
❏ Supplements of 10g of fish oil taken daily over a six-week period have been shown to improve symptoms of schizophrenia.
❏ Supplements of folic acid and vitamins E, C, and B_3 may help to prevent the increased neurological and behavioral problems associated with schizophrenia in some people.

DEMENTIA

KEY FOODS

BANANAS
page 90

PROGRESSIVE LOSS OF MENTAL FUNCTION is usually caused by brain disease. Conditions associated with dementia include Alzheimer's disease, arteriosclerotic dementia, Parkinson's disease, multiple sclerosis, and Down syndrome.

✪ SYMPTOMS Intellectual functioning gradually declines, and confusion, paranoia, agitation, and depression may develop.

✚ CONVENTIONAL TREATMENT Drug treatment for the underlying cause of the dementia is necessary. Antidepressant and antipsychotic drugs are commonly used.

✔ BENEFICIAL FOODS
People with progressive dementia are at risk of losing weight if they lose interest in food. They may experience a decline in their senses of smell and taste. Swallowing may become difficult.
Bananas, sandwiches, and other finger foods may help those who find using utensils difficult.
Jellies, puddings, and custards provide liquids in a form that is not too loose or souplike. This helps to avoid the risk of choking.

Casseroles or stews served in a single dish may help to minimize confusion at mealtimes and are preferable to having to cope with different kinds of food served on the same plate.
Cold drinks should be in good supply and within easy reach. Those who experience loss of thirst may forget to take drinks unless they are readily available and easy to take.

✘ FOODS TO AVOID
Tough and crunchy foods, and foods with a mixture of textures, such as pear slices in gelatin or minestrone soup, may be difficult to swallow.

⊘ OTHER MEASURES
❏ Distractions, such as television, should be minimized at mealtimes.
❏ Portion sizes should be appropriate for the individual. Large portions can be overwhelming and difficult to deal with.
❏ Plate guards and adapted utensils may be helpful to encourage independence when eating.

See Also Alzheimer's Disease, page 241

MIGRAINE

KEY FOODS

POULTRY
page 124

APPLES &
PEARS
pages 74–75

OATS
page 95

LEGUMES
pages 58–60

MORE THAN JUST A HEADACHE, the typical migraine lasts for 24–48 hours and the person usually feels exhausted for one or two days afterward. Migraines tend to run in families and are three times more common in women than in men. The exact cause remains unknown but research suggests that attacks are linked to chemical changes in the body.

✪ SYMPTOMS The common migraine consists of a severe, throbbing headache, usually located on one side, and often accompanied by loss of appetite, nausea, vomiting, or dislike of food. There may be sensitivity to smell, light, and noise that leads the person to rest in a quiet, darkened room. A "classical" migraine consists of a severe headache that is preceded by visual disturbances, such as flashing lights, blind spots, and, less commonly, tingling in the face or limbs.

In the first phase of a migraine attack, blood vessels throughout the body become constricted. In the second phase, they dilate more than normal. It is this expansion of the vessels in the brain that causes the pain.

✚ CONVENTIONAL TREATMENT Doctors advise avoiding common triggers for migraines. These include stress, lack of sleep, too much sleep, extreme emotions, missed meals, and in some cases, certain foods. An attack may be treated with painkillers, such as aspirin or acetaminophen, and antinausea medication. The two can be combined in one tablet. Prescription migraine tablets can be taken to reduce the number of attacks. These drugs help to boost a naturally occurring chemical called 5 H-T, which is low during migraine attacks. Low 5 H-T causes dilation of arteries in the brain. In many cases, constricting the arteries with drugs can control migraine attacks.

✔ BENEFICIAL FOODS

Chicken and turkey are low-fat foods that are also rich in protein. Protein foods do not lead to swings in blood sugar levels. Low blood sugar levels are thought to be among the common triggers for migraines. Protein, such as eggs, beef, and legumes, should be included at every mealtime. Snacks that are rich in protein are also helpful.
Apples, pears, cherries, grapes, and apricots are fruits that raise blood sugar levels in a regulated way, making them good between-meal snacks for maintaining blood sugar control.
Oatmeal oats, rye bread, and legumes, such as red kidney beans, red and green lentils, chickpeas, and lima beans, all contain soluble fiber and help to keep blood sugar levels steady. These foods are good sources of carbohydrate and, in the case of legumes, good protein sources.

✖ FOODS TO AVOID

Certain foods contain "vasoactive amines" which appear to trigger the constriction of blood vessels in the brain. Tyramine and phenylethylamine are the two main substances suspected of causing the problem, although other amines may have similar effects. Dietary factors, when combined with lifestyle and environmental factors, may be responsible for migraines. It may be wise to exclude the following foods from the diet.
Alcohol, chocolate, ripe cheese, and other dairy products contain tyramine and other amines. In a survey of 500 people, these foods were the worst dietary culprits for triggering migraines. Pickled herrings, sausages, sour cream, avocados, and yeast extract also contain tyramine and may cause migraines.
Nuts, chocolate, wheat germ, and shellfish are sources of copper. It is thought that copper is involved with the metabolism of vasoactive amines and increases the likelihood of attack.
Oranges, grapefruits, and satsumas should be excluded from the diet. Citrus fruits increase the intestinal absorption of copper and may play a part in the migraine-triggering process.
Fried and fatty foods, onions, pork, and seafood have been cited as common triggers.
Hot dogs and cured meats contain nitrites that have been added as preservatives, and they may trigger migraines in susceptible people.

◐ OTHER MEASURES

❑ Fish oil supplements, in doses of 1oz a day, give significant migraine relief to some people.
❑ Magnesium supplements may be helpful for women who experience premenstrually related migraines and headaches.
❑ Regular meals and snacks are an important part of the dietary management of migraines.
❑ Relaxation techniques, such as yoga, may help.
❑ Suddenly giving up tea and coffee, both of which contain caffeine, may act as a trigger for migraine in certain people.
❑ Keeping a diary recording every activity and everything consumed during the 24 hours before an attack is useful, as there may be common features that are responsible for the migraine.

See Also Stress & Anxiety, page 231

EATING PLAN FOR MIGRAINE

Eating regularly is important for anyone who is trying to avoid migraine attacks. Avoiding sugary carbohydrates, such as cakes and pastries, which tend to cause a rapid rise in blood sugar levels, is advisable. Individual "trigger" foods must also be excluded from the eating plan.

BREAKFASTS	LIGHT MEALS	MAIN MEALS	SNACKS
Oatmeal with honey and nectarine slices	Ham salad sandwich on wholewheat bread	Rosemary turkey kebabs with whole-grain rice and a green salad	Bowl of cereal with soy milk
◆	Fresh grape and pear salad	Caramelized pears	◆
Scrambled eggs on toasted rye bread and broiled tomatoes	◆	◆	Medium-ripe banana
◆	Chicken and watercress sandwich	Roast monkfish on tagliatelle and a bed of julienne carrots	◆
Whole-grain wheat flakes with chopped, "ready-to-eat" apricots and skim milk or soy milk	Cherries	Fruit-filled crêpes	Oatcakes
	◆	◆	◆
	Baked potato with baked beans and a diced cucumber salad	Pan-fried beefsteak with zucchini and baked potato	Rye bread with slice of ham
		Baked apple with custard	

EPILEPSY

KEY FOODS

WHOLE GRAINS
pages 92–99

OILY FISH
page 118

VEGETABLES
pages 42–71

DAIRY
PRODUCTS
pages 126–128

THE NEUROMUSCULAR DISORDER in which abnormal electrical impulses in the brain cause recurrent transient seizures is known as epilepsy. Seizures often appear to be spontaneous, but may be set off by external factors, such as flashing lights. Epilepsy can be linked to traumatic birth, brain infections, head injuries, stroke, brain tumors, and alcohol or drug withdrawal.

SYMPTOMS "Petit mal" seizures are mild. These may cause the person to stare into space or twitch slightly. "Grand mal" seizures are more extreme and the person can fall to the ground, become unconscious, and have convulsions.

CONVENTIONAL TREATMENT
Epileptic attacks can be controlled by a variety of anticonvulsant drugs. The medication prescribed relates to the particular type of epilepsy.

BENEFICIAL FOODS
Some foods can help to reduce the side effects of anticonvulsant drugs used in epilepsy.
Whole-grain breads, breakfast cereals, brown rice, and wholewheat pasta are rich in insoluble fiber. By bulking up the stools, these foods can help to relieve constipation, which is a side effect of the drug phenytoin used to treat epilepsy.
Dry crackers, plain biscuits, rice cakes, and dry toast may help symptoms of nausea brought on by the drugs phenytoin, phenobarbital, carbamazepine, ethosuximide, and valproic acid.
Herrings, kippers, sardines, pilchards, tuna, and eggs supply vitamin D, which is metabolized more quickly than normal when taking phenytoin and phenobarbital.
Brussels sprouts, kale, beets, black-eyed peas, foods fortified with folic acid, such as some breakfast cereals and breads, and yeast extract help to enhance levels of folic acid, which may be depleted through the use of phenytoin.
Milk, yogurt, cheese, fromage frais, tofu, tahini, dark green vegetables, and sardines or pilchards eaten with their softened bones are good sources of calcium, which is depleted through the use of phenytoin.

FOODS TO AVOID
Strong-smelling foods, such as cooked cabbage and percolated coffee, and fried and fatty foods, rich cakes, and cookies may increase feelings of nausea in those who are taking drugs for epilepsy.

OTHER MEASURES
❑ Food supplements may be useful if there is a deficiency of certain nutrients in the diet.
❑ Stressful situations need to be avoided.

See Also Stress & Anxiety, page 231

HYPERACTIVITY

KEY FOODS

SEEDS
pages 103–105

OILY FISH
page 118

WHOLE GRAINS
pages 92–99

LEAN MEATS
page 122

FISH
pages 118–121

POULTRY
page 124

EGGS
page 129

LEGUMES
pages 58–60

THIS CONDITION AFFECTS mainly children and is also known as attention deficit disorder (ADD) and learning disorder. The causes of hyperactivity are not yet determined. Factors that have been suggested include genetic tendencies, a mother who smoked during pregnancy, parental styles of upbringing, and food allergies. The best method of diagnosing the condition has yet to be established.

⊗ SYMPTOMS
Hyperactive children are overactive and have short attention spans. Other symptoms may include social, learning, and behavioral problems, thirst, anxiety, aggression, and poor eating and sleeping habits. A hyperactive child may be easily distracted and impulsive, unaffectionate, clumsy and poorly coordinated, fidget constantly, talk too fast or be difficult to understand, and have sudden mood changes and temper tantrums.

✚ CONVENTIONAL TREATMENT
Once a diagnosis has been made, treatment of the condition is by drugs, diet, or behavior therapy, or often a combination of all three. The drugs given are, paradoxically, stimulants. It has been estimated that about 20 percent of cases of hyperactivity are due to a true food allergy. The removal of food additives from the diet does seem to help to lessen symptoms in many children. The Feingold diet, developed in 1975 by Dr. Ben Feingold of San Francisco, forms the basis of some dietary approaches. It involves the avoidance of food and drink containing substances called salicylates, which are related to aspirin.

✔ BENEFICIAL FOODS
Sesame, pumpkin, and sunflower seeds are good sources of omega-6 fatty acids. There is evidence that hyperactivity is improved by increasing intakes of essential fats, which have been found to be in short supply in many hyperactive children. Essential fats are needed for the normal transmission of messages along nerves and for the laying down of memory.

Mackerel, salmon, kippers, sardines, pilchards, anchovies, pumpkin seeds, and flaxseed oil all supply omega-3 fatty acids, which are crucial to nerve function. These foods should be consumed regularly in order to maintain normal nerve functioning.

Breakfast cereals, bread, oats, rice cakes, rice, pasta, and potatoes are acceptable starchy foods that can be eaten without adverse effects.

Lean meats, fish, poultry, eggs, and legumes are acceptable sources of protein.

✖ FOODS TO AVOID
No dietary manipulation of a child's diet should be carried out without the guidance of a doctor and a dietician. Removing important foods from the diet results in the removal of certain nutrients; these have to be replaced through other foods in order to avoid deficiencies.

Sugar, sweetened drinks, and foods containing sugar, such as cookies, cakes, pastries, and candies produce rapid increases in blood sugar levels. These can trigger hyperactivity in some children and adults.

Almonds, apples, apricots, currants, peaches, plums, prunes, oranges, berries, tomatoes, and cucumbers contain natural salicylates. These are aspirinlike substances that need to be removed from the diets of hyperactive children.

Tartrazine is an orange coloring used as a food additive. It may contribute to hyperactivity. It is frequently found in packaged convenience foods, the rinds of cheeses, smoked cod and haddock, chewing gum, candies, lime and lemon sodas, seafood dressings, mint sauce, dessert toppings, canned fruits, pie fillings, canned peas, salad dressing, prepackaged cakes, marzipan, maple-flavored syrup, and carbonated drinks.

Benzoic acid is an additive that may contribute to hyperactivity. It is used as a preservative and is found in many jams, dessert sauces, flavoring syrups, fruit pulp and purée, fruit juices, marinated herring and mackerel, pickles, salad dressings, and fruit yogurt.

Carbonated drinks contain high levels of phosphorus, which is capable of disturbing the calcium and magnesium balance in the body and can lead to hyperactivity.

Coffee, tea, cola, and other drinks containing caffeine may worsen the symptoms.

⊘ OTHER MEASURES
❏ Evening primrose and fish oil combinations have been tested clinically, and have been shown to bring about a positive effect on the symptoms of hyperactivity in children and clumsiness associated with this condition.

❏ Valerian is an herb with known calming influences. A medical herbalist should be consulted in order to determine the most suitable dose and form in which to administer this herb.

❏ Alternative relaxation therapies such as massage, reflexology, and aromatherapy may be beneficial for this condition.

See Also Children & Nutrition, page 136

ALZHEIMER'S DISEASE

KEY FOODS

OILY FISH
page 118

CITRUS
FRUITS
pages 86–88

BERRIES
pages 82–85

GREEN
VEGETABLES
pages 44–50

AVOCADOS
page 51

NUTS &
SEEDS
pages 100–105

A FORM OF progressive dementia, Alzheimer's disease is characterized by nerve-cell degeneration in the memory center of the brain. In effect, the brain's circuits become disconnected and, as a result, the transfer and communication of information is disrupted. The cause of Alzheimer's remains unknown. There appears to be a genetic component and aluminum toxicity may be involved.

✪ SYMPTOMS

In the early stages of the disease there is increasing forgetfulness and anxious depression. This progresses to loss of memory of recent events, disorientation, and personality changes. Eventually, there is extreme confusion, feeding problems, and psychosis. In the later stages of Alzheimer's there may be weight loss, swallowing difficulties and, in some people, a refusal to eat. Confinement to bed may be necessary.

✚ CONVENTIONAL TREATMENT

There is, as yet, no treatment for this disease, although tranquilizers may be given for behavioral problems and sleeping difficulties. People with Alzheimer's disease must be kept well-nourished. Eventually, it will be necessary for all their daily needs to be attended to in order for them to sustain life.

✪ BENEFICIAL FOODS

Salmon, sardines, mackerel, anchovies, pumpkin seeds, and flaxseed oil all supply the body with omega-3 fatty acids. Pumpkin, sesame, and sunflower seeds also provide omega-6 fatty acids. Fatty acid deficiency has been noted in people with Alzheimer's. The lack of these substances in the brain could be a reason for the nerve damage involved in Alzheimer's disease. Regular intakes of foods that are rich in fatty acids may be beneficial.

Oranges, grapefruits and other citrus fruits, and berries, peppers, sweet potatoes, and green leafy vegetables are all rich sources of vitamin C. Daily intakes of this natural antioxidant may help to protect against nerve damage. Further research into this area of nutritional therapy is required.

Wheat germ, avocados, nuts, seeds, and green leafy vegetables supply vitamin E. Increasing dietary intakes of this vitamin may help to delay the deterioration that takes place in people with Alzheimer's in the later stages of the disease.

Milk-based meal-replacement drinks can make good between-meal snacks. Most of these drinks are fortified with vitamins and minerals and they therefore boost intakes of essential nutrients.

Sandwiches, biscuits, buns, and malt loaf are nourishing snacks that can be offered to Alzheimer's patients who are underweight.

Toast with peanut butter, toasted sandwiches, and other "finger foods" can improve energy intakes if use of utensils is difficult.

✖ FOODS TO AVOID

Soups, casseroles, and other foods that have a loose consistency and are messy to handle are best avoided by those with Alzheimer's.

Individual nuts and sweets may be difficult for people with Alzheimer's to swallow.

Foods and drinks that are packed in aluminum containers, drinking water with aluminum levels exceeding 15mcg per quart, and foods cooked in aluminum pans are not recommended by some experts. Aluminum consumed in large quantities is known to be toxic to the brain. High levels of aluminum have been found in some people with Alzheimer's and population studies suggest that the disease is most common in areas with high concentrations of aluminum in the drinking water. Results of such research are controversial.

Rhubarb contains oxalic acid, which can dissolve aluminum if it is cooked in aluminum skillets. There is some evidence that people with Alzheimer's are prone to aluminum poisoning from food and environmental sources.

◉ OTHER MEASURES

❑ Supplements of vitamin E may help to slow the progression of Alzheimer's. In some cases, this vitamin may help to delay the need for those with moderate dementia to be hospitalized.

❑ Some research has revealed that supplements of omega-3 and omega-6 fatty acids may be useful. Improvements in mood, appetite, sleep, and short-term memory have been reported.

❑ Brain levels of substances that are related to vitamin B_1 have been found to be deficient in people with Alzheimer's. Improvements in symptoms were noted after these people were given supplements of vitamin B_1.

❑ It may be helpful to provide the main meal of the day at lunchtime, since peak brain functioning occurs at about midday.

❑ Toothpastes and antacid tablets containing aluminum are best avoided by those with a family history of Alzheimer's.

See Also Depression, page 233; The Elderly & Nutrition, page 144; Stress & Anxiety, page 231

FOOD SAFETY

BASIC FOOD SAFETY

In order to reduce the risk of food poisoning, make sure that you only buy fresh food. It is also wise to:

- **BUY FROM** a reputable retailer.
- **AVOID FOODS** that are packaged in damaged containers.
- **AVOID FOODS** that have passed their "use-by" or "best before" dates.
- **TAKE REFRIGERATED** and frozen food home as quickly as possible.
- **STORE COOKED** and uncooked foods separately. Use plastic wrap to protect foods.
- **MAKE SURE** that your hands, kitchen utensils, and surfaces are kept clean.

FOOD & TRAVEL

Extra care should be taken with food and drink when traveling abroad. Unfamiliar foods or poor hygiene in food preparation can cause discomfort or illness.

- **WATER** in some countries is not safe to drink. Always drink bottled or boiled water when traveling abroad.
- **STREET VENDORS** often have low hygiene standards. It is therefore best to avoid buying food from them.
- **MEAT AND SEAFOOD** dishes may cause food poisoning or diarrhea.
- **WASH FRUITS AND VEGETABLES** in boiled water or peel them before eating in order to avoid the risk of taking in contaminated water.

GONE ARE THE DAYS WHEN people ate foods that they grew themselves. Today we depend on supermarkets to supply our "daily bread." Much of these foods are mass produced, and may contain a range of chemicals that flavor and preserve them. Careful, hygienic storage and handling of foods goes a long way to ensuring food safety. However, other issues, such as genetic modification, may also concern the consumer.

FOOD ADDITIVES

Substances are added to foods to aid preservation, to prevent bacterial and mold growth, to improve the texture, color, taste, or nutritional content of a food, or as a processing aid, such as raising agents or emulsifiers. To qualify for usage, an additive must be proven to be safe, effective, and necessary. Only after satisfying these criteria is its use permitted. Although additives improve safety and variety for the consumer, they may also be responsible for adverse reactions.

Fortified with vitamins
Extra vitamins have been added during processing

Calories
Number of calories, or kilojoules per serving

Sodium
Amount of sodium in an average serving

Sugars
Products may contain several types of sugar

Vitamins
Milligrams or micrograms of vitamins per serving

Recommedations
Serving related to recommended daily amounts of nutrients

LOW SODIUM
FORTIFIED WITH VITAMINS

NUTRITION FACTS
Servings per pack: Approx 12 (30g)

Amount per 30g serving with whole milk (125ml)

Calories 173 k/cal	
Total fat 3.1g	
Saturated Fat 1.4g	
Sodium 0.3g	
Total Carbohydrates 29.8g	
Sugars 16.6g	
Protein 6.4g	
Vitamin C	16.4mg
Vitamin B$_1$	0.4mg
Vitamin B$_2$	0.6mg
Niacin	4.7mg
Vitamin B$_6$	0.5mg
Folic Acid	51.0mcg
Vitamin B$_{12}$	0.6mcg
Pantothenic Acid	1.9mg
Iron	3.6mg

•A 30g serving provides 25% of the RDA of these 8 vitamins and Iron.

INGREDIENTS: Cereal Grains (Whole-grain Oats, Whole-grain Wheat, Whole-grain Barley, Whole-grain Rice, Whole-grain Maize), Sugar, Starch, Honey, Partially Inverted Brown Sugar Syrup, Ground Almonds, Salt, Calcium Carbonate, Trisodium Phosphate, Antioxidant: Tocopherols, Flavoring.

Low sodium
Contains less than 140mg of salt per serving

Amounts
Nutrient quantities calculated for one serving

Fat
Fat content broken down to show how much of the fat is saturated

Carbohydrates
Total carbohydrate content is shown

Protein
Protein content must be shown even if there is very little or none

Iron
The iron content must be shown even if there is very little or none

Ingredients
These substances must be listed individually, in order of quantity, with the largest constituent first

Food irritants
Lists of ingredients need to be checked by those people who suffer an allergic reaction to such foods as nuts or wheat

FOOD LABELS
There are laws regulating the information given on food labels. Amounts must relate to a serving size, and terms such as "light" and "low-fat" must not be used to mislead the consumer. Some processed foods, such as refined bread, are required to list additional nutrients. The label for this product, a breakfast cereal, shows it has been fortified with vitamins, possibly to replace nutrients lost in production.

ANTIBIOTICS & PESTICIDES

Antibiotics are used to prevent and treat infections in farm animals. Hormones are frequently given to beef cattle and chickens to promote growth and possibly to dairy cows to promote milk yields. Pesticides are used to safeguard crops from molds, weeds, and other pests. The level of pesticides, antibiotics, and other chemicals used in food production is monitored by official bodies, although some people believe that the recommended levels are too high.

NATURAL TOXINS

Just because food is natural does not mean that it is necessarily safe. Some foods contain naturally occurring poisons. Eating large amounts of the green parts, eyes, and sprouts of potatoes, for example, can cause diarrhea, stomachaches, breathing problems, or even death. Legumes contain hemaglutinins, natural toxins that are killed if the beans are boiled for 20 minutes, but cause severe illness if the beans are soaked but not cooked. Nutmeg, mace, and dill contain myristicin, which, in large amounts, may cause vomiting and colic.

BIOTECHNOLOGY & FOODS

The genetic modification (GM) of foods involves moving a single gene from one species to another in order to produce crops with new features, such as greater resistance to viruses, fungi, or insects. In animals reared for food, biotechnology can help with the development of new vaccines and in the production of disease- and parasite-resistant animals. Although the regulation of GM crops is stringent, there is concern that not enough research has been done in this area. In some countries, all GM foods must be labeled by law.

ORGANIC FOODS

People who do not wish to eat foods that are produced with the assistance of chemicals may choose to buy organic foods. Organic farming prohibits the use of genetically modified species, artificial fertilizers, and pesticides. In livestock production, feed additives and growth regulators are not permitted, and there are strict guidelines concerning animal welfare. Regulations concerning organic food production are enforced through inspections by authorized bodies. Foods that meet their standards carry certification symbols from qualifying bodies such as the UK Register of Organic Foods in the UK and the Quarantine Inspection Service in Australia.

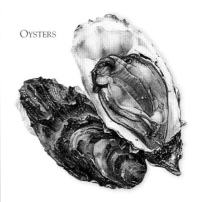

OYSTERS

FOOD POISONING

Certain foods, such as shellfish, meats, and poultry, may cause food poisoning if they have been infected by bacteria, molds, or parasites. The most common types of food poisoning and their sources and symptoms are listed below:

• LISTERIOSIS Symptoms are influenza-like, but *Listeriosis* can also result in premature birth or miscarriage. Found in unpasteurized milk, contaminated pâté, and precooked poultry. Avoid this by handling and storing foods appropriately and eating them within "use-by" dates.

• SALMONELLA Symptoms may include nausea, stomachaches, fever, diarrhea, and vomiting. Found in poultry, eggs, meat products, and milk products. Avoid by storing foods appropriately and eating them within "use-by" dates.

• CLOSTRIDIUM BOTULINUM Symptoms can include difficulty in swallowing and breathing, blurred vision, and respiratory or cardiac failure. Found in "blown" canned or vacuum-packed foods. This form of food poisoning is very rare, but avoid buying dented or rusty cans.

• ESCHERICHIA COLI Symptoms include stomachaches, fever, diarrhea, and vomiting, usually within 24 hours of infection. Found in foods contaminated by those with poor personal hygiene. Over-the-counter foods, such as sandwiches, salads, and undercooked chicken, can be risky. Avoid this by storing and preparing foods hygienically, and by not buying foods from outlets that appear to be unclean.

• STAPHYLOCCUS AUREUS Symptoms include excessive salivation, nausea, vomiting, stomach cramps, and diarrhea. Found in foods contaminated by those with poor personal hygiene. Avoid by storing and preparing foods hygenically, and by not buying foods from outlets that appear to be unclean.

• MOLDS Stomach cramps and diarrhea may result from eating foods that appear to be moldy. Throw away foods with obvious mold growth as well as any that are past their "use-by" dates.

NUTRITION & DIET

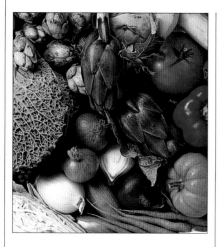

T HERE ARE SEVERAL OPTIONS available to a person requiring advice about diet and nutrition. It is possible to consult a conventional medical practitioner, or a practitioner of complementary medicine. Each has its benefits, and the methods of treatment may vary widely, from the prescription of a diet to a range of herbal remedies aimed at supplementing any nutrients that may be deficient in the diet.

CONSULTING A DIETICIAN

Consultation with a dietician is usually by doctor's referral. Dieticians are trained to degree level in nutritional science and have to complete a supervised placement in a hospital, working with patients, before qualifying to practice. A dietician's practical training includes learning about nutrition for individuals of all ages and with many different kinds of specific requirements, and the construction of special diets aimed at preventing or treating disease.

Dieticians are able to advise people on a wide range of conditions, from acute kidney failure and liver disease to diabetes, allergies, and weight problems, recommending dietary changes based on an individual's particular conditions and lifestyle. Their work is a sideline of conventional medicine, and they may work hand in hand with the medical profession. Before consulting a dietician, always ensure that he or she is officially registered with the appropriate governing body.

NUTRITIONAL THERAPISTS

Nutritional therapy is a form of complementary medicine that is different from the practice of dietetics or nutritional advice from nutritionists. Nutritional therapists have not had hospital-based training; instead, they are likely to have trained in a number of areas such as naturopathy, nutrition, physiology, and biochemistry. Training programs for nutritional therapists may vary from country to country. These practitioners are, however, often trained to degree level with a solid grounding in the sciences.

Nutritional therapists take a holistic view of the body, and are likely to focus on the circumstances, symptoms, and state of mind of the individual, rather than giving treatments that respond to the ailment alone. The advice of a nutritional therapist is not always based on scientific theory, and is likely to have elements in common with traditional medical practice such as Chinese medicine.

VEGETARIAN DIETS

When carefully planned, vegetarian diets can be nutritious and capable of supporting good health. In fact, studies show that vegetarianism appears to reduce the likelihood of illnesses such as heart disease, high blood pressure, and cancer of the colon. There are different kinds of vegetarian diet, some of which cut out many traditional sources of nutrients, such as dairy products. Vegetarians should take particular care to ensure that their nutritional needs are being met.

• LACTO-OVO VEGETARIAN DIET This diet excludes meats, poultry, fish and shellfish, and animal products such as gelatin, but includes milk and milk products, such as cheese, as well as eggs. Vegetarians following this diet need to ensure that they include iron-rich plant foods and that they do not rely too heavily on high-fat dairy foods as their main source of protein.

• VEGAN DIET Vegans exclude all animal products, including milk, eggs, and honey, from the diet. Animal products such as whey, lecithin, and vitamin D_3 obtained from fish oils are also avoided. Vegans need to ensure that adequate amounts of protein and iron are consumed, as well as taking vitamin B_{12} either as supplements or in fortified foods, since it virtually only occurs in animal foods. Vitamin D deficiency may also be a problem if little time is spent outdoors with the skin exposed to the sun. Vitamin D_2, the nonanimal form of this vitamin, may be added to soy milk and soy cheese.

The methods of diagnosis used by a nutritional therapist to identify a person's problems and seek solutions are varied. They may include hair analysis, iridology or analysis of the eye, vega testing of electrical resistance in the skin, hormone profiling, sweat tests, chemical testing for candida antibodies indicating yeast infections, kinesiology to assess energy flow, blood pressure tests, or urine, sweat, and stool tests.

Elimination diets, high-dosage nutritional supplements, and the promotion of optimum nutrition (*see page 13*) are some of the therapeutic options offered by nutritional therapists, who, in spite of the tendency of conventional medical and dietetic practitioners to dismiss this approach, often achieve good results. It is worth noting that conventional medicine tends to be more accepting of the role that nutritional therapy can play in the prevention of illness than in its ability to treat illness.

NUTRITIONISTS

A nutritionist is trained in nutrition to degree level or higher but has not had hospital-based training. Nutritionists focus on the science of nutrition, and apply their knowledge to health promotion and education, conducting dietary surveys, and research. Nutritionists may be consulted during the production of health or cookbooks, for example, or they may be called upon as experts in television documentary programs on health.

Nutritionists tend not to give consultations to people with dietary needs or problems. If they do, they will generally focus on helping an individual to get the most out of their food, and may offer general advice on low-level supplementation if the diet is obviously deficient in certain vitamins and minerals. In this capacity there is little difference between a nutritionist and a dietician.

OTHER HEALTH PROFESSIONALS

Some dietitians undergo further specialized training to qualify them to give specific advice to athletes, both amateurs and professionals, about their dietary needs. Sports dieticians may also advise athletes on foods that they can eat to help the body defend itself against illness and injury, and to promote healing after injury.

Doctors, nurses, and other health workers are easy to see without referrals. Although these people are not nutritional specialists, they can be a good source of general information and advice about diet and nutrition.

EXCLUSION DIETS

A range of exclusion diets can be followed in order to discover if certain foods are the cause of sensitivities and intolerances. All exclusion diets need to be organized and overseen by a qualified dietician or nutritionist.

• **SIMPLE EXCLUSION DIET** A simple exclusion diet excludes a single food or food constituent from the diet. This food may be easy to remove, such as strawberries or shellfish, or may be a more staple food, such as wheat, milk, or eggs, which can be more difficult to avoid, especially in prepackaged foods.

• **MULTIPLE EXCLUSION DIET** This type of diet excludes several foods that are commonly known to be responsible for adverse reactions. These foods might include milk, wheat, nuts, fish, azo dyes, and, in some cases, coffee, chocolate, and citrus fruits.

• **THE FEW FOODS DIET** The few foods diet is a restrictive exclusion diet comprised of a small group of foods that are rarely known to cause sensitivity reactions. Typically, these include turkey and rabbit; plain meats, with the exception of pork; carrots, cauliflower, and broccoli; rice, rice cakes, and puffed rice; sweet potatoes, tapioca, sago, and buckwheat; pears and peaches; sunflower, safflower, olive, and rapeseed oils; milk-free margarine; mineral, tap, and soda water; salt; sugar, syrup, molasses, and honey; and, for babies and children, a suitable milk substitute. Vitamin and mineral supplements may be required.

• **EXTREME EXCLUSION DIET** The most extreme exclusion diet removes all foods and instead provides nourishment via a formula diet. This may be appropriate for people with Crohn's disease or severe eczema. Symptoms must be monitored throughout an extreme exclusion diet, and food must be reintroduced under the supervision of a doctor who will recommend a suitable maintenance diet.

FEW FOODS DIET INCLUDES OLIVE OIL, PEARS, AND MEATS

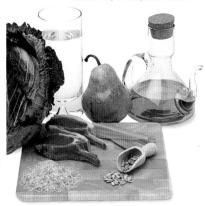

GLOSSARY

Words in *italics* within the text are defined elsewhere in the glossary.

A

Acetic acid a simple organic acid used for preserving foods

Adrenaline a *hormone* secreted by the body in response to stress

Ajone a garlic extract

Alcohol dehydrogenase an *enzyme* that breaks down alcohol in the stomach and liver

Alginic acid a *polysaccharide* found in seaweeds and used as a thickening and binding agent in foods

Alkaloid an organic substance found in plants which is involved in the maintenance of body systems

Allicin a substance found in garlic, leeks, and onions

Alpha carotene a type of *carotene*

Alpha-linolenic acid the name of the *omega-3 fatty acid*

Alpha tocopherol the main type of *vitamin* E found in human tissue

Amine the organic base of body chemicals such as histamine

Amino acids compounds of carbon, hydrogen, oxygen, and nitrogen, which combine to make *proteins*

Anthocyanidin a violet, red, or blue, water-soluble, *antioxidant* pigment

Antibody a substance produced in the blood in response to an *antigen*

Antigen a substance that can stimulate production of *antibodies*

Antioxidants substances that protect against the action of *free radicals*

Arachidonic acid an acid *metabolite* of the *omega-3* and *omega-6 fatty acids*

Ascorbic acid the chemical name given to *vitamin* C

B

Bacteria a group of *micro-organisms*, some of which cause disease

Beta carotene a pigment in orange-yellow vegetables, such as carrots, that is converted into *vitamin* A

Bifidobacteria beneficial *bacteria* added to foods to help regulate the numbers of intestinal micro-organisms, and to enhance immunity

Bioflavonoids see *flavonoids*

Biotin a B *vitamin* needed by the body for *metabolism*

Blood sugar sugar in the blood, in the form of *glucose*, from which the body produces energy

C

Caffeic acid an *antioxidant* found in many plants

Calcitonin a *hormone* that is essential for healthy bones

Calcium a *mineral* essential for a healthy skeleton

Calorie a measure of energy

Capsaicin the constituent in chilies that produces a burning sensation

Carbohydrates a group of simple or complex compounds in foods and a major source of energy in the diet

Carcinogen a substance that is potentially cancer-causing

Carotene a yellow-red pigment found in plants, such as *beta carotene*

Carotenoids a group of yellow-red pigments, including *carotenes*

Cellulose the supporting cell structure of plants, consisting of long chains of *glucose* units

Chlorophyll the green *antioxidant* pigment found in plants

Cholecalciferol the chemical name given to *vitamin* D

Cholesterol a fatty, crystalline substance carried in the blood by *proteins* and essential for many *metabolic* functions

Cholorogenic acid a substance found in various fruits and vegetables that has anticancerous benefits

Chylomicron a form of *lipoprotein*

Citric acid an organic acid found in plant and animal tissue

CLA conjugated linoleic acid, a *fat* thought to prevent the formation of cancer and hardening of the arteries

Cobalamin the chemical name given to *vitamin* B$_{12}$

Collagen the main constituent of white, fibrous tissue in the body

Conjugated linoleic acid see *CLA*

Coumarins plant *nutrients* believed to help thin the blood and to help prevent cancer

Cruciferous vegetables a plant group that includes broccoli, cabbages, kale, cress, cauliflower, and turnips

Curcumin an *antioxidant* found in corn, mustard, and turmeric

D

Daidzien an *isoflavone*

Deoxyribonucleic acid see *DNA*

DHA docosahexenoic acid, an *omega-3 fatty acid* found in oily fish

Diallyl disulfide an antibacterial substance found in garlic

Dietetics the feeding of individuals according to nutritional principles

Diosgenin an active plant *nutrient* found in fenugreek

Diuretic a dietary agent that increases the flow of urine

DNA deoxyribonucleic acid, the main constituent of chromosomes that carries information concerning an organism's genetic makeup

Docosahexenoic acid see *DHA*

Dopamine a *neurotransmitter* related to *adrenaline* and *noradrenaline*

E

EAR Estimated Average Requirement, a guideline of recommended daily energy requirements, or *calories*

Echinacea a plant extract with antiviral and antibacterial qualities

Eicosapentenoic acid see *EPA*

Electrolyte a solution of a substance able to conduct electricity

Ellagic acid a *phenolic* substance found in berries that has *antioxidant* properties

Endosperm the inner, starchy part of cereal grains

Enterobacteria *bacteria* that enter the body via the digestive tract

Enterococcus a type of *bacterium* that commonly causes food poisoning

Enzymes types of *protein* that act as catalysts for reactions in the body

EPA eicosapentenoic acid, an *omega-3 fatty acid* found in oily fish

Ergocalciferol the chemical name given to *vitamin* D$_2$

Escherichia coli (E-coli) a type of *bacterium* that causes food poisoning and urinary infections

Essential fatty acids the *fats* linoleic acid, *alpha-linolenic acid*, and *arachidonic acid* needed in the diets of all animals

Ester a compound produced by the reaction between an acid and alcohol

Estimated Average Requirement see *EAR*; see also *RDA* and *RNI*

Estrogen a *hormone* produced by the ovaries

Ethyl alcohol or **ethanol** forms of alcohol

Ethylene a gas, found in bananas, that has the effect of ripening fruits

F

Fats a group of *nutrients* that supply the body with its most concentrated form of energy

Fatty acids a group of more than 40 natural acids, of which three are *essential fatty acids*

Fiber a type of *carbohydrate* in foods that may be soluble and digestible or insoluble and indigestible

Flavone a compound found in plants

Flavonoids a group of more than 4,000 *antioxidants* found in fruits, vegetables, and other plants

Folate a B *vitamin* needed for healthy blood and body tissues

Folic acid the synthetic form of *folate*

Free radicals unstable, reactive substances found in the body and in the environment, thought to be the triggers of cancer and heart disease

Fructose a sugar found in fruits

G

Galanin a *neurotransmitter* in the brain that appears to play a role in the desire for *fat* in the diet

Gamma-linolenic acid see *GLA*

Gelatin a water-soluble *protein*

Genistein a type of *isoflavone* that has weak *estrogen*-like properties

GI glycemic index, a system of ranking foods according to their effects on *blood sugar* levels

GLA gamma-linolenic acid, a *metabolite* of the *omega-6 essential fatty acid*, linoleic acid

Glucose a simple sugar formed by the breakdown of starch

Glucosinolate a plant *nutrient* with anticancerous effects

Glutathione-s-transferase an *enzyme* with detoxifying properties

Gluten a *protein* complex found in wheat and rye

Glycemic index see *GI*

Glycerol a colorless, odorless, liquid used as a sweetener in foods

Glycogen the form in which *carbohydrate* is stored in the body

H

Haem iron a form of *iron* found in red meats and meat products that is easily absorbed by the body

HDL high-density lipoprotein, a form of *lipoprotein*

Helicobacter pylori a *bacterium* that causes stomach ulcers

Hemoglobin the respiratory pigment in red blood cells that is able to bind and release oxygen

Heparin an acid in the liver and lungs which, if injected intravenously, inhibits blood coagulation

Hesperidin the main *flavonoid* that is thought to strengthen blood capillary walls

Heterocyclic aromatic amines a family of compounds, found in various cooked meats and fish, that may cause cancer

High-density lipoprotein see *HDL*

Homocysteine a substance created by *methionine* in the body in order to repair damaged tissues

Hormone a chemical secreted by the endocrine glands and carried in the blood to regulate the functions of tissues and organs

Hydrochloric acid an acid secreted by the stomach to help kill *bacteria*

Hydroxyphenylisatin a substance in prunes that stimulates the smooth-muscle cells of the colon wall

Hyericin the active extract from St. John's Wort that increases levels of *serotonin* in the brain

Hypericum the botanical name for St. John's Wort

IJK

Indoles substances present in cruciferous vegetables, such as broccoli, that are believed to reduce the risk of some cancers

Insulin a *hormone* produced by the pancreas to regulate *blood sugar* levels

Interleukin a substance that greatly boosts the immune system

Intrinsic factor a *protein* released by stomach glands that is essential for the absorption of *vitamin* B$_{12}$

Inulin a complex *carbohydrate* composed of *fructose* units

Iodine a *trace element* present in seafood and needed by the body to make the *hormone* thyroxine

Iron an essential *trace element* needed by the body to carry oxygen in the blood and to prevent anemia

Isoflavones plant *nutrients* that have mild *estrogen*like effects

Isothiocyanates (ITCs) plant *nutrients* that appear to reduce the risk of some cancers

ITCs *see isothiocyanates*

Kaempferol a *flavonoid* in vegetables

L

Lactalbumin the more easily digested of two *proteins* found in milk

Lactobacillus a type of beneficial *bacterium*

Lactose the *carbohydrate* found in milk, also known as milk sugar

Lactucarium a sedativelike substance found in lettuce stems

LDL low-density lipoprotein, a form of *lipoprotein*

Lecithin a fatty substance in the blood that helps to transport *fats*

Lentinan a *phytonutrient* found in mushrooms and thought to fight cancer

Leucotriene a substance produced by the breakdown of *essential fatty acids*

Lignan a plant *nutrient* that has *antioxidant* effects

Limonoid a *flavone* found in citrus fruits, especially in the seeds

Linoleic acid the essential *omega-6 fatty acid* found in pumpkins and flax seeds

Linolenic acid *see alpha-linolenic acid*

Lipoprotein a substance combining *fat* and *protein* that carries *cholesterol* in the blood

Long-chain fatty acids *essential fatty acids*, such as *linoleic acid*, that consist of chains of between 16 and 18 carbon atoms

Low-density lipoprotein *see LDL*

L-tyrosine an *amino acid*

Lutein a yellow–orange *carotene* with *antioxidant* effects

Lycopene the red *antioxidant* pigment present in tomatoes

Lysine an essential *amino acid*

M

Macronutrients the main *nutrients*: *proteins*, *carbohydrates*, and *fats*

Malic acid an organic acid found in fruits such as apples

Metabolic rate the rate at which the body burns energy

Metabolite a substance produced during *metabolism*

Metabolism the series of chemical changes in the body by which foods and drinks are broken down into simpler substances

Methionine an essential *amino acid*

Microbe a microscopic organism, such as a *bacterium*

Micro-organism a microscopic organism, such as a *bacterium*

Micronutrients *vitamins*, *minerals*, or *trace elements*

Minerals substances that originate in nonliving materials, are found in foods, and are essential to life

Molecule the smallest, simplest unit of a chemical compound

Monosaccharide a type of easily digested *carbohydrate* consisting of a single sugar, such as *glucose*

Mucin the substance found in figs that is responsible for their laxative effect

Myoglobin a complex *protein* that stores oxygen in muscle cells

N

Neurotransmitter a chemical that transmits messages between nerves

Niacin a B *vitamin* needed in *metabolism*, and the name given to nicotinic acid and nicotinamide

Nicotine-derived nitrosaminoketone *see NNK*

Nitrate a component of plants

Nitrite a substance found in plant foods, and used in food processing such as meat preservation

Nitrosamine a substance produced by the reaction between *amines* and *nitrites* or *nitrates* in the diet, and which may cause cancer

N-nitroso compounds substances found in foods that may lead to stomach cancer

NNK nicotine-derived nitrosaminoketone, the cancerous substance in tobacco smoke

Nobiletin a *flavone* found in orange peel that may be anticancerous

Non haem iron a form of *iron* found in plant foods, that is more difficult for the body to absorb than *haem iron*

Noradrenaline a *hormone* secreted by the nervous system that constricts blood vessels

Nucleoprotein a compound within a cell nucleus consisting of *protein* bound to a nucleic acid

Nutrients essential dietary constituents, such as *vitamins*, *minerals*, *proteins*, and *fats*

O

Oleic acid an unsaturated, *long-chain fatty acid* found in human fat

Omega-3 and omega-6 fatty acids fats that are essential for many cellular and *metabolic* processes

Organic goitrogen a substance in plants that causes a swelling of the thyroid gland known as goiter

Oxalate a salt of *oxalic acid*

Oxalic acid an acid that blocks the absorption of *calcium*

P

P-coumaric acid a *polyphenol* that helps to prevent the formation of cancer-causing *nitrosamines*

Pantothenic acid a B *vitamin* needed for *metabolism*

Pectin a soluble *fiber* found in fruits that is used as a setting agent in jam

PEITC an *isothiocyanate* found in watercress that detoxifies *NNK*

pH a standard measure of the relative acidity or alkalinity of a substance

Phenolic compounds *antioxidant* agents in fruits and vegetables

Phytates substances in plants that appear to bind to *calcium*, *iron*, and *zinc*, and which may reduce their absorption from foods by the body

Phytochemicals *see phytonutrients*

Phytoene a *carotene* found in pumpkins, mangoes, and papayas

Phytofluene a *carotene* found in apricots and peaches

Phytonutrients chemical compounds, or phytochemicals, found in plants and known to have beneficial effects on human health

Phytosterol a substance that can mimic the *hormone estrogen*

Polyphenolic flavonol an *antioxidant* found in tea

Polyphenol a *flavonoid* found in plants

Polysaccharide a complex *carbohydrate*, such as *cellulose*, made up of many sugar *molecules*

Proanthocyanadin a *bioflavonoid* found in berries

Probiotic a type of *bacterium* that grows in the intestine

Proteins complex nitrogenous compounds found in all animal and vegetable tissue, and needed in the human diet for the growth and repair of body tissue and organs

Psoralen an active plant constituent found in parsley

Purine a constituent of *nucleoproteins* from which *uric acid* is derived

Pyridoxine the chemical name given to *vitamin* B$_6$

QR

Quercetin a *polyphenol*, found in tea, onions, and apples, that has *antioxidant* properties

Quinones active plant constituents

Radioallergosorbent test *see RAST*

Raffinose a *carbohydrate* found in legumes that is hard to digest

RAST radioallergosorbent test, used to identify food allergens

RDA Recommended Daily Allowance, suggested intake of *nutrients* for the maintenance of good nutrition in the average person

Recommended Daily Allowance *see RDA*

Reference Nutrient Intake *see RNI*

Resting (basal) metabolic rate the amount of *calories* that the human body uses when at rest

Retinol the chemical name given to *vitamin* A

Riboflavin the chemical name given to *vitamin* B$_{12}$

RNI Reference Nutrient Intake, a guideline of recommended amounts of *nutrients* that should be included daily in the diet of the average person

Rutin a *flavonoid*

S

St. John's Wort (hypericum) a plant from which *hyericin* is extracted that may relieve depression

Salicylates aspirinlike substances found in foods

Salmonella a type of *bacterium* that commonly causes food poisoning

Saponins a group of substances in plants that emulsifies oils

Selenium a *trace element* with *antioxidant* properties that plays a role in reducing the risk of cancer

Serotonin a brain chemical that promotes a feeling of well-being and helps to control appetite

Short-chain fatty acids *fatty acids* that consist of chains of carbon atoms with fewer carbon atoms than *long-chain fatty acids*

Silymarin milk thistle, an herb that encourages liver-cell renewal

Sodium chloride an electrolyte, commonly known as salt, that is essential to human health

Solanine an *alkaloid* found in potatoes that have turned green, which causes nausea and vomiting and can be fatal when ingested

Stacchyose a *carbohydrate* found in legumes that is not easily digested

Staphylococcus a type of *bacterium* that may cause food poisoning

Sulforaphane a plant *nutrient* that may suppress tumor growth

T

Tangeretin a *flavone* that may have anticancer properties

Tannin a substance that gives foods an astringent effect in the mouth

Tartaric acid an acid found in fruits, and used to flavor lemonade

Terpene a component of the essential oils in citrus fruits

Thiamine the chemical name given to *vitamin* B$_1$

Tocopherol the synthetic form of *vitamin* E

Trace elements organic substances essential to human health, and including *iron*, *zinc*, and *selenium*

Trehalose a sugar found in mushrooms

Triglycerides *esters* of *glycerol* combined with fatty acids

Tryptophan an essential *amino acid* needed to produce *serotonin*

TVP textured vegetable *protein* that is used to simulate meat

Tyrosine a nonessential *amino acid* made in the body and used to make *dopamine* and *noradrenaline*

UV

Uric acid an acid formed during the breakdown of *nucleoproteins* in body tissues and excreted in the urine

Vasoactive amines *amines* capable of affecting constriction and dilation of veins

Vitamins organic substances containing carbon, hydrogen, and oxygen, that are present in foods and are essential for good health

Volatile oil an oil with therapeutic properties found in herbs and in spices, such as ginger

XYZ

Xanthophyll a yellow *carotene* with *antioxidant* functions

Xylitol a sugar substitute that protects against tooth decay

Zeathanxin a *carotene* found in corn and egg yolk

Zein a *protein* obtained from corn and of poor nutritional value

Zinc a *trace element* needed for a healthy immune system and for reproduction

Zingiberene a component of the *volatile oil* found in ginger

Zingerols a group of active ingredients found in ginger

BIBLIOGRAPHY

Balch, James & Phyllis *Prescription for Nutritional Healing: A Practical A-Z Reference to Drug-Free Remedies Using Vitamins, Minerals, Herbs & Food Supplements*, Avery, US, 1993.

Bean, Anita *Food for Fitness: Nutrition Guide, Eating Plans, Recipes*, A. & C. Black, UK, 1988.

Beling, Stephanie *Power Foods: Good Food, Good Health with Phytochemicals, Nature's Own Energy Boosters*, Harper Collins, US, 1997.

Bender, Arnold E. *Dictionary of Nutrition & Food Technology*, Butterworths, UK, 1984.

Brewer, Dr. Sarah *The Complete Book of Men's Health*, Thorsons, UK, 1995.

British Nutrition Foundation *Diet and Heart Disease: A Round Table of Factors*, Chapman & Hall, UK, 1995.

Carruthers, Dr. Malcolm *Maximising Manhood: Beating the Male Menopause*, Harper Collins, UK, 1996.

Garrow, J.F. & James, W.P.T. *Human Nutrition & Dietetics*, Churchill Livingstone, UK, 1994.

Grigson, Jane *Jane Grigson's Vegetable Book*, Penguin, UK, 1980; *Jane Grigson's Fruit Book*, Penguin, UK, 1982.

Guyton, A.C. *Textbook of Medical Physiology*, Saunders, US, 1991.

Herbert, Victor & Subak-Sharpe, Genell J. (ed.) *Total Nutrition: The Only Guide You'll Ever Need*, St. Martin's Griffin, US, 1994.

Holford, Patrick *The Optimum Nutrition Bible*, Piatkus, UK, 1997.

Holland, B., Brown, J. & Buss, D.H. *Third Supplement to McCance & Widdowson's The Composition of Foods: Fish & Fish Products*, Royal Society of Chemistry, UK, 1993.

Holland, B., Unwin, I.D. & Buss, D.H. *Fourth Supplement to McCance & Widdowson's The Composition of Foods: Milk Products & Eggs*, Royal Society of Chemistry, UK, 1989.

Holland, B., Unwin, I.D. & Buss, D.H. *Fifth Supplement to McCance & Widdowson's The Composition of Foods: Vegetables, Herbs & Spices*, Royal Society of Chemistry, UK, 1991.

Johns, Timothy & Romeo, John T. Functionality of Food Phytochemicals, *Recent Advances in Phytochemistry Volume 31*, Plenum Press, US, 1997.

Leeds, Dr. Anthony & Miller, Jennie Brand *The Glucose Revolution Pocket Guide to the Top 100 Low Glycemic Foods*, Hodder & Stoughton, UK, 1996.

Marieb, Elaine N. *Human Anatomy & Physiology*, The Benjamin Cummings Publishing Co. Inc., US, 1991.

McArdle, William, Katch, Frank & Katch, Victor *Exercise Physiology, Energy, Nutrition & Human Performance*, Lea & Febiger, US, 1991.

McCance, R.A. *Immigrant Foods (The Composition of Foods, Second Supplement)* HMSO, UK, 1985.

Ministry of Agriculture, Fisheries & Foods *Fatty Acids: Seventh Supplement to Fifth Edition of McCance & Widdowson's The Composition of Foods*, HMSO, UK, 1982.

Morrison, Judith H. *The Book of Ayurveda: A Holistic Approach to Health and Longevity*, Gaia Books, UK, 1995.

Newall, Carol A., Anderson, Linda A. & Phillipson, J. David *Herbal Medicines: A Guide for Health Care Professionals*, The Pharmaceutical Press, UK, 1996.

Ody, Penelope *The Herb Society's Complete Medicinal Herbal*, Dorling Kindersley, UK, 1994.

Ornish, Dr. Dean *Dr. Dean Ornish's Program for Reversing Heart Disease*, Century, US, 1991.

Paul, A.A., Southgate, D.A.T. & Pitchford, Paul *Healing with Whole Foods – Oriental Traditions & Modern Nutrition*, North Atlantic Books, US, 1993.

Royal Society of Chemistry & Ministry of Agriculture, Fisheries & Foods *McCance & Widdowson's The Composition of Foods*, Royal Society of Chemistry, UK, 1991.

Sheldon Margen, M.D. *The Wellness Encyclopedia of Food and Nutrition: How to Buy, Store, and Prepare Every Variety of Fresh Food*, Rebus, US, 1992.

Stoppard, Dr. Miriam *Menopause*, Dorling Kindersley, UK, 1995.

Tannahill, Reay *Food in History*, Penguin, UK, 1998.

Vaughan, J.G. & Geissler, C.A. *The New Oxford Book of Food Plants*, Oxford, UK, 1997.

Werbach, Melvin *Nutritional Influences on Illness*, Third Line Press, US, 1993.

Williams, S. *Nutrition & Diet Therapy*, Mosby, US, 1997.

World Cancer Research Fund & American Institute for Cancer Research Food *Nutrition & the Prevention of Cancer*, World Cancer Research Fund & American Institute for Cancer Research Food, US, 1997.

ACKNOWLEDGMENTS

Author's appreciation I would like to thank Mrs. Chapman, my Home Economics teacher who sparked my interest in nutrition through her inspirational teaching in the 1970s, and all those who encouraged me along the way – Professor Bender, Pat Judd, Edith Elliot, Kristina Zaremba, Peter Duckworth, Maurice Hanssen, Geoffrey Canon, and my parents.

I would like to thank Richard Norman and Jennifer Dickson for their tremendous help in sourcing so many of the hundreds of clinical papers that I used when researching this book (and my mom for painstakingly filing them). Lots of luck to you both once you finish your studies. Also, thanks to Julie Dean.

The Healing Power of Food would not have been possible without the support and encouragement of Daphne Razazan and Krystyna Mayer at Dorling Kindersley – thank you both. A very special thank you goes to Christiane Gunzi, my long-suffering editor at Picthall & Gunzi.

Your sense of humor, patience, and understanding were very much appreciated. I couldn't have done it without you!

A special thank you, as always, goes to Ian Wilson, whose wisdom, judgement, and friendship mean the world to me. Finally, a huge thanks to Nick for encouraging me to sit and write when I would rather have been in Greece and Cuba with him, and for being so tolerant about giving up our weekends.

Photography Leslie J. Borg, A-Z Botanical Collection, p.61 (*middle*); Ian O'Leary (pages 8–9, 40–41, 130–31, 148–49); Nigel Caitlin, Holt Studios, p.92 (*top left*); Inga Spence, Holt Studios, p.72 (*top left*). All other photography by Sarah Ashun, Martin Cameron, Andy Crawford, Philip Dowell, Philip Garward, Steve Gorton, Clive Streeter, Dave King, David Murray, Stephen Oliver, Stephen Shott, Jane Stockman, and Andrew Whittuck.

Illustrations AKG, London, Erich Lessing p.10 (*top left*); Katz pictures, Mansell Collection, p.12 (*top left*). Anatomical illustrations by Phil Wilson and Debbie Maizels; *Key Food* icons by Sarah Young; additional artworks from *Complete Home Medical Guide* and *The DK Children's Illustrated Encyclopedia*, published by Dorling Kindersley.

Models for anatomical illustrations, Natalie Creary, Julian Evans, and Flavia Taylor.

Picthall & Gunzi would like to thank Dominic Zwemmer for design help; John Bates, Anna Crago, and Jill Somerscales for editorial help; and Lynn Bresler for the index.

Dorling Kindersley would like to thank Dr. Naomi Craft for her helpful comments on the ailments section.

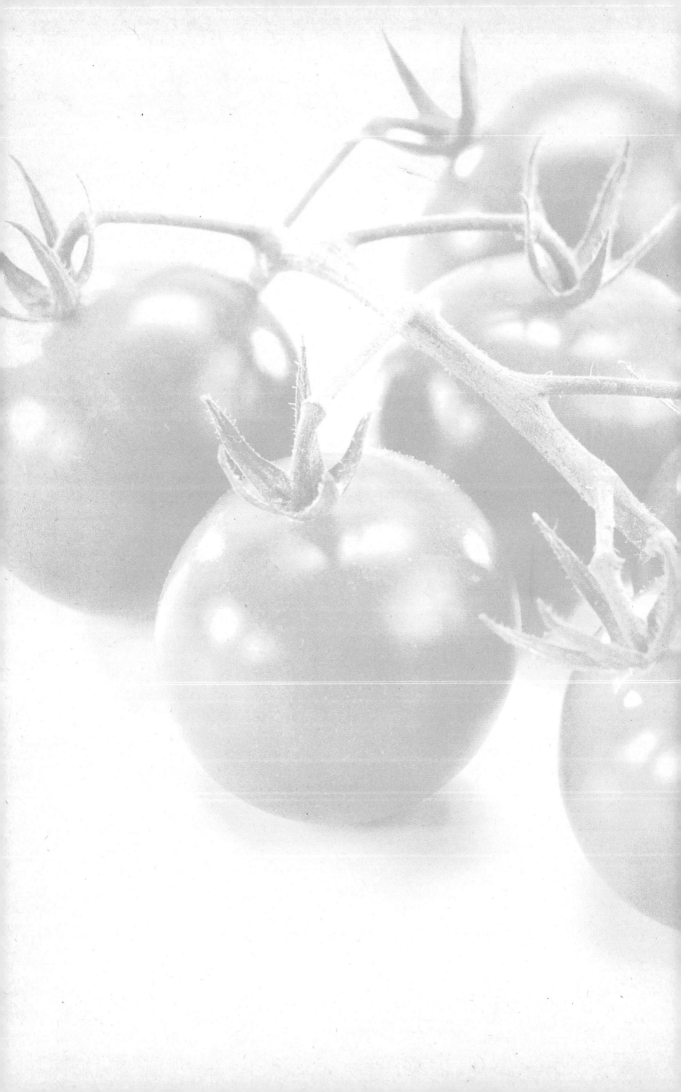